PET SKIN and HAIRCOAT PROBLEMS

TESTS AND TREATMENTS

For Veterinary Technicians

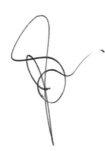

Lowell Ackerman, DVM

Diplomate, American College of Veterinary Dermatology

Mesa Veterinary Hospital, Ltd.

Mesa, Arizona

Designed and Published by Veterinary Learning Systems

Credits:
Cover photo: Michael Slack

The following material originally appeared in Nesbitt GH, Ackerman LJ (eds): *Dermatology for the Small Animal Practitioner.* Trenton, NJ, Veterinary Learning Systems, 1991:
     Figures 1-1, 2-1 through 2-4, 2-6, 2-7, 4-2, 4-4, 4-5 (panels A through I), 4-8, 4-10 through 4-13, 7-1, and 7-2
     Tables 1-2, 2-2, 3-1, 3-3, 4-3, 5-1 through 5-4, and 8-1
     Boxes on pp. 152, 153, 156, and 158
     Appendix on pp. 26–30
     Illustrations in Color Plates I through VI and VIII

Library of Congress Card Number: 93-85305

ISBN 1-884254-03-9

Introduction

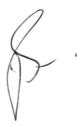

*D*ermatologic disorders in dogs and cats are one of the primary reasons for presentation of a pet to a veterinary practice. Moreover, as the volume of information concerning dermatology continues to expand, it has become increasingly difficult for veterinary professionals to keep abreast with the most current material available in this field. *Pet Skin and Haircoat Problems* represents a complete practical reference to dermatologic diseases in dogs and cats written specifically with the veterinary technician in mind.

A related text, *Dermatology for the Small Animal Practitioner*, edited by Gene H. Nesbitt and Lowell Ackerman, was published in 1991. This earlier title was enthusiastically received by the general practitioners and veterinary students for whom it had been written. Its success served as the inspiration for *Pet Skin and Haircoat Problems*.

CONTENTS

CHAPTER THREE

Diagnosis and Management of Bacterial Skin Diseases   73

CHAPTER FOUR

Diagnosis and Management of Fungal Skin Diseases   91

CHAPTER FIVE

Diagnosis and Management of Immunologic   113
Skin Diseases

CHAPTER SIX

Diagnosis and Management of Endocrine Skin Disorders

CHAPTER SEVEN

Cytology, Histopathology, and Immunopathology

CHAPTER EIGHT

Specific Therapies

CHAPTER NINE

Client Counseling

CHAPTER ONE
Introduction

*T*he skin, the largest organ of the body, interacts extensively with other organ systems. Moreover, the skin has its own branch of the immune system.

The maintenance of skin and haircoat places a phenomenal nutritional drain on animals. Hair growth is closely associated with a variety of circulating hormones. Also, the skin can serve as a suitable environment for the proliferation of a variety of bacteria, fungi, and parasites.

There has been a virtual explosion of information in the field of dermatology. Clearly, continuing education is more critical now than it ever has been. Veterinarians and veterinary hospital staff are under pressure to keep up to date with all this new information.

TERMINOLOGY

Dermatology has a language all its own, and it is important that everyone involved with dermatologic cases be familiar with the same language. The following terms are basic to communicating about dermatologic lesions of dogs and cats.

Primary lesions are those that arise first on the skin. Secondary lesions are a reflection of changes that have occurred on the skin. For example, a blister or pustule is a primary lesion; once it ruptures, it leaves an erosion or ulcer, both secondary lesions. A dog may have a macule or papule (each a primary lesion) associated with flea bites. In time, rubbing and chewing may lead to crusting, excoriations, lichenification, and hyperpigmentation, all secondary lesions.

Refer to Figure 1-1 for examples of a number of primary and secondary lesions and to the Appendix on pp. 26–30 for a list of cutaneous lesions and their morphologic classifications.

Primary Lesions

Macule	A circumscribed, flat discoloration of the skin up to 1 cm in diameter.
Patch	Macules greater than 1 cm in diameter.
Papule	A circumscribed, elevated, superficial solid lesion up to 1 cm in diameter. A bump.
Plaque	A circumscribed, elevated, superficial solid lesion greater than 1 cm in diameter.
Wheal	An edematous, transitory papule or plaque. A hive.
Nodule	A solid lesion that extends beneath the skin surface. A papule that has enlarged in three dimensions.
Vesicle	A circumscribed elevation of the skin, up to 1 cm in diameter. A blister.
Bulla	A vesicle greater than 1 cm in diameter.
Pustule	A circumscribed elevation of skin containing purulent fluid. A pimple.
Petechia	A circumscribed deposit of blood or blood pigment up to 1 cm in diameter.
Purpura	A circumscribed deposit of blood or blood pigment greater than 1 cm in diameter. A bruise.

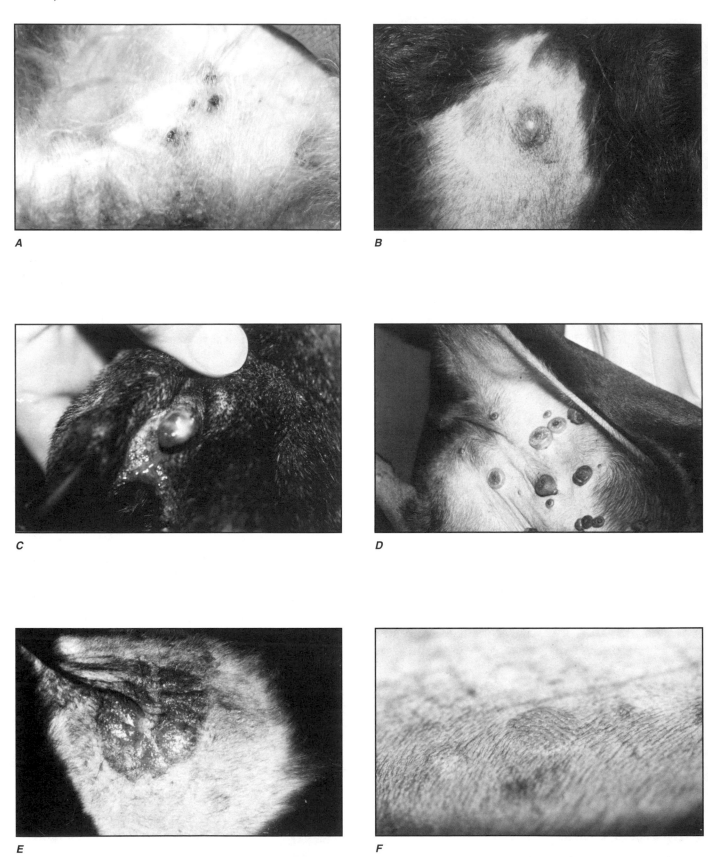

Figure 1-1. Primary and secondary lesions. **A,** *Maculopapular eruption on the ventrum associated with fleabite dermatitis.* **B,** *Pustular eruption consisting of a fluid-filled structure containing purulent material.* **C,** *Nodule, a palpable solid mass.* **D,** *Tumor, a nodule containing neoplastic cells; these are papillomas.* **E,** *Plaque, a large, flat-topped lesion; erythematous in this case.* **F,** *Wheal, a superficial elevation with a smooth, rounded surface resulting from edema; this one is an allergy test site.* **G,** *An erosive to ulcerative dermatosis seen in association with pyotraumatic dermatitis.* **H,** *Pronounced scaling in a dog with epidermal dysplasia.* **I,** *Facial crusting in a puppy with dermatomyositis.*

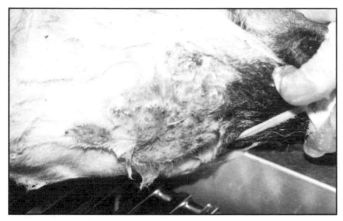

G

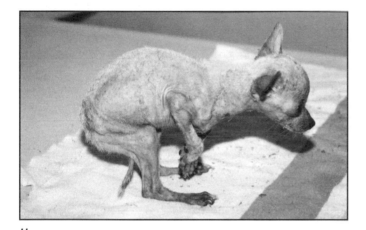

H

Figure 1-1. Cont'd.

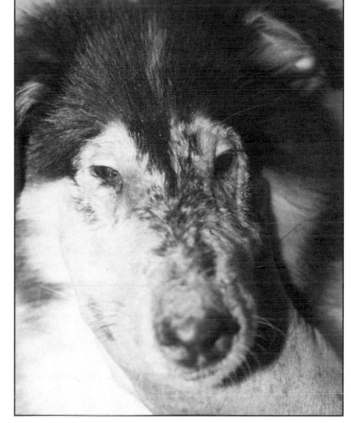

I

Secondary Lesions

Scale	Dead epidermal cells, which may be dry or greasy, that are shed.
Crust	Variously colored collection of skin exudates. A scab.
Excoriation	Abrasion of the skin, usually superficial and traumatic in nature.
Fissure	A linear break in the skin, sharply defined with abrupt walls.
Erosion	An excavation in the skin limited to the epidermis and not breaking the integrity of the dermal-epidermal junction. Usually the result of a burst pustule or vesicle.
Ulcer	An irregularly sized and shaped cavity in the skin that goes deeper than just the epidermis.

Scar	A formation of connective tissue that replaces tissue lost through injury or disease.
Lichenification	A diffuse area of thickening and scaling, in which the surface lines and markings on the skin become exaggerated.
Induration	Palpable thickening of the skin.
Sclerosis	Hardening of the skin.

Descriptive Terms Used in Dermatology

Abscess	A cavity filled with pus.
Acral	Relating to the peripheral parts of the body, usually the legs.
Allergen	A substance capable of causing an allergy.

Alopecia Hair loss.

Anthropophilic Organisms adapted specifically to living in or on humans, such as certain species of ringworm fungi.

Antibody A substance produced by plasma cells that protects the body.

Antigen A substance that results in antibody production.

Antimicrobial A substance that kills or inhibits microbes.

Antiseptic A substance that kills or inhibits microbes on living tissues.

Autogenous Originating from one's own body. For example, autogenous bacterins are made from microbes isolated directly from the patient to be treated.

Autoimmune Referring to a condition in which the body makes antibodies against some of its own tissues.

Bacillus A rod-shaped bacterium.

Cellulitis Inflammation of the connective tissue that does not form a discrete abscess.

Cerumen A wax-like secretion found in the ear canal.

Ceruminolytic A substance that dissolves earwax.

Chemotherapy The treatment of diseases with chemical substances or drugs.

Chlamydospore A form of thallospore, a fungal spore.

Chrysotherapy Treatment of disease with gold compounds.

Coccus A round bacterium.

Congenital Appearing since birth.

Conidia A fungal spore that is produced asexually. **Macroconidia** are large spores; **microconidia** are small spores.

Depigmentation Loss of color (pigment) from the skin.

Eczema A poorly defined term commonly used to refer to inflammatory rashes with various other clinical features. Not a specific diagnosis.

Emollient An agent that softens the skin or soothes irritation.

Endocrine Hormonal.

Erythema Redness.

Erythroderma An inflammatory reaction in the skin often accompanied by redness and scaling.

Exfoliate To shed.

Exudation Oozing of material through the skin.

Fistula An abnormal passage leading from a site of infection to the surface of the skin.

Fomites Objects, such as bedding and grooming instruments, capable of transmitting infections.

Geophilic Specifically adapted to living in the soil, such as certain species of ringworm fungi.

Hematoma A bruise.

Heritable Referring to a trait that can be inherited.

Hyperpigmentation Increased pigmentation.

Iatrogenic A problem induced by medical treatment.

Immunotherapy Treatment directed at promoting appropriate immune responses.

Infection A microbial condition on or within the body.

Infestation A condition in which parasites live on the skin surface.

Inflammation A tissue reaction characterized by redness, heat, pain, and, sometimes, loss of function.

Keratin The proteins forming the top layers of the skin.

Keratinization	The process of forming keratin on the skin surface.
Lesion	Any abnormal change.
Leukotrichia	Whitening of the hair.
Metastasis	Spreading of disease from one part of the body to another.
Necrolysis	A breakdown of tissue as a result of cell death.
Necrosis	The death of cells or tissues in a living animal.
Neoplasia	Cancer, either benign or malignant.
Photodermatitis	An inflammatory reaction in the skin resulting from exposure to sunlight.
Poliosis	Depigmentation of the hairs; greying.
Polydipsia	Increased thirst.
Polyphagia	Increased hunger.
Polyuria	Increased urination.
Prognosis	A forecast of the probable outcome of a disease.
Pruritus	Itchiness.
Sebum	The waxy, oily product of the sebaceous glands excreted into the hair follicles.
Spongiosis	Intercellular edema in the epidermis.
Sporangium	A fungal organ that contains asexual spores.
Tardive	An inherited trait not manifested at birth but appearing at a later time.
Tumor	A swelling, usually used to describe a neoplasm.
Urticaria	Hives.
Xerosis	Dryness.
Xerostomia	Dry mouth.
Zoonosis	A disease that may be transmitted between animals and humans.

ANATOMY OF THE SKIN (Figure 1-2)

Anatomically, the skin is divided into the epidermis, the dermis, and the hypodermis (panniculus or subcutaneous tissue) and the contents therein. The thin surface layer is the epidermis, which consists of keratinocytes that rise to a transitional zone, die, and then form the surface scale. Beneath the epidermis is the dermis; the dividing line between these two layers is the dermal-epidermal junction or the basement membrane zone. The dermis contains collagen, elastin fibers, blood vessels, and blood cells. It is the source of nutrition for the overlying epidermis, which has no blood supply of its own. Beneath the dermis is a zone of fat, the subcutaneous tissue. It acts as a shock absorber to the wear and tear of everyday life.

The hair follicles are formed from epidermal appendages that grow down into the dermis, where they have access to a nutritive source (dermal papilla) in the dermis. After birth, no new hair follicles are formed. Dogs and cats have compound hair follicles, which means that more than one hair can exit through a pore. Each hair follicle is associated with grape-like sebaceous glands to form a pilosebaceous unit. Apocrine glands, a form of sweat gland, are found in the deep dermis and hypodermis. Eccrine glands, the common sweat glands of humans, are only found in the footpads and nose of dogs and cats.

In dogs and cats, hairs do not grow continuously; rather, they grow in cycles. Each cycle starts with a growing stage (anagen), then a transitional stage (catagen), and, finally, a resting stage (telogen). Many factors affect the hair growth cycle, but the most important are photoperiod, hormones, temperature, and nutritional status.

THE KERATINIZATION PROCESS (EPIDERMAL RENEWAL)

The keratinization process describes the turnover of epidermal cells from living keratinocytes to dead surface scale. The process is a critical one, because disorders of keratinization (also referred to as seborrhea) are very common in dogs and cats. It is difficult to manage these cases effectively without understanding the processes involved.

The bottom layer of the epidermis is known as the basal cell layer. This layer is responsible for creating daughter cells that rise through the ranks in an orderly fashion through the spinous cell layer (the stratum spinosum) to a transitional zone (the stratum granulosum). All the while, the epidermal cells produce keratin, a very important protein. Keratin is a tough protein; the combination of keratin and intercellular lipids forms a protective, water-tight barrier to the environment. Most of the intercellular lipids come from specialized organelles within keratinocytes, called lamellar

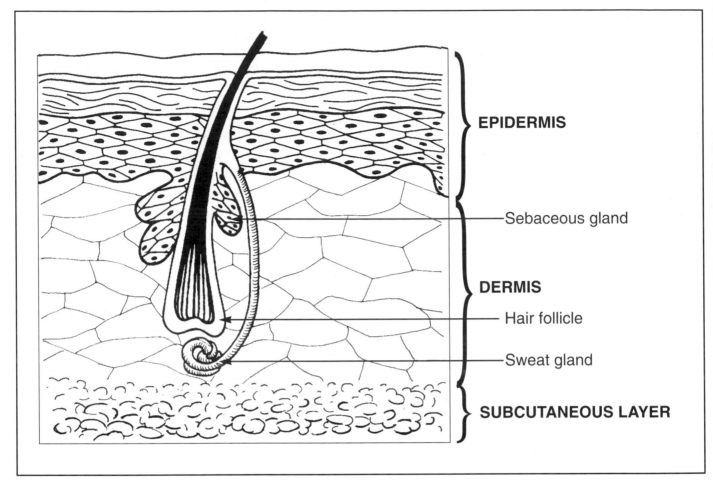

Figure 1-2. Anatomy of the skin.

bodies. Keratin filaments form the backbone of the keratinocytes in the stratum spinosum, and keratin is the primary protein in surface scale. A cystine-rich protein called filaggrin directs the aggregation of keratin filaments and their conversion into the inert keratin protein of surface scale. At the transitional zone, the epidermal cells normally die, flatten out, discharge lipids from the lamellar bodies, and form the surface layer of scale (the stratum corneum). In most dogs it takes about 3 weeks from the creation of cells in the basal cell layer to the time they reach the transitional zone. Another 3 weeks pass before the cells in the stratum corneum are shed into the environment.

DISORDERS OF KERATINIZATION

Disorders of keratinization refer to those conditions in which the epidermal renewal process is less than orderly. Much of the time, the problem involves an accelerated cycle. When a cycle is completed in 4 to 10 days, rather than the normal 21 days, build-up of scale on the skin surface results. This condition is commonly labeled as seborrhea, but there are many other problems that can result in a keratinization disorder.

Most causes of keratinization disorders are the result of genetic abnormalities in the keratinization process; thus they can be managed but they cannot be cured (e.g., the typical "seborrheic" cocker spaniel has an inborn error in its keratinization process). On the other hand, if a dog suddenly develops "seborrhea" as an adult, diagnostic efforts should be directed against "acquired" keratinization defects that may involve allergies, nutritionally related conditions, or even some cancers.

Of the many different processes that can lead to keratinization disorders, some are primary (usually genetic in origin) but the majority are secondary to other underlying disorders.

Secondary Keratinization Disorders

Secondary keratinization disorders are usually referred to as seborrhea because they tend to be scaly, dry, or greasy. In fact, it is not sebum that makes the skin seem greasy but rather the cholesterol and lipid derivatives of the surface skin cells (keratinocytes). The increase in surface keratin and lipids creates an excellent environment for the growth of numerous bacteria and yeasts. When surface microbes break down these compounds, a rancid odor is produced. This is the clinical syndrome that most veterinarians recognize as seborrhea.

Some common conditions that can result in secondary keratinization disorders include:

- Allergies
- Infestation with ectoparasites
- Dermatophytes
- Endocrinopathies
- Nutritional disorders
- Metabolic disorders
- Immune-mediated conditions
- Environmental conditions
- Certain neoplasias

Clinically, this might result in scaling, greasiness, dryness of the skin, and ceruminous otitis externa.

The diagnostic approach to secondary keratinization disorders requires much testing, because so many different conditions must be considered. All animals with keratinization disorders should have multiple skin scrapings and dermatophyte cultures. If allergies are the likely cause, hypoallergenic diet trials and therapeutic trials with parasiticides may facilitate the diagnosis. Thyroid function tests and biochemical profiles should be performed if an endocrine-related or metabolic disorder is suspected. All cats should be evaluated with a viral profile (for feline leukemia virus and feline immunodeficiency virus) in addition to a complete blood count and biochemical profile. Finally, skin biopsies may aid in the characterization of the problem even if they rarely provide an absolute diagnosis.

Specific Keratinization Disorders
Seborrhea

Seborrhea is a hyperproliferative disorder of keratinocytes seen in cocker spaniels. Other breeds with similar syndromes include springer spaniels, Irish setters, basset hounds, West Highland white terriers, Doberman pinschers, Chinese Shar peis, and Labrador retrievers. Recently, it has been shown that the actual defect is limited to the epidermal cell population and does not involve an underlying metabolic prob-

lem. If seborrheic skin is grafted onto a normal animal, it remains seborrheic. If normal skin is grafted onto a seborrheic dog, it remains normal. Affected dogs frequently have dry and scaling or greasy skin, secondary pyoderma, and, often, ceruminous otitis externa. Other commonly involved areas are the periocular and interdigital regions, the axillae, and the perineum. Diagnosis can be confirmed by biopsies. Treatment includes the following:

- Frequent (twice weekly) antiseborrheic shampooing
- Dietary supplementation with omega-3 and omega-6 fatty acid supplements
- In selected cases treatment with etretinate (Tegison®—Roche Dermatologics), a retinoid used in the treatment of human psoriasis (dosage = 1 mg/kg daily)

Monitoring of blood counts and liver function are mandatory. None of the retinoids are currently licensed for use in dogs and cats.

Zinc-Related Dermatoses

Zinc-related dermatoses include at least three different syndromes:

- Zinc deficiency
- Zinc-responsive dermatosis
- Generic dog food disease

The fact is, however, that anything that interferes with the absorption of zinc, affects its longevity or function in the body, enhances its excretion, or causes general body wasting also reduces the body stores of zinc.

Zinc Deficiency

Some Siberian huskies, malamutes, Samoyeds, and perhaps Great Danes and Doberman pinschers have a genetic defect that decreases the body's ability to absorb zinc from the intestine. Therefore the problem is not necessarily caused by a dietary deficiency of zinc. Even though these animals may ingest normal amounts of zinc, it is not being adequately absorbed. The most commonly affected areas are the top of the nose, the footpads, elbows, and hocks. The areas are typically red and are covered with tenacious crusts. Pruritus may or may not develop.

Zinc-Responsive Dermatosis (see Plate I-1)

In young, rapidly growing dogs, the contents of high calcium diets, calcium supplements, or high fiber diets may compete with zinc for absorption, thus reducing zinc stores. This too is not a true zinc deficiency. Clinically, signs of this condition include:

- Focal crusts and plaques over the head, trunk, and extremities
- Crusty, thickened, and fissured areas around the footpads and top of the nose
- Moderately enlarged lymph nodes in affected areas

Generic Dog Food Disease

Generic dog food disease is a poorly understood phenomenon. The occurrence of extensive crusting and scaling was reported 2 to 4 weeks after dogs were given generic diets as the sole food source. The predominant sites of involvement include the feet, face, pressure points, mucocutaneous junctions, and trunk. It is presumed that the high cereal (i.e., high fiber) content of these diets results in a zinc imbalance, because analysis of these diets often reveals adequate zinc content.

* * *

There are no absolute tests to diagnose these syndromes. Blood levels of zinc are rarely diagnostic. Biopsies are helpful in many cases but may not be able to confirm the diagnosis in all cases. Treatment, however, is relatively straightforward and involves:

- Dietary management
- Zinc supplementation (selected cases only)
- Symptomatic treatment if warranted

Dietary management consists of putting the animals on a good plane of nutrition, removing any and all dietary supplements, and ensuring the animal is fed a brand name dog food. The problem should resolve within 6 to 8 weeks. An animal that requires zinc supplementation usually benefits from administration of zinc sulfate, zinc gluconate, zinc picolinate, or zinc methionine (1.1 mg elemental zinc/kg twice daily). It is important that doses be based on amounts of elemental zinc. For instance, zinc sulfate contains about 22% zinc by weight. Therefore, a 100 mg tablet of zinc sulfate provides 22 mg of elemental zinc. A 100 mg tablet of zinc gluconate (13% zinc) provides 13 mg of elemental zinc. Most forms purchased in pharmacies list the content of elemental zinc on their label (e.g., 10 mg or 50 mg tablets). Recent research has shown that a plant-based enzyme supplement (Prozyme™—The Prozyme Company, Elk Grove Village, Illinois) increases absorption of dietary zinc by as much as 30%. Blood levels of cis-linoleic acid, selenium, and pyridoxine are also enhanced. Symptomatic treatment with antiseborrheic shampoos, emollient rinses, and antibiotics may also be indicated.

Vitamin A–Responsive Dermatosis

Vitamin A–responsive dermatosis is not a vitamin A deficiency but a condition that responds to high supplemental doses of the vitamin, well above maintenance levels. The disorder is usually seen in the cocker spaniel, but other breeds of dog (e.g., Labrador retriever, cairn terrier) may be affected. The condition is characterized by scaling, hair loss, and pinpoint crusting. The crusts originate in the hair follicles and are properly described as follicular hyperkeratosis. Diagnosis is supported by biopsy findings, namely follicular hyperkeratosis and abnormal keratinization (dyskeratosis). Therapy includes megadose vitamin A therapy, usually involving doses of 500 to 1000 IU/kg/day. Most affected cocker spaniels benefit from supplements of 10,000 IU once or twice daily. Because vitamin A is stored in the liver, liver function evaluation should be an important component of any monitoring program.

Sebaceous Adenitis

Sebaceous adenitis is a periappendageal dermatitis (see Plate I-2) in which hair follicles and the glands that supply them are involved in an inflammatory process. It is most commonly reported in standard poodles, but Akitas, Irish setters, golden retrievers, vizslas, yellow Labrador retrievers, and collies may also be affected.

The first clinical signs include noninflammatory hair loss and scaling, usually beginning on the back. As the condition progresses, more areas are affected and infection and pruritus may become evident. Most dogs are less than 5 years of age when first affected. Diagnosis can only be confirmed by histopathologic evaluation of skin biopsies. Samples should be collected from normal, mildly affected, and severely affected skin.

Because sebaceous adenitis is likely a collection of disorders rather than just one disorder, it is not surprising that a single treatment approach is not sufficient for all cases. Initially, corticosteroids may be helpful in stopping the progression of the disorder. Later, frequent antiseborrheic shampooing and application of emollients (e.g., propylene glycol and water, urea, lactic acid) may be beneficial. The propylene glycol can be mixed in a 50:50 combination with water and used as a daily spray. This helps increase the water content of the surface skin, making it more pliable and facilitating the shedding of dead skin. High dose treatment with fish oil or other omega-3 fatty acid sources may offset some of the abnormalities of the surface lipid film that occurs with this disorder. Treatment with isotretinoin (1 mg/kg once or twice daily) is effective in some animals but is not licensed for this purpose. Similarly cyclosporine (Sandimmune®—Sandoz Pharmaceuticals) has been used at oral dosages of 5 mg/kg bid, but side effects must be anticipated. Akitas with this condition appear to be the most refractory to treatment.

Epidermal Dysplasia (see Plate I-3)

Epidermal dysplasia is a severe keratinization disorder seen in West Highland white terriers. It is presumed to be genetic in nature but this is yet to be confirmed. The process starts in dogs less than 1 year of age; the skin of affected animals becomes increasingly scaly, with associated hair loss. Many of these dogs are initially misdiagnosed as having allergies. In time, there is severe erythema, pruritus, hair loss, hyperpigmentation, lichenification and ceruminous otitis. These dogs have been nicknamed "armadillo westies" because of the severity of the skin changes. Infection with the yeast *Malassezia pachydermatis* is a common sequela as is bacterial pyoderma.

The diagnosis is confirmed by skin biopsy, which may also reveal the presence of *Malassezia* yeasts. If not, yeast preparations (see Chapter 4) should be performed to uncover yeasts that may exist elsewhere. Although treatment of the primary condition is universally unsuccessful, management procedures can make the situation bearable. *Malassezia* infection should be treated with ketoconazole (10 mg/kg/day) for a month and twice weekly treatments with ketoconazole shampoo (Nizoral® shampoo—Janssen), miconazole shampoo (e.g., Dermazole—Allerderm/Virbac) or selenium disulfide preparations. This treatment is also effective in many cases in which yeasts are not isolated. Additional therapies include application of propylene glycol and water (50:50) or other emol-

lient sprays on a daily basis. Drugs affecting the keratinization process such as corticosteroids and retinoids, may offer temporary, initial benefit.

Follicular Dysplasia (see Plate I-4)

Types of follicular dysplasia include:

- Color dilution alopecia
- Follicular dystrophy
- Black hair follicular dysplasia
- Focal adnexal dysplasia
- Spiculosis

Color Dilution Alopecia

Color dilution alopecia (color mutant alopecia), probably the most common form of follicular dysplasia, is seen in blue and fawn color dilutions of Doberman pinschers, miniature pinschers, Irish setters, dachshunds, chow chows, poodles, Great Danes, whippets, Yorkshire terriers, Newfoundlands, Chihuahuas, Italian greyhounds, salukis, and mixed breed dogs. The progressive hair loss is only noted in areas of abnormal color; other regions remain normal. Bacterial folliculitis may occur in affected areas. The diagnosis can be made by histopathologic assessment of biopsies. Treatment is symptomatic and includes follicle-flushing shampoos (e.g., benzoyl peroxide), emollient rinses and sprays, and, when bacterial infections are evident, antibiotic therapy.

Follicular Dystrophy

Follicular dystrophy is a similar condition seen in Doberman pinschers, Siberian huskies, English springer spaniels, and rottweilers. These dogs fail to completely shed their puppy coat and the guard hairs become dry and brittle. The result is progressive balding. The remaining coat often has a reddish discoloration. Biopsies are critical in these cases because often the hair follicles are caught in the transitory catagen stage. This "trichilemmal keratinization"—often referred to as "flame follicles"—shares many features with the sex steroid endocrine skin diseases, suggesting that a hormonal imbalance may be involved. Because most affected animals are males, this supposition is worth exploring. A heritable predisposition has also been proposed. No therapies have been successful to date; if a sex hormone link is established, however, treatments like those used for growth hormone–responsive dermatosis may be helpful.

Black Hair Follicular Dysplasia

Black hair follicular dysplasia is a tardive hereditary alopecia in black and white–spotted dogs, especially papillons, dachshunds, and some mongrels. Dysplasia of the follicle in the alopecic areas of black skin results in abnormal hair development, shedding, and scaling. The white skin is not affected. Diagnosis is confirmed by biopsy. No treatments are currently available, but the condition does not cause any medical problems other than dry skin and hair loss.

Focal Adnexal Dysplasia

Focal adnexal dysplasia is a relatively common but poorly studied entity in which firm plaques and nodules develop, usually on the limbs. The hair follicles are thickened and become dilated. Large lesions may become cystic, rupture, and cause a more severe inflammatory reaction. The cause is unknown, and no treatments are available. Antibiotics may be needed to treat cellulitis and furunculosis if the lesions rupture.

Spiculosis

Spiculosis is a dysplastic reaction of hair bulbs in which the hairs become thick and brittle. It has been reported in Kerry blue terriers. The thick, hard, irregular hair shafts (spicules) arise from papules on affected skin. If the diagnosis is suspected based on clinical findings, it can be confirmed by biopsy. The treatment of choice is isotretinoin (Accutane®—Roche Dermatologics) at 1 mg/kg/day or conscious neglect.

Ichthyosis (see Plate I-5)

Ichthyosis is a rare hereditary disease that results in extreme scaling and crusting. If the condition in companion animals is anything like that affecting humans, there are actually several different variants. Most of the affected breeds reported in the literature are terriers or terrier crossbreeds; affected Cavalier King Charles littermates have also been studied. Typically, young dogs have excessive scaling, which progresses with age. The footpads are thickened with large accumulations of keratin at the margins of the pads. The diagnosis is confirmed by biopsies. Treatment is palliative and consists of warm water soaks, antiseborrheic shampooing, and emollient rinses. Etretinate (Tegison®—Roche Dermatologics) may be beneficial in some cases.

Acne (see Plates I-6 and I-7)

Acne is a follicular keratinization defect that affects certain breeds, such as the Great Dane, Doberman pinscher, bulldog, and bull terrier. Bacterial infection is a consequence, not the cause, of the disorder. The condition begins with the development of comedones (blackheads) as the hair follicles first become plugged. Later, as the follicles distend with keratin, they can become nodular and infected and may be accompanied by draining tracts. In dogs the most common areas for involvement are the chin, muzzle, and lip margins; in cats acne lesions are characterized by comedones on the chin and lower lips. The diagnosis can be confirmed by biopsy, but clinical presentation is usually sufficiently suggestive. Treatment is aimed at flushing the hair follicles and keeping them open and clean. Benzoyl peroxide washes are the treatment of choice. Antibiotics are only needed to control secondary bacterial invasion. Canine lesions are often contaminated with staphylococci, whereas cultures from cats usually reveal *Pasteurella multocida* of beta-hemolytic streptococci. If lesions are nodular in nature, intralesional injections of corticosteroids may be needed. Retinoids such as topical tretinoin cream (Retin-A® 0.05%—Ortho Pharmaceutical) are helpful for localized conditions while oral isotretinoin (Accutane®—Roche Dermatologics) is used initially for more generalized problems.

Schnauzer Comedo Syndrome

Schnauzer comedo syndrome is a common, presumably hereditary disorder of follicular keratinization. Affected schnauzers have small crusts on the back, which initially cause little or no discomfort. If crusts become overly distended and secondarily infected, however, other clinical signs become apparent. The diagnosis can frequently be based on clinical signs, but biopsies can confirm the diagnosis if there is any doubt. The treatment of choice initially is twice weekly benzoyl peroxide shampoos, which can be tapered to be given every 2 to 3 weeks for maintenance. Daily alcohol rubs are also helpful at cleansing follicles. For very localized problems, topical tretinoin cream (Retin-A® 0.05%—Ortho Pharmaceutical) can be helpful.

Callus

Calluses develop over pressure points subjected to repeated trauma. They are most commonly seen on the elbows and hocks of large breeds of dogs, and occasionally on the sternum of others (e.g., dachshunds). As dogs drop their weight onto hard surfaces, such as concrete or wood, the repeated impact of these body parts can traumatize the skin and drive hairs and debris into the deeper dermal tissues. This results in callus pyoderma with deep infection and, often, draining tracts.

Most calluses are harmless and require no treatment. For minor problems, application of skin softeners, emollients, and keratolytics (e.g., KeraSolv Gel—DVM Pharmaceuticals) is sufficient. For large calluses and callus pyoderma, the use of antibiotics and protective padding is warranted. Surgery is often an unsatisfactory option because of the sites involved.

Localized Hyperkeratotic Conditions

Several different conditions can result in the localized accumulation of keratin. These include:

- Footpad hyperkeratosis
- Nasodigital hyperkeratosis
- Keratoses
- Lichenoid-psoriasiform dermatosis
- Large plaque parapsoriasis

Footpad Hyperkeratosis (see Plate I-8)

Footpad hyperkeratosis is the localized accumulation of keratin on the footpads such that they become thickened, cracked, and scaly. The most common causes are pemphigus foliaceus, distemper infection (hard pad disease), zinc-related dermatosis, and generalized keratinization disorders. Parasitism, bacterial infections, fungal infections, contact eruptions, other autoimmune diseases, other nutritional conditions, congenitohereditary diseases, and even some cancers might be involved. Initial diagnostic efforts should include skin scrapings, fungal culture, complete blood counts, and, in many cases, biopsies. In cats viral profiles (especially for feline leukemia virus) are mandatory.

Nasodigital Hyperkeratosis

Nasodigital hyperkeratosis is a keratinization disorder in which excess keratin accumulates on the planum nasale (top of nose) and/or footpads. Although any dog can be affected, cocker spaniels, English springer spaniels, and old dogs are most

commonly reported. The accumulated keratin causes dryness, cracking, and ulceration in affected areas. Nasal dermatitis is associated with many systemic and cutaneous diseases, including autoimmune disorders, nutritionally related conditions, metabolic problems, and solar damage, so diagnosis is not simple. Biopsies are helpful in directing further efforts. Treatment should target the underlying cause whenever possible. Symptomatic therapy includes water soaks and sealing in moisture with petroleum jelly. Topical keratolytics such as a combination of salicylic acid, lactic acid, and urea (KeraSolv Gel—DVM Pharmaceuticals) may be helpful in removing surface crusts.

Canine Ear Margin Dermatosis

Canine ear margin dermatosis is a rare keratinization defect seen principally in dachshunds. Affected animals have many greasy plugs that are tightly adherent to the skin surface and hair shafts along the ear edges. No other areas are involved. The cause is unknown, but severe cases can progress to ulceration and necrosis of the pinnae. Diagnosis can be confirmed by biopsy if necessary. Treatment is symptomatic and includes keratolytic shampoos and gels and, in severe cases, topical corticosteroids.

Keratoses

Keratoses are localized accumulations of keratin. They can be further defined as seborrheic, actinic, or proliferative, based on their histopathologic appearance. Actinic keratoses are important because they may represent precancerous lesions. Proliferative keratoses (cutaneous horns) form over tumors, virus-induced lesions (especially feline leukemia virus), and other keratoses. Treatment is symptomatic.

Lichenoid Dermatoses

Lichenoid dermatoses are uncommon disorders in dogs and include idiopathic lichenoid dermatitis, lichenoid keratosis, and lichenoid-psoriasiform dermatitis. Lichenoid-psoriasiform dermatitis (see Plate I-9) affects young springer spaniels and results in scaling plaques that usually are limited to the inner pinnae but sometimes are seen on the abdominal skin. Affected animals are completely asymptomatic, and treatment is not necessary.

Large Plaque Parapsoriasis

Large plaque parapsoriasis is extremely rare. This focal scaling condition of papules, plaques, and crusts may be associated with hyperpigmentation and hair loss. Skin biopsies are needed for diagnosis but may not be confirmatory in all cases. Treatment is attempted with antiseborrheic shampoos, emollients, and corticosteroids. Prednisone (2.2 mg/kg/day) usually results in remission; maintenance doses of 1.1 mg/kg on alternate days are usually sufficient.

IMMUNOLOGY AND SKIN DISEASE

The immune system is a remarkable protective mechanism that helps keep animals and humans safe from a variety of invaders and diseases. The immune system does not consist of one organ but is a complex array of interrelated cells and organs that function in a balanced and integrated fashion.

Immunity refers to all the mechanisms used by the body as protection against environmental agents that are foreign to the body. These foreign substances include drugs, microbes, foods, chemicals, and various inhalants (e.g., pollens).

Although an individual is born with the capacity to mount the defenses provided by the immune system, immunity is only acquired after exposure to the foreign agent. For instance, pets are not born with immunity to rabies. It must be introduced to their system so that they can mount an appropriate, and hopefully protective, response. The substance that triggers the response is known as an "antigen," and the protective protein produced by the immune system is called an "antibody."

Animals receive some passive immunity from their mothers during nursing. The most important period is the first 24 hours after birth, during which colostrum, an antibody-rich portion of the milk, is produced. This immunity is called "passive" rather than "active" because the immunity was actively produced by the mother and then passively transferred to the young; the offspring therefore have received some short-lived protection from their mother but have yet to produce antibodies themselves. This provides some residual protection to the newborn for the first few months of life. Vaccination schedules are established to augment this passive immunity by stimulating antibody production by the young at a time when maternally provided antibody levels are waning. As the antibody protection derived from the mother begins to dwindle, vaccination stimulates the young to start producing their own antibodies.

The normal immune system can falter for a number of reasons, and the outcomes can be quite variable:

- The immune systems may be compromised by drugs or disease (immune suppression).
- It may be impaired (immune dysfunction).
- It may not function properly (immune incompetence).

Some of these problems are inherited, whereas others are acquired.

On the other hand, if the immune system responds excessively, this can also cause damage to the body. These disorders are referred to as immune-mediated diseases. Some animals may actually produce antibodies to parts of themselves in conditions known as autoimmune diseases. In general, each of these immune-mediated diseases can be categorized as one of four hypersensitivity reactions based on the immunologic mechanism involved (Table 1-1). Granulomatous reactions, sometimes listed as type V reactions, are also included in the table.

All of the hypersensitivity reactions are caused by either antibody reactions or immunoreactive cells, especially lymphocytes. In very general terms, differentiation between the two systems (antibody-mediated versus cell-mediated) is based on the type of lymphocyte involved:

- B-lymphocytes (so named because they were first identified in the bursa of chickens) later evolve into antibody-producing cells known as plasma cells. Antibodies are produced in response to specific agents.
- T-lymphocytes are named because they are programmed in the thymus and are responsible for patrolling the body perimeter and searching for invaders.

The first three types of hypersensitivity reactions involve antibodies. Antibody and foreign agent (antigen) fit together like a lock and key so that the antibody-antigen complex can be removed by other scavenging cells of the immune system. Sometimes the antibody response is sufficient to control disease, and other times it is not.

TABLE 1-1

HYPERSENSITIVITY REACTIONS

TYPE	MECHANISM	EFFECTOR	EXAMPLE
I	Immediate	Antibody (IgE, IgG)	Atopy
II	Cytotoxic	Antibody (IgG) ± complement	Pemphigus
III	Immune complex	Antigen-antibody ± complement	Lupus
IV	Delayed	Lymphocyte (lymphokine)	Contact allergy
V	Granulomatous	Histiocyte	Mycobacteriosis

Immunoglobulins

Antibodies are special proteins that are also known as immunoglobulins (Igs). In general, immunoglobulins can be subdivided into different types, identified as IgG, IgM, IgA, and IgE.

Immunoglobulin G

IgG is the most common immunoglobulin found in the bloodstream of animals and humans. When pets are vaccinated, it is this antibody (IgG) that is most often produced, and the antibody is specific for the particular disease agent (e.g., rabies, distemper, feline panleukopenia). Most antibodies latch onto the agent when it is encountered and allow it to be cleared from the body by the rest of the immune system.

Immunoglobulin M

IgM, the first antibody produced, is very large but is rapidly replaced by levels of IgG.

Immunoglobulin A

IgA is responsible for resistance to disease in those parts of the body directly communicating with the environment, such as the respiratory, digestive, integumentary (skin), and urinary / reproductive systems. It is a surface-acting antibody that helps control infections at these important boundaries to the outside world. Vaccines that are introduced via the nose (given intranasally) as a spray—such as the ones for tracheobronchitis (canine cough) and feline infectious peritonitis (FIP)—try to stimulate the production of specific IgA rather than IgG to catch the infection in the respiratory passages before it reaches the bloodstream. Also, IgG does not achieve as high a level in respiratory secretions as does IgA. Several breeds of dog with IgA deficiency have been recognized, the most common of which is the Chinese Shar pei.

Immunoglobulin E

IgE is a specific antibody that is involved in the development of allergy. In an evolutionary sense, this antibody was probably important as a response to parasites, but current hygiene and medical treatment has made this immunoglobulin unnecessary and even problematic. Dogs have a much higher level of IgE in their bloodstream than humans. It is suspected that cats produce IgE as well, but this has not yet been conclusively proven.

* * *

It can therefore be seen that there are many different classes of immunoglobulins and a limitless number of specific antibodies that can be produced in response to disease-causing agents. Unfortunately, the B-cell system may become overactive and produce unnecessary antibodies that may harm the system. In allergic patients, special types of antibodies are produced to a variety of agents (e.g., pollens, molds, house dust, food), causing some disturbing signs. In autoimmune diseases, autoantibodies are produced that selectively attack parts of the animal's own body.

The T-lymphocytes help modulate the immune response, and some may enhance or suppress the effects of B-lymphocytes. T-lymphocytes perform a variety of functions, depending on their type:

• T-helper cells help B-cells make antibody.

- T suppressor cells suppress the production of antibody.
- Some T-lymphocytes directly attack target cells.
- Other T-lymphocytes mediate delayed hypersensitivity reactions (e.g., contact allergy).

The T-lymphocytes also have a direct effect by producing special substances (lymphokines) rather than antibodies.

Every cell in the body bears a unique marker that informs the T-cell system that it belongs; everything else the T-cells encounter is considered foreign and destroyed. This process poses some problems to transplant patients, because T-cells attempt to destroy the transplanted organ (commonly known as organ "rejection"). T-lymphocytes perform important patrol functions for the immune system and offer surveillance against surface attack. T-lymphocyte function becomes deficient in humans with acquired immunodeficiency syndrome (AIDS) and in cats with feline immunodeficiency virus (FIV) infections. Dogs born with defects in their T-cell systems are prone to develop demodicosis.

The skin has its own immune apparatus, referred to as skin-associated lymphoid tissue (SALT) and skin immune system (SIS). The epidermal cells (keratinocytes) produce several important cytokines (proteins involved in regulating the immune response), including interleukins and growth factors; cytokines play a significant role in mediating inflammation and immune responses in the skin. Interleukins serve as communicators between different leukocytes. Most interleukins are classified as lymphokines (produced by lymphocytes) or monokines (produced by monocytes and macrophages). In addition to T-lymphocytes, keratinocytes, and a variety of white blood cells, the skin has Langerhans cells that reside in the lower epidermis. When stimulated by antigen, these dendritic cells migrate through the dermis and then to the lymphatics, initiating an immunologic cascade.

White Blood Cells

The B- and T-lymphocytes are the most important white blood cells (leukocytes) of the immune system. Most of the lymphocytes in the SIS are T-lymphocytes. Although they circulate in the bloodstream, they are found most of the time in the dermis. Also of importance are cells of the mononuclear-phagocyte system.

Mononuclear-Phagocyte System

The mononuclear-phagocyte system is a rather confusing array of cells in many different organ systems that act as an immunologic net and data processing unit. These cells process immunologic information, relay this information to the appropriate cells, and produce a variety of factors and proteins that enhance this action. They are also capable of scavenging foreign material and not only dispose of the invaders but remember the episode to respond to future attacks.

Neutrophils

Neutrophils, sometimes referred to as pus cells, are commonly recruited to fight bacterial infections. They produce a number of enzymes and factors to help with this task and then engulf the microbes to ingest them. These cells are produced in the bone marrow, and their numbers are increased in blood counts taken from patients with infection.

Eosinophils

Eosinophils are white blood cells primarily responsible for downgrading the immune response. They release granules to cause this effect. Eosinophils are most prominent in conditions involving an immune reaction or parasites.

Mast Cells

Mast cells recruit other inflammatory cells, mainly by releasing their contents of inflammatory mediators, such as histamine, protein-breaking enzymes, leukotrienes, and heparin. They are most important in allergic disorders. Basophils are related cells that circulate in the bloodstream.

* * *

Mediator substances—such as leukotrienes, prostaglandins, complement, lymphokines, free radicals, adaptagens, and other factors—are also important in the inflammatory process. Many protein factors are also involved in inflammation and immunity. Most are produced by either lymphocytes or members of the mononuclear-phagocyte system.

IMMUNODEFICIENCY DISEASES

Immunodeficiency syndromes may be primary or secondary:

- The primary immunodeficiencies—most of which are heritable disorders—are caused by underlying defects of the T-cells, B-cells, or neutrophils.
- Secondary immunodeficiencies—which are acquired—are usually attributable to underlying infectious, nutritional, metabolic, or parasitic disorders.

Most primary immunodeficiency diseases are seen in young animals, and there is often a striking breed or species predisposition. On the other hand, secondary immunodeficiencies are usually seen in adult animals, as a consequence of some other problem. The two syndromes are difficult to distinguish clinically, because both result in recurrent infections.

IgA Deficiency

IgA deficiency is the most common specific immunoglobulin deficiency in dogs. Affected animals suffer from a specific lack of IgA, which is important in protecting the body surfaces, especially the skin, respiratory tract, digestive system, and reproductive system. It is most commonly seen in the beagle, Chinese Shar pei, dachshund, chow chow, dalmatian, miniature schnauzer, West Highland white terrier, and German shepherd.

Clinically, IgA deficiency can manifest as surface infections, including recurrent respiratory infections, urinary tract infections, and skin infections. Most dogs have a history of problems from a young age. There is no sex predilection. Concurrent skin problems include allergies, otitis externa, hypothyroidism, or demodicosis. A deficiency of IgA predisposes animals to infections, the development of allergies, and immune-mediated diseases.

Diagnosis is confirmed by submitting serum samples for immunoglobulin analysis (IgA, IgG, IgM). It is not unusual that affected dogs might have high levels of IgG and/or IgM as the body attempts to compensate for the deficient immunoglobulin. It is important to perform blood counts and thyroid profiles on all affected dogs to discount concurrent problems that might affect the response to treatment. Allergy testing is necessary in a significant number of cases.

The treatment of choice for IgA deficiency is nonspecific immune stimulation. This may be done with staphylococcal bacterins such as Staphage lysate (SPL)® (Delmont Laboratories), thymic hormones, or other immunostimulants.

Response is variable. IgA levels should be monitored every 6 months thereafter.

Combined Immunodeficiency

Combined immunodeficiency (CID) is a rare disorder that was first reported in basset hounds. It is inherited as a sex-linked trait in this breed. Pups develop recurrent infections between 3 and 6 months of age when their immunity is waning. These dogs have defective T-cells and hypoplasia of the thymus and lymphoid glands. Commonly, IgG and IgA levels are low as well. Diagnosis can be suspected based on blood tests for immunoglobulin and lymphocyte levels. Confirmation can be made by testing for T-cell function (lymphocyte blastogenesis, delayed-type hypersensitivity testing). There is no adequate treatment. Most die at a young age (9 to 12 months).

Lethal Acrodermatitis

Lethal acrodermatitis is an inherited condition of bull terriers characterized by a marked deficiency of T-cells and impaired cell-mediated immune responsiveness. It appears to be transmitted as an autosomal recessive trait. Affected pups are lighter colored at birth than littermates and develop diarrhea and recurrent respiratory and skin infections. They develop a stilted gait; interdigital dermatitis and footpad lesions are commonplace. Most succumb to pneumonia. On postmortem examination, profound thymic hypoplasia is noted. Most treatments are ineffective, but there are some anecdotal reports about successes using ketoconazole therapy (10 mg/kg bid). Etretinate therapy is also being explored.

Thymic Hypoplasia

Thymic hypoplasia shares many similarities with lethal acrodermatitis. It is seen in weimaraners and is believed to be associated with a growth hormone deficiency. Affected dogs are dwarfed and suffer from recurrent infections. Diagnosis can be confirmed in dwarfed animals by finding growth hormone deficiency with concurrent thymic hypoplasia. Treatment can be attempted with growth hormone and thymic hormone (i.e., thymosin).

Cell-Mediated Immunodeficiency

Cell-mediated immunodeficiency has been documented in German shepherds with chronic recurring pyodermas. These dogs have deep pyoderma and cellulitis associated with abnormal lymphocyte transformation (blastogenesis) assays. In many cases the immunoglobulin levels are elevated but the immune response is ineffective and unbalanced. Occasionally, affected dogs respond to immunomodulatory therapy (e.g., with bacterins, thymic hormones, and levamisole). In Europe successes have been reported with an autogenous vaccine, formulated by combining formalinized discharge with fresh heparinized blood from the patient.

Cyclic Hematopoiesis

Cyclic hematopoiesis is a congenital disorder of grey collies (grey collie syndrome) and is associated with the mutant gene for silver-grey (blue) haircoat. This disorder is caused by an autosomal recessive trait and is lethal to dogs by 6 months of age if treatment is not instituted. Affected pups have the coat color change and are weak, stunted, and subject to recurrent infections. Systemic amyloidosis is a common finding. Diagnosis is made by evaluating blood counts every few days for a 2 week period. The disorder is characterized by a rise and fall of blood cells over an 11 to 14 day interval. Neutropenia is the most common finding, and the condition was once referred to as "cyclic neutropenia." Treatment can be attempted with daily endotoxin or lithium. The dose of lithium citrate (Lithonate-S—Rowell Laboratories) is 21 mg/kg/day in divided doses to reach a desired serum level of 0.05 to 1.0 mEq/L. This preparation is toxic to cats. Bone marrow transplants have also been used experimentally to correct the stem cell defect.

Canine Granulocytopathy Syndrome

Canine granulocytopathy syndrome is an inherited defect of neutrophil function that has been reported in Irish setters. A slightly different but related condition (bactericidal defect) has been reported in Doberman pinschers. Affected dogs have no problem making neutrophils, but these cells do not function properly. Recurrent fever, pyoderma, gingivitis, and other evidence of infection are commonplace. Blood counts reveal persistently high levels of neutrophils (perhaps 10 times normal) with hyperpigmentation and regenerative left shift.

Complement Deficiency

Complement (C3) deficiency is a rare immune deficit that is transmitted as an autosomal recessive trait in humans and Brittany spaniels. Although carriers appear unaffected, homozygotes for the condition have recurrent infections that can be life threatening. Diagnosis is made by assessing C3 levels, which are 10% of normal in affected dogs and 30% to 50% of normal in carrier animals. No treatment options are currently available other than managing the recurrent infections.

Immunoincompetence

Sometimes, dogs and cats have recurrent infections for no apparent reason. Undoubtedly, many are due to immune deficits that we do not have the abilities to measure. Others may be due to suppressive actions of drugs, environmental pollutants, dietary additives, concurrent diseases, or other stressors. The term "immunoincompetence" is acceptable in these cases because there may not be a clear-cut deficiency or visible evidence of immune suppression.

These animals are often diagnostic enigmas because they never respond completely to therapy or infections recur once treatment has concluded. Also, diagnostic tests often are not conclusive (e.g., thyroid levels are borderline or immunoglobulin levels are low normal or marginal). These cases, commonly seen in practice, do not fit neatly into any specific category.

The diagnostic approach to these cases should involve a complete physical examination, thyroid profile, complete blood count (CBC), and determination of immunoglobulin levels. Most cases yield equivocal results. Treatment may be attempted with long-term antibiotic therapy, and immunomodulatory therapy (discussed below) may be warranted.

TESTS OF IMMUNE FUNCTION

The diagnosis of immunodeficiency disorders is complicated by the following:

- The conditions are relatively rare.
- The tests needed to confirm a diagnosis are not universally available.
- These conditions have been described only recently; many veterinarians may not be familiar with the conditions or the tests needed to diagnose them.

The candidate for an immune function work-up is a dog or cat with recurrent infections for no apparent reason. Primary immunodeficiencies are found in young animals, usually less than 6 months of age. Secondary immunodeficiencies often follow infections or infestations, especially demodicosis in dogs and feline immunodeficiency virus and feline leukemia virus in cats.

A basic assessment of the immune response should evaluate the B-cell system, the T-cell system, and neutrophil function. Complement studies are rarely needed. The first test to be performed in all cases is a CBC with careful leukogram assessment. This is helpful in evaluating the T-cell system as well as neutrophil function.

Measuring the T-Cell System

Lymphopenia is a useful (albeit imprecise) measure of T-cell numbers because about 75% of the circulating lymphocytes are T-cells. Therefore a drop in total lymphocyte numbers usually implies a loss of T-cells.

Lymphocyte stimulation (blastogenesis) is a test that can be performed by specialized laboratories. A sample of peripheral blood lymphocytes (most of which are T cells) are stimulated by phytohemagglutinin (PHA) or concanavalin A. Tritiated thymidine is used as a radioactive marker of cell division (stimulation). Blood from a normal dog or cat must also be submitted to serve as a control sample.

A similar test that can be performed in the clinic is a delayed-type hypersensitivity test. This is performed like a regular allergy test; PHA is injected intradermally, and the reaction is monitored in 24 to 48 hours. Technically, this is similar to a tuberculin test. The difference is that PHA causes reactions in most normal animals. Those that do not respond likely have some defect in their T-cell–mediated immune response. Unlike humans, however, dogs have weak responses to most stimulants, and results must be cautiously evaluated in this species.

Other sophisticated tests of T-cell function are levels of T-helper cells (CD4+) and T-suppressor cells (CD8+), total T-lymphocyte counts, and ratio of T-helper to T-suppressor cells. These are only available on an experimental basis and are not performed at most veterinary laboratories.

Measuring the B-Cell System

It is possible to measure total B-cell numbers in a blood sample, because B-cells (unlike T-cells) have immunoglobulin molecules on their surface. It is not practical to perform this evaluation with current assays, however. What can be done and is of more importance is measuring levels of the specific immunoglobulin families in blood samples. IgG, IgM, and IgA can all be measured from a single blood sample. IgE levels are not needed because they only constitute a small percentage of circulating immunoglobulins and because IgE deficiencies (agammaglobulinemia E) do not cause medical problems. The most simple and reliable method of quantitating immunoglobulin levels is by quantitative radial immunodiffusion (RID). This test is performed by specialized laboratories.

Specific aspects of the immune system can also be measured. To measure response to a particular antigen, (e.g., vaccine), a blood sample is collected and the levels of antibody are compared to those in a sample drawn 10 days after vaccination. An increase in titer implies immunologic recognition and immunoglobulin production.

Measuring Neutrophil Numbers and Function

Neutrophil numbers can be simply evaluated by careful assessment of a leukogram. Neutropenia is defined as less than 3000 neutrophils/µl of blood in dogs and less than 2500/µl of blood in cats. The numbers of neutrophils counted reflect the circulating neutrophil pool (CNP). Another population of neutrophils known as the marginal neutrophil pool (MNP) contains roughly the same number of cells in dogs. In this species, therefore, the actual total neutrophil count is twice that of the leukogram. In the cat the circulating pool is small such that the ratio of circulating to marginal neutrophils is about 1:3. Obviously, shifts in the CNP and the MNP affect neutrophil counts more profoundly in cats than dogs.

Measuring neutrophil function is more difficult than counting neutrophils on a leukogram. To function properly a neutrophil must be able to respond to stimuli, engulf the organism, and kill it. Chemotactic assays, phagocytic index, bactericidal activity, chemiluminescence, and the nitroblue-tetrazolium (NBT) assay can be performed by specialized laboratories for those rare cases that warrant them.

Measuring Complement Levels

Complement plays a role in certain autoimmune and hypersensitivity disorders by binding

TABLE 1-2

IMMUNE STIMULANTS

DRUG	DOSAGE/ADMINISTRATION		
Staphage lysate (SPL)® (Delmont Laboratories)	Day 1: 0.2 ml SC Day 2: 0.4 ml SC Day 3: 0.6 ml SC Day 4: 0.8 ml SC Day 5: 1.0 ml SC Day 12: 1.5 ml SC Weekly: 1.5 ml SC or 0.5 ml SC every 3–4 days		
Staphoid® A-B (Coopers Animal Health) or Lysigin® (Bio-Ceutic)	Day 1: 0.1 ml ID; 0.15 ml SC Day 2: 0.1 ml ID; 0.40 ml SC Day 3: 0.1 ml ID; 0.65 ml SC Day 4: 0.1 ml ID; 0.90 ml SC Day 5: 0.1 ml ID; 1.15 ml SC Day 12: 0.1 ml ID; 1.40 ml SC Day 19: 0.1 ml ID; 1.65 ml SC Day 26: 0.1 ml ID; 1.90 ml SC Monthly: 0.1 ml ID; 1.90 ml SC		
Levamisole	2.2 mg/kg 3 times/wk		

ImmunoRegulin® (ImmunoVet)	Weight	Dose	Frequency
	<17 lb (<8 kg)	0.25 ml IV	Injections are given twice weekly for 2 weeks, then weekly until good clinical response
	17–33 lb (8–15 kg)	0.50 ml IV	
	34–88 lb (16–40 kg)	0.75 ml IV	
	>88 lb (>40 kg)	1.00 ml IV	

to immune complexes and initiating an inflammatory reaction. Levels of complement, especially C3, can be measured by specialized laboratories. Currently, evaluation of complement in dogs and cats is not routine.

IMMUNOMODULATORY THERAPY

Immunomodulatory therapy is used in an attempt to "normalize" the immune process. Although gamma globulin therapy (100 mg/kg IM once monthly) can be used for B-cell defects, no specific therapy is available for most immunodeficiency and immunoincompetence cases. Treatment options involve "nonspecific" immune stimulation using bacterins, levamisole, or thymic hormones (Table 1-2).

Bacterins are suspensions of bacteria used as vaccines to stimulate the immune response. They can be prepared from the bacteria from individual animals (autogenous bacterins) or purchased commercially. Staphage lysate (SPL)® (Delmont Laboratories), Staphoid® A-B (Coopers Animal Health), and Lysigin® (Bio-Ceutic) are derived from staphylococci, whereas ImmunoRegulin® (ImmunoVet) is derived from *Propionibacterium acnes.* The staphylococcal preparations can be given subcutaneously, but ImmunoRegulin® must be given intravenously or intraperitoneally. Staphage lysate (SPL)® appears to be the preparation of choice for nonspecific immune stimulation.

Levamisole is an anthelmintic used in large animals but has been shown to potentiate the immune system at dosages of 2.2 mg/kg three times weekly. Unfortunately, it can cause a number of severe side effects, including depression, inappetence, ataxia, hepatic degeneration, hemolytic anemia, gastric upset, cardiac arrhythmias, respiratory distress, and convulsions. Use of levamisole as an immune stimulant warrants care-

NUTRIENTS THAT MAY BE BENEFICIAL FOR PETS WITH SKIN DISEASES	
Vitamins	**Fatty Acids**
Vitamin A	cis-Linoleic acid
Pyridoxine	Eicosapentaenoic acid
Riboflavin	gamma-Linolenic acid
Pantothenic acid	
Ascorbic acid	**Amino Acids**
Vitamin E	Methionine
	Cysteine
Minerals	Cystine
Zinc	
Selenium	

DIETARY CAUSES OF SKIN DISEASE

Deficiency

Increased requirement

Imbalance

Hypersensitivity or intolerance

Nutritionally responsive disorder

ful and routine monitoring of blood counts and biochemical profiles.

Natural immune stimulants can also be helpful in dogs and cats but have been less intensively studied than chemotherapeutic approaches. Thymic hormones have been used experimentally to try to stimulate the immune system with some successes. Nevertheless, these products are expensive and difficult to acquire. Commercial desiccated thymus gland extracts contain undetermined amounts of these hormones and are commercially available and relatively inexpensive. Few clinical trials have been performed to demonstrate their usefulness, however. Vitamin E and selenium have been clearly demonstrated to augment the immune system, but there is insufficient evidence that they result in appreciable immune stimulation. Most research has shown that deficiencies adversely affect the immune system, but little has been done to show the effect of supplementation on immunodeficiency not associated with nutritional deficiency.

As progress is made in the study of immunology in dogs and cats, cytokines likely will prove useful in the management of recurrent infections. This is already being explored for respiratory disease resistance in cattle and pigs. As mentioned, cytokines are just proteins involved in regulating the immune response. To date, granulocyte colony-stimulating factor (G-CSF) has been cloned in dogs, and tumor necrosis factor (TNF-alpha) and interferon-alpha have been cloned in cats. Much attention had been originally focused on interferon, but interleukin research holds the most promise today.

NUTRITION AND SKIN DISEASE

Few topics stir debate among veterinarians, technicians, breeders, pet supply professionals, and pet owners as much as the subject of nutrition. When a pet has skin problems, most pet owners are tempted to change the diet and they are encouraged in this process by most breeders, pet store employees, and other pet owners. On the other hand, most veterinarians tend to downplay the role of nutrition in skin diseases if owners are feeding one of the commercially prominent diets.

Nutritional supplements for pets abound in the marketplace, yet few actually meet the requirements of a pet with a skin problem. Animals have a certain maintenance requirement for essential amino acids, essential fatty acids, vitamins, and minerals. During growth and times of stress, this requirement is essentially doubled. Skin disease is a definite form of stress because a high percentage of dietary nutrients are needed to maintain the skin and haircoat on a daily basis. The need for additional nutrients is not generalized, however. Certain vitamins, minerals, fatty acids and amino acids are more likely to be beneficial than others (see box at left).

There are several different circumstances under which diet can have an impact on skin problems (see box above). Veterinarians tend to concentrate on deficiency disorders but these are relatively rare in pets fed commercial rations. It is important that diets exceed National Research Council (NRC) requirements because these levels only indicate amounts that prevent deficiency. These requirements are much different than recommended daily allowances (RDAs) or Optimal Daily Allowances (ODAs). For minimum requirements in the United States diets should meet daily requirements based on American Association of Feed Control Officials (AAFCO) feeding trials for specific life stages. In Canada diets should be certified as acceptable by the Canadian Veterinary Medical Association.

Much more common than dietary deficiencies are nutritional imbalances. Some of these are the fault of commercial diets, but, more often, the problem is the result of supplementation by pet owners. For example, calcium supplements can interfere with the absorption of zinc, leading to deficiency-type syndromes, even when there is adequate zinc in the ration. Cheap diets, especially generic dog foods, may have a high percentage of cereal and fiber that can also result in decreased absorption of zinc. With oversupplementation of fatty acids, the requirement for additional vitamin E is also increased. Therefore dietary supplements should be discouraged unless there is a medically important reason for them.

There are relevant reasons to consider supplementation in some circumstances:

- The various processing methods of pet food are very exacting and potentially destructive to nutrients such as vitamins.
- The exposure of vitamins to light, oxygen, wide pH changes, heat, and moisture can result in significant losses of vitamin potency.
- Vitamins and minerals may be poorly balanced in homemade rations.
- Some pets, show dogs and cats, and competitive dogs may benefit from more "optimal" nutrient sources than the average pet.

The concept of nutritional supplementation to achieve a healthier skin and haircoat is easy to appreciate, yet there is scant evidence supporting this practice.

Most experts in the field of pet nutrition agree that animals on a good basic plane of nutrition achieve little benefit from supplementation; most commercially prominent diets provide considerably more of all the required vitamins and minerals than needed by pets on a daily basis. Still, several skin disorders have been recognized that have responded to increased amounts of specific nutrients in the diet.

Protein

Proteins are needed as a source of amino acids, the building blocks of body proteins. The skin and hair require 25% to 30% of the animal's total daily protein intake for maintenance; a minimum of 12% of the caloric intake (usually 22% on a dry basis) should be made up of protein in canine diets. Dogs and cats do not have a specific protein requirement, however. They need specific "essential amino acids" in their diets. The percentage of protein in the diet is less important than is the presence of all the essential amino acids in the correct balance. The high protein requirement of the cat (24% on a dry basis) does not seem to be related to an elevated requirement for any one amino acid. Cats fed dog foods may become protein deficient because the protein requirement for dogs is much less. Cats have a very real requirement for taurine and arginine, two important amino acids, but deficiencies rarely manifest as skin and haircoat problems. Protein quality is more important than the actual percentage of protein in the diet. If the source of protein cannot be digested, absorbed, and utilized, the actual percentage listed on the package is irrelevant.

Because most commercial pet foods have more than adequate amounts of protein, protein deficiency is rare in animals and only seen in individuals fed a poor quality diet or those animals that are ill and unable to take adequate feedings. Clinical signs include a dry and brittle haircoat, scaling, patchy hair loss, and, perhaps, crusting. Treatment consists of providing a good quality diet that contains adequate protein. Changing to a better quality diet is more realistic than trying to supplement a poorly formulated homemade or commercial diet.

Fatty Acids

Fats usually make up 5% to 20% of the dry matter of pet foods and may provide 25% to 50% of the daily caloric needs of the animal. Fats are a great source of fuel and supply 2.25 times more energy than either proteins or carbohydrates. They also provide essential fatty acids (EFAs), increase the palatability of feeds, and provide a vehicle for absorption of fat-soluble vitamins. Though linoleic, alpha-linolenic, and arachidonic acids are all considered essential fatty acids, linoleic acid is truly essential in the dog; if it is adequately provided in the diet, the other two fatty acids can be synthesized within the body. In cats arachidonic acid must also be supplied.

Linoleic acid is the major unsaturated fatty acid in most vegetable oils and makes up 15% to 25% of poultry and pork fat. Essential fatty acids should constitute at least 1% of the diet or 2% of the caloric intake. Because animals tend to regulate their food intake by energy needs, fats should not constitute more than 20% of the diet or the animal will not consume enough to meet maintenance requirements for other nutrients.

Poor quality pet foods may be deficient in fatty acids. Dry foods in particular are limited in the amount of fats that can be incorporated without causing rancidity. Antioxidants are normally added to foods to delay this process, but foods stored for long periods, especially at high temperatures, can lose their fatty acid content. Medical conditions that limit the body's ability to absorb or metabolize ingested fats can also result in fatty acid deficiency. Animals must normally be fed a fatty acid–deficient diet for many months before they begin to show signs. A dry, lusterless coat and prominent dandruff are often the first signs evident. Bacterial infections can further affect the skin and haircoat.

Therapy involves feeding a good quality food with adequate fat content and supplementing the diet with a suitable fatty acid compound. This fatty acid supplement may be purchased commercially or formulated by adding adequate sources of linoleic acid (and arachidonic acid in the cat) to the diet. The best sources of linoleic acid are safflower oil and flaxseed oil. Arachidonic acid is only found in animals (the cat is an obligate carnivore); fish, meat, and egg yolks are good sources. Some fatty acid supplements (e.g., sunflower oil, olive oil) may alter serum and cutaneous fatty acid concentrations in dogs and are more useful than saturated fats as supplements. Plant-based enzyme supplements (e.g., Prozyme™—The Prozyme Company, Elk Grove Village, Illinois) have also been shown to significantly increase blood levels of cis-linoleic acid and alpha-linolenic acid and so offer a nonfat alternative to increasing fatty acid levels in the blood. Fat supplements should be given cautiously to animals with pancreatitis, gallbladder disease, or malabsorption syndromes, in which increased dietary fat can have medical consequences. Excessively high levels of fatty acids can interfere with the metabolism of vitamin E. Topical applications of essential fatty acids also result in some absorption directly through the skin.

Omega-3 and Omega-6 Fatty Acids

Essential fatty acids are polyunsaturated fatty acids of which two series have been described:

- The omega-3 (n3) series is derived from alpha-linolenic acid.
- The omega-6 (n6) series is derived from cis-linoleic acid.

alpha-Linolenic acid and cis-linoleic acid have no biologic activity other than their capacity to provide energy like other fats. To function as EFAs, they must be biochemically transformed in the body. Specific enzymes are required to convert alpha-linolenic acid to eicosapentaenoic acid and cis-linoleic acid to gamma-linolenic acid. The resulting products have biologic activities as essential fatty acids and continue along different biochemical pathways.

The omega-3 fatty acids include:

- Eicosapentaenoic acid (EPA)
- Docosapentaenoic acid (DPA)
- Docosahexaenoic acid (DHA)

All are derivatives of linolenate and originate in phytoplankton and algae, which are consumed by larger marine life, such as fish. Some fish (e.g., herring, mackerel, salmon) store these fatty acids in their muscles, whereas others (e.g., cod) store them in the liver. Cod liver oil, with 9% to 20% EPA, is rarely used in animals because oversupplementation can result in toxicity from fat-soluble vitamins. The omega-3 fatty acids may be helpful supplements in pets with allergies, keratinization disorders (seborrhea), arthritis, heart disease, and hyperlipidemia.

The most important omega-6 fatty acid is gamma-linolenic acid. Evening primrose (*Oenothera biennis*) oil, borage oil (*Borago officinalis*), and blackcurrant (*Ribes nigrum*) seed oil are major sources.

The positive effects of omega fatty acids are probably related to enzyme bypass rather than correction of any immune defect. Such products as DermCaps (DVM) and EFA-Z Plus® (Allerderm/Virbac) contain a combination of omega-3 and omega-6 fatty acids. These differ from most vegetable oils sold in retail outlets, which contain linoleic and alpha-linolenic acids but not their omega-3 and omega-6 derivatives.

Zinc

Zinc is a cofactor in many enzymes, nucleic acid metabolism, and immune function. Some dog food ingredients and supplements such as calcium (Ca), phytates (fiber), iron (Fe), tin (Sn), and copper (Cu) decrease zinc (Zn) absorption. This is another reason why general supplements that include a multitude of nutrients may actually do more harm than good. Anything that interferes with the absorption of zinc, affects its longevity or function in the body, enhances its excretion, or causes general body wasting and catabolism also reduces the body stores of zinc.

Zinc-responsive dermatoses have been recognized in dogs (see Plate I-1):

- One syndrome has been recognized in rapidly growing puppies.
- Another syndrome appears to affect mainly the sled dog breeds.

These animals have a higher than normal requirement for zinc, and their blood zinc levels are normal.

The first syndrome involves dietary supplementation, especially with calcium and phytate-containing products, in young, rapidly growing dogs. These dogs therefore suffer from a functional zinc imbalance. This is another reason why calcium supplements are potentially harmful more often than they are helpful in the rapidly growing dog.

The clinical presentation is usually one of tenacious crusts, redness, and a variable degree of itchiness; the most affected areas include the face, footpads, elbows, and hocks. It is quite likely that the condition formerly known as "dry pyoderma" was really zinc-responsive dermatosis. Young, rapidly growing dogs whose diets have been oversupplemented (especially with calcium) may also have stunted growth, bone deformities, and a poor appetite. Signs of zinc deficiency in kittens include scaling, reduced weight gains, and impaired testicular function.

The second syndrome affects some Siberian huskies, malamutes, Samoyeds and, perhaps, Great Danes and Doberman pinschers. These dogs may have a genetic defect that results in a decreased ability to absorb zinc from the intestine. This may also result in impaired metabolism of zinc.

Treatment is straightforward and relatively easy. Animals whose diets have been oversupplemented respond to elimination of the supplementation and provision of a balanced diet. Animals with inherited defects probably require some form of zinc supplementation (1 mg/kg of elemental zinc once or twice daily) for life (see box at right). Most forms purchased in pharmacies list the content of elemental zinc on their labels. Recent research has shown that a plant-based enzyme supplement (Prozyme™—The Prozyme Company, Elk Grove Village, Illinois) increases absorption of dietary zinc by as much as 30%. Blood lev-

---

SUITABLE FORMULATIONS FOR ZINC SUPPLEMENTATION	
Zinc sulfate	Zinc methionine
Zinc gluconate	Zinc picolinate

---

els of cis-linoleic acid, selenium, and pyridoxine are also enhanced. Animals that absorb zinc poorly from the digestive tract must be given zinc intravenously if treatment is to be successful.

Another condition known as "generic dog food disease" may also reflect a zinc imbalance, but this has not been decidedly proven. These dogs usually develop clinical signs between 2 and 4 weeks after being given a generic diet as the sole food source. Affected animals are often healthy on physical examination but lethargic and depressed. Extensive crusting and scaling are noted; predominant sites of involvement include the distal extremities, face, pressure points, lips, nailbeds, and trunk.

Diagnosis is often made by careful physical examination, attention to feeding history, pathologic evaluation of biopsies, and response to diet correction. Treatment involves dietary management only; usually, switching to a brand name diet is sufficient to correct the situation in 6 to 8 weeks. Ongoing dietary supplementation is unnecessary in these cases.

Vitamin A

Vitamin A has important roles in maintaining the integrity of the skin, maintaining the architecture of the skin, and regulating immune function. Anything that interferes with the absorption of vitamin A or enhances its excretion can result in a relative deficiency. Most animals can form vitamin A in their bodies if provided with beta-carotene, but cats require preformed vitamin A.

A vitamin A–responsive dermatosis has been reported in dogs. This is not a deficiency syndrome but rather a skin condition that responds to large doses of vitamin A supplementation. The disorder is usually seen in the cocker spaniel, but other breeds (e.g., Labrador retriever, cairn terrier) may also be affected. The condition is characterized by dandruff, hair loss and marked crusting, especially on the back. The scaling and crusting (follicular keratosis) originate in the hair follicles.

In the cat vitamin A deficiency has resulted in night blindness, loss of hair, rough coat, and muscle weakness. Cats fed dog foods can become deficient in vitamin A because they require vitamin A preformed and cannot synthesize it from beta carotene. It is also clear that vitamin A toxicity is a much larger threat to cats than vitamin A deficiency because many organs (especially the liver and heart) contain exceptionally high levels of vitamin A.

Diagnosis is based on the history, clinical signs, and histopathologic evaluation of biopsies. Therapy includes megadose vitamin A administration (10,000 to 50,000 IU once or twice daily), usually for life. Twice daily administration may be necessary initially to effect remission. Doses should then be tapered to the minimal amount on which the patient can be maintained with few or no lesions. Use of large doses of vitamin A should not be viewed lightly in view of reports of toxicities. Because vitamin A is stored in the liver, liver function evaluation should be an important component of any monitoring program.

Vitamin E

Vitamin E is a fat-soluble vitamin that acts as a natural antioxidant and is a mild anti-inflammatory agent. Good natural sources include wheat germ, soybeans, vegetable oils, enriched flour, whole wheat, whole grain cereals, and eggs.

Dogs with experimentally induced vitamin E deficiency show scaling (dandruff), increased susceptibility to infection, redness of the skin, and visual defects resembling progressive retinal atrophy. These observations have only been made under experimental conditions, and vitamin E deficiency is extremely rare in pets fed good quality commercial diets.

Vitamin E deficiency causes steatitis (yellow fat disease), retinal disease, and impaired reproduction in the cat. This deficiency was a major problem when cats were fed predominantly fish diets that were not protected with antioxidants. Although antioxidants such as ethoxyquin have received a degree of notoriety lately, their use in diets has made vitamin E deficiency almost nonexistent.

Excessive supplementation with fatty acids can actually reduce the availability of vitamin E in the body. The stability of vitamin E varies considerably among the different forms available. At therapeutic levels (200 to 800 IU twice daily) vitamin E has been used in treatment of discoid and systemic lupus erythematosus, demodicosis, acanthosis nigricans, dermatomyositis, and epidermol-

ysis bullosa simplex. Vitamin E is rarely successful alone in the management of these conditions but can be a relatively nontoxic aid to therapy.

GENETICS AND SKIN DISEASE

There are many breed-related skin diseases, but relatively few have been studied in great detail. Most of these conditions tend to run in families (the result of familial traits) rather than being clear-cut genetic disorders. Therefore conditions such as inhalant allergies (atopy) can be prevalent in certain breeds, but the outcome of specific matings may be difficult to predict. Several conditions with a genetic basis are discussed in different parts of this book. For example, lethal acrodermatitis is covered under immunodeficiency disorders and several inherited scaling disorders are covered as keratinization disorders.

Cutaneous Asthenia (see Plates I-10 and I-11)

Cutaneous asthenia (Ehlers-Danlos syndrome) is a biochemical disorder that causes the skin to be overly fragile and stretchable. Affected breeds include the beagle, dachshund, boxer, St. Bernard, German shepherd, English springer spaniel, greyhound, schnauzer, and mongrels. The genetic nature of the condition is complex, but there is much evidence to suggest a dominant trend. An autosomal recessive form of the disease has been described in Himalayan cats. Another form in domestic short-haired cats is transmitted by autosomal dominant inheritance and is lethal in homozygotes. Cutaneous asthenia is an inherited disorder of connective tissue characterized primarily by skin fragility, skin hyperextensibility, joint hypermobility, and vascular fragility. In dogs the tensile strength of the skin is only one twenty-seventh of that of nonaffected littermates. There are 11 different types of cutaneous asthenia in humans, but studies in animals have not been as thorough.

The diagnosis of cutaneous asthenia is usually made clinically, but it is also helpful to calculate a skin extensibility index, as follows:

$$\frac{\text{Height of fold of skin over lumbar region (cm)}}{\text{Distance from occiput to base of tail (cm)}} \times 100$$

A skin extensibility of greater than 14.5 in dogs and 19 in cats is highly suggestive of cutaneous asthenia. Biopsies can also be helpful, but not all cases have diagnostic changes evident on regularly prepared specimens. Some diagnostic changes can only be uncovered with electron microscopy, which is not commonly available to general practitioners.

No treatments are available for cutaneous asthenia, but dogs and cats with this disease can have a normal life span provided they are protected from trauma. Affected animals should not be used for breeding.

Dermatomyositis (see Plate I-12)

Dermatomyositis is seen mostly in collies, Shetland sheepdogs, and their crossbreeds but has also been reported in an Australian cattle dogs, basset hounds, and Pembroke Welsh collies. It is an inflammatory disease of skin, muscle, and, sometimes, blood vessels. The condition is presumed to be inherited as an autosomal dominant trait, with variable expressivity. It has recently been proposed that a genetic predilection complicated by an infectious agent (likely a virus) may actually initiate clinical disease. It has also been proposed that the multisystemic nature of dermatomyositis suggests an immune-mediated process. Clearly, the condition requires further investigation.

Animals first begin to show signs at about 12 weeks of age, including erosions, ulcers, scars, and crusts on the face, ears, elbows, hocks, and other friction points. There is associated hair loss. In later stages muscle wasting may be evident. The first sign of myositis is usually temporal muscle wasting on the forehead. More severely affected dogs may have difficulty drinking, eating, and swallowing; megaesophagus can result in aspiration pneumonia. Many affected dogs experience stunted growth. Although rare, adult onset dermatomyositis has been seen, particularly in the Shetland sheepdog. Some of these dogs may have had subtle lesions as pups, with the overt disease precipitated by stressful events such as whelping, lactation, estrus, trauma, or exposure to intense sunlight.

Diagnosis is suspected based on clinical findings, and histopathologic assessment of biopsies is often supportive. Electromyographic (EMG) studies may show abnormalities in the muscles as well. Basic hematologic and biochemical profiles usually reveal no abnormalities. Serum concentrations of IgG and circulating immune complexes (CICs) are usually elevated in the face of normal IgA and IgM levels. The degree of elevation of IgG and CIC often correlates positively with disease severity. Occasionally, antiglobulin (Coombs') and rheumatoid factor tests are positive. Serum antibody titers to calicivirus and other viruses have been isolated in affected dogs, suggesting the possibility that an infectious agent may contribute to the pathogenesis of dermatomyositis.

There are no specific treatments for dermatomyositis. Both vitamin E (200 to 800 IU/day) and corticosteroids (0.5 mg/kg daily or on alternate days) have been used to relieve scaling and scarring, but neither can cure the condition. Some animals appear to go into remission spontaneously around puberty, whereas others get progressively worse. Animals that have recovered and their parents should not be bred. Insufficient data have been collected to permit reliable pedigree analysis. Pentoxifylline (Trental®—Hoechst-Roussel Pharmaceuticals) is being evaluated for the management of severe cases, but optimal doses have not yet been established.

Disorders of Pigmentation
Dalmation Bronzing Syndrome

Dalmatian bronzing syndrome likely represents an inherited defect in metabolism of uric acid (in humans accumulation of uric acid results in gout). Dalmatians with this defect for development of urinary stones suffer from recurrent urinary tract infections; these dogs may develop a "moth-eaten" coat that becomes secondarily infected and may even change color to a bronze hue, especially along the back. The diagnosis can be confirmed by biopsy or suspected based on blood tests for uric acid and analysis of urine for urate crystals. Because most dalmatians have higher uric acid levels than other breeds, diagnosis must be made cautiously on the basis of significantly elevated levels. The condition can easily be controlled by limiting the amount of specific proteins (purines) in the diet and/or by treating with drugs (i.e., allopurinol) that lower blood uric acid levels. Commercial prescription diets are available (e.g., Prescription Diet® Canine u/d®—Hill's); alternatively, recipes for diets are available that substitute eggs and vegetables for meats (which are particularly high in purines).

Acquired Aurotrichia (Gilding Syndrome)

Acquired aurotrichia (gilding syndrome) is seen in miniature schnauzers; the coat color of affected animals changes from normal to golden, especially along the topline. Most of these dogs are fairly young (average age of 2½ years when first detected). Diagnosis is confirmed by biopsy findings of a loss of pigment in the primary (guard) hairs and the relative atrophy of secondary hairs. Approximately half of these dogs eventually regain their normal color without medical intervention. Affected dogs should not be bred but are unlikely to suffer from any medical problems as a result of this condition.

Pigmentary Loss Syndromes

Pigmentary loss syndromes include:

- Vitiligo—patchy loss of pigment
- Leukotrichia—whitening of the hairs
- Poliosis—greying of the hairs

In general, vitiligo refers to white patches that occur on the surface of the skin. A heritable form of vitiligo may be seen in Belgian Tervurens, Labrador retrievers, rottweilers, and Doberman pinschers. A similar loss of pigment in chow chows is the result of an inherited deficiency of tyrosinase, an enzyme important in pigment production.

Leukotrichia was reported in Labrador retrievers, which started to show whitening of the hairs on the face, back, and legs by 8 weeks of age. Apparently the condition resolved on its own by 14 weeks of age, with no need for treatment. It is recommended that biopsies and blood profiles be done on all cases of pigmentary change to differentiate genetic and nongenetic causes.

Albinism

Albinism is relatively rare in dogs and cats. In cats the albino series is composed of a dominant normal color gene and several recessive mutant alleles that are incompletely dominant and result in silver, Burmese, Maltese, and Siamese dilutions. The Chédiak-Higashi syndrome is an autosomal recessive genetic disorder seen in blue smoke Persian cats with yellow rather than copper-colored eyes. This partial form of albinism is associated with an increased susceptibility to infection, a bleeding tendency, and photophobia. Affected cats have enlarged intracytoplasmic granules in many neutrophils, which appear eosinophilic with most common blood stains. Ophthalmic examination and coagulation profiles are also indicated. Cats with Waardenburg's syndrome are not albinos. This syndrome is characterized by white fur, blue eyes, and hearing loss. The hearing loss may be unilateral or bilateral, and long-haired animals are afflicted with hearing loss more often than short-haired animals.

Lentigo

Lentigo (lentiginosis profusa) is a rare condition in which black macules and patches are found on the skin. The pug is predisposed to this condition, and the mode of inheritance is believe to be autosomal dominant. The general health status of these dogs remains unaffected by the hyperpigmentation.

Hair Follicle Defects

Many of the hair follicle defects seen in dogs and cats (e.g., follicular dysplasia, grey collie syndrome, aurotrichia) have been described elsewhere in this chapter. Congenital hypotrichosis (alopecia) is rare but has been reported in the cocker spaniel, Belgian shepherd, toy poodle, whippet, bichon frise, basset hound, Labrador retriever, and beagle. Hereditary hypotrichosis has been recognized in the Siamese, Devon Rex, and a rare breed of Mexican cat. Affected animals are often born with a fairly normal haircoat but have generalized permanent hair loss by 4 to 6 months of age.

In cats hairless breeds have arisen as spontaneous mutations that were encouraged to reproduce and breed true. These include the Sphinx cat (Canadian hairless cat) and Birman cat. At least two mutations give rise to hairless cats, one of which has normal whiskers and the other attenuated whiskers. Hairless breeds of dog include the Mexican hairless and xoloitzcuintl. Hairless cats and dogs tend to develop oily skin and nail folds, and the hair follicle may foster blackhead (comedo) formation. Symptomatic therapy requires antiseborrheic shampooing once or twice weekly and routine cleaning of the nail beds.

Acral Mutilation Syndrome

Acral mutilation syndrome is a bizarre condition reported in German short-haired pointer and English pointer pups. It is probably inherited as an autosomal recessive trait and results in a sensory neuropathy. Affected pups chew at their feet to the point of mutilation. The condition first appears in animals at 3 to 5 months of age as a loss of pain sensation. Diagnosis can be rendered by EMG and histopathologic examination. No treatment is available.

Dermoid Sinus

Dermoid sinus is an abnormal congenital tract that connects the skin surface with the underlying spine. The tract is lined with skin and sebum; hair and debris eventually fill the channel and cause inflammation. Though the condition is most common in the Rhodesian ridgeback, it has also been reported in the boxer and Shih tzu. Diagnosis can be confirmed by biopsy and by injecting contrast media into the tract and taking appropriate radiographic studies.

Benign Familial Pemphigus (Hailey-Hailey Disease)

Benign familial pemphigus (Hailey-Hailey disease) has been recently reported in English setter puppies. Despite the name, the condition is not related to immune-mediated pemphigus variants. The disease starts within the first few months of age and small papules enlarge into proliferative, alopecic lesions with overlying crusts. Diagnosis is by biopsy. No treatments are available. An autosomal dominant form of inheritance with variable expressivity is presumed.

Familial Vasculopathy

Familial vasculopathy is a recently described disorder seen in young German shepherds. By 6 to 8 weeks of age, dogs had problems including lethargy, fever, and joint swelling. There was swelling of the nose, crusting and ulceration of ear margins and tail tip, and swelling and ulceration of the footpads. It is presumed, but not proven, that some impairment of immune responsiveness may be responsible. Lesions may be induced or may worsen shortly after vaccination. Diagnosis is confirmed by biopsy. No medications have been reported to be helpful, but the condition may spontaneously improve.

Mechanobullous Diseases

Mechanobullous diseases represent several different disorders that result in blisters and ulcerations wherever the skin is mechanically traumatized. An epidermolysis bullosa-like syndrome has been described in the beaçeron (Berger de Beauce) similar to epidermolysis bullosa dystrophica in humans. Junctional epidermolysis bullosa has also been described in dogs. In cats a hereditary junctional mechanobullous disease was found to be the cause of a nail shedding disorder. Diagnosis relies on histopathologic findings. No treatments are available other than symptomatic management.

Mucopolysaccharidosis

Mucopolysaccharidosis is a rare disease that results from a defect in the supporting substances (glycosaminoglycans) of the dermis. Mucopolysaccharidosis VI (Maroteaux-Lamy syndrome) has been documented in cats, especially the Siamese. The condition has an autosomal recessive mode of inheritance. Affected cats develop a broad, flat face, small ears, and diffuse corneal clouding. Inclusion bodies may be seen within neutrophils. Mucopolysaccharidosis I (Hurler syndrome), which has been reported as well, is associated with progressive lameness, broad face, small ears, corneal clouding, and bone dysplasia.

**APPENDIX:
MORPHOLOGIC CLASSIFICATION OF CUTANEOUS LESIONS**

	DIFFERENTIAL DIAGNOSIS		
CATEGORY	CANINE/FELINE	CANINE ONLY	FELINE ONLY
Maculopapular			
Macular	Allergic inhalant dermatitis	Acanthosis nigricans	
	Food allergy		
	Allergic contact dermatitis		
	Irritant contact dermatitis		
	Drug eruption		
	Erythema multiforme		
	Lupus erythematosus		
	Alopecia areata		
	Parasitism		

Cont'd.

CATEGORY	DIFFERENTIAL DIAGNOSIS		
	CANINE/FELINE	CANINE ONLY	FELINE ONLY

Papular	Parasitic dermatoses
	Bacterial folliculitis
	Drug eruption
	Food allergy
	Dermatophytosis
	Comedones/Acne
	Erythema multiforme
		Vitamin A–responsive
		  dermatosis
		Dermatitis herpetiformis
		Hormonal hypersensitivity
			Miliary dermatitis
			Hypereosinophilic
			  syndrome

Papulonodular Nodular	Parasitism Deep pyoderma Atypical pyoderma Dermatophytosis Intermediate mycoses Deep mycoses Lupus profundus Neoplastic Dermoid cyst Nodular panniculitis Juvenile cellulitis Mucinosis Eosinophilic granuloma Sebaceous adenitis Sterile pyogranuloma Calcinosis circumscripta	Intermediate pyoderma	Abscess Acne Panniculitis
Plaques	Dermatophytosis Urticaria Lymphoma	Bacterial hypersensitivity Lupus profundus Viral papillomatosis Calcinosis cutis Calcinosis circumscripta Histiocytoma Histiocytosis Keratoses Nevi Lichenoid dermatoses Mucinosis Erythema multiforme Acanthosis nigricans Dermatitis herpetiformis	Sporotrichosis Eosinophilic plaque Mast cell tumor Linear granuloma Vitamin E deficiency Mucopolysaccharidosis Xanthomatosis Tumoral calcinosis

Vegetative		Pemphigus vegetans
		Mast cell tumor
		Cutaneous papilloma
		Sebaceous gland
		  hyperplasia
		Squamous cell carcinoma
		Transmissible venereal
		  tumor
		Fibroma
		Nevi	

Cont'd.

APPENDIX—Cont'd

CATEGORY	DIFFERENTIAL DIAGNOSIS		
	CANINE/FELINE	CANINE ONLY	FELINE ONLY
Vesiculopustular			
Vesicular	Pemphigus	Dermatomyositis	Lupus erythematosus
	Pemphigoid	Epidermolysis bullosa	
	Erythema multiforme	simplex	
		Dermatitis herpetiformis	
Pustular	Demodicosis	Subcorneal pustular	Abscess
	Bacterial pyoderma	dermatosis	Acne
	Dermatophytosis	Sterile eosinophilic	Feline immunodeficiency
		pustules	virus (FIV) infection
		Lupus erythematosus	
		pustulosis	
Alopecia			
Focal/Multifocal	Demodicosis	Scleroderma	
	Bacterial pyoderma		
	Dermatophytosis		
	Alopecia areata		
	Cutaneous asthenia		
Patchy	Demodicosis	Protein deficiency	Hyperadrenocorticism
	Lice infestation	Bronzing syndrome	
	Cheyletiellosis	Color-mutant alopecia	
	Dermatophytosis	Spiculosis	
	Drug eruption		
	Lupus erythematosus		
	Telogen defluxion		
Regional	Discoid lupus	Growth hormone	Feline endocrine alopecia
	erythematosus	responsive	Psychogenic alopecia
	Hypothyroidism	Hyperestrogenism	
	Hyperadrenocorticism	Hypoestrogenism	
		Pattern baldness	
		Testicular neoplasia	
		Dermatomyositis	
		Follicular dysplasia	
		Toxicity	
Generalized	Dermatophytosis	Demodicosis	Alopecia universalis
	Systemic lupus		Hypotrichosis
	erythematosus		
	Drug eruption		
Erosive-ulcerative			
Parasitic		Fleas	
		Demodicosis	
		Sarcoptic mange	
Microbial		Skin fold pyoderma	Superficial pyoderma
		Pyotraumatic dermatitis	Systemic mycosis
		Perianal pyoderma	Cat pox infection
		Bacterial granuloma	FIV infection
			Mycetoma
			Atypical mycobacteriosis

Cont'd.

APPENDIX—Cont'd

CATEGORY	DIFFERENTIAL DIAGNOSIS		
	CANINE/FELINE	CANINE ONLY	FELINE ONLY
Immune mediated	Pemphigus Pemphigoid Cutaneous vasculitis Toxic epidermal necrolysis Drug eruption		
Miscellaneous		Superficial necrolytic dermatitis	Indolent ulcer Squamous cell carcinoma Fleabite reactions

Exfoliative
Patchy
	Ectoparasitism
	Dermatophytosis
	Drug eruption
	Pemphigus foliaceus
	Fatty acid deficiency
		Pagetoid reticulosis
		Sjögren's syndrome
		Color-mutant alopecia
		Hyperestrogenism
		Vitamin A–responsive
		  dermatosis
		Periappendageal
		  dermatosis
		Generic dog food disease
		Subcorneal pustular
		  dermatosis
		Chronic maculopapular
		  dermatoses
		Parapsoriasis
		Food hypersensitivity
		Hypothyroidism
			Protein deficiency
			Vitamin A deficiency
			Vitamin E deficiency
			Biotin deficiency
			Lynxacariasis

Regional	Pemphigus foliaceus
	Pemphigus erythematosus
	Discoid lupus
	  erythematosus
		Hypothyroidism
		Zinc-responsive
		  dermatosis
		Tyrosinemia
		Nasodigital hyperkeratosis
			Cheyletiellosis

Generalized	Dermatophytosis
	Drug eruption
	Systemic lupus
	  erythematosus
	Pemphigus foliaceus
	Keratinization disorders
		Demodicosis
		Hypothyroidism
		Vitamin E deficiency
		Ichthyosis
		Lymphoma
		Metabolic disorders
			Cheyletiellosis
			Hypereosinophilic
			  syndrome
			Lynxacariasis

Indurated Turgid	Urticaria Angioedema	Myxedema Mucinosis Juvenile cellulitis	Growth hormone– secreting tumor Mucopolysaccharidosis

Cont'd.

APPENDIX—Cont'd

DIFFERENTIAL DIAGNOSIS

CATEGORY	CANINE/FELINE	CANINE ONLY	FELINE ONLY

Solid	Cellulitis
	Bacterial granuloma
	Fungal granuloma
	Calcinosis cutis
	Tumoral calcinosis
	Neoplasia
		Scar
		Amyloidosis
		Intermediate mycoses
		Scleroderma
		Periappendageal
		  dermatitis
		Chronic maculopapular
		  dermatoses
		  (lichenification)	

Pigmented Red	Drug eruption Petechiae Purpura Vasculitis Contact dermatoses Lupus erythematosus Photodermatitis Erythema multiforme	Fold pyoderma Pyotraumatic dermatosis Histiocytoma Demodicosis	Eosinophilic plaque Linear granuloma

White	Systemic lupus
	  erythematosus
	Albinism
		Vogt-Koyanagi-Harada
		  syndrome
		Scleroderma
		Vitiligo
		Tyrosinase deficiency
			Waardenburg's syndrome
			Chédiak-Higashi syndrome

Dark	Basal cell tumor Melanoma	Postinflammatory reaction Hypothyroidism Hyperadrenocorticism Growth hormone responsive Acanthosis nigricans Lentigines Melanoma Vascular nevi Hemangioma Hemangiosarcoma Organoid nevus Melanocytic nevus	
Skin colored	Scleroderma Papilloma Sebaceous gland hyperplasia Callus Epidermal nevus Sebaceous nevus		

Adapted with permission from Ackerman LJ: *Practical Canine Dermatology,* ed 3. Goleta CA, American Veterinary Publications, 1989, pp 12–19; and from Ackerman LJ: *Practical Feline Dermatology,* ed 3. Goleta, CA, American Veterinary Publications, 1989, pp 13–16.

RECOMMENDED READINGS

Ackerman L: Basic guide to the immune system. *Pet Focus* 3(4):7–9, 1991.

Campbell KL, Dorn GP: Effects of oral sunflower oil and olive oil on serum and cutaneous fatty acid concentrations in dogs. *Res Vet Sci* 53:172–178, 1992.

Campbell KL, Neitzel C, Zuckermann FA: Immunoglobulin A deficiency in the dog. *Canine Pract* 16(4):7–11, 1991.

Carothers MA, Kwochka KW, Rojko JL: Cyclosporine-responsive granulomatous sebaceous adenitis in a dog. *JAVMA* 198(9):1645–1648, 1991.

Codner EC, Thatcher CD: Nutritional management of skin disease. *Compend Contin Educ Pract Vet* 15(3):411–423, 1993.

Dodds WJ: Immune deficiency diseases. *Pet Focus* 3(4):10–12, 1991.

Elmslie RE, Dow SW, Ogilvie GK: Interleukins: Biological properties and therapeutical potential. *J Vet Intern Med* 5:283–293, 1991.

Freeman LJ, Hegreberg GA, Robinette JD: Ehlers-Danlos syndrome in dogs and cats. *Semin Vet Med Surg (Small Anim)* 2(3):221–227, 1987.

Gershwin LJ: Immunologic evaluation of the small animal patient. Proceedings of the 10th ACVIM Forum, San Diego, 1992, pp 83–85.

Hargis AM, Mundell AC: Familial canine dermatomyositis. *Compend Contin Educ Pract Vet* 14(7):855–864, 1992.

Kunkle GA: Canine dermatomyositis: A disease with an infectious origin. *Compend Contin Educ Pract Vet* 14(7):866–871, 1992.

Kwochka KW: Cell proliferation kinetics in the hair root matrix of dogs with healthy skin and dogs with idiopathic seborrhea. *Am J Vet Res* 51(10):1570–1573, 1990.

McKeever PJ, Torres SMF, O'Brien TD: Spiculosis. *JAAHA* 28(3):257–262, 1992.

Miller WH Jr: Colour dilution alopecia in Doberman pinschers with blue or fawn coat colours: A study on the incidence and histopathology of this disorder. *Vet Dermatol* 1:113–122, 1990.

Miller WH Jr: Alopecia associated with coat color dilution in two Yorkshire terriers, one saluki, and one mix-breed dog. *JAAHA* 27(1):39–43, 1991.

Miller WH Jr: Deep pyoderma in German shepherd dogs associated with a cell-mediated immunodeficiency. *JAAHA* 27(5):513–517, 1991.

Power HT, Ihrke PJ, Stannard AA, Backus KQ: Use of etretinate for treatment of primary keratinization disorders (idiopathic seborrhea) in cocker spaniels, West Highland white terriers, and basset hounds. *JAVMA* 201(3):419–429, 1992.

Schmeitzel LP: Canine dermatomyositis: An immune-mediated disease with a link to canine lupus erythematosus. *Compend Contin Educ Pract Vet* 14(7):866–871, 1992.

Scott DW: Vitiligo in the rottweiler. *Canine Pract* 15(3):22–25, 1990.

Scott DW, Miller WH Jr: Epidermal dysplasia and *Malassezia pachydermatis* infection in West Highland white terriers. *Vet Dermatol* 1:25–36, 1989.

Stewart LJ, White SD, Carpenter JL: Isotretinoin in the treatment of sebaceous adenitis in two vizslas. *JAAHA* 27(1):65–71, 1991.

White PD: Essential fatty acids: Use in management of canine atopy. *Compend Contin Educ Pract Vet* 15(3):451–457, 1993.

White SD, Batch S: Leukotrichia in a litter of Labrador retrievers. *JAAHA* 26(3):319–321, 1990.

White SD, Shelton GD, Sisson A, et al: Dermatomyositis in an adult Pembroke Welsh corgi. *JAAHA* 28(5):398–401, 1992.

CHAPTER TWO

Diagnosis and Management of Parasitic Skin Diseases

There are a number of parasites that affect dogs and cats (Table 2-1 and Figure 2-1). Fleas and ticks are most commonly discussed, but mites, lice, nematodes, flies, and protozoa can all be troublesome.

FLEAS

Flea control represents one of the most important challenges to veterinarians and veterinary technicians. Many misconceptions need to be addressed so that appropriate treatment can be implemented.

Fleas are wingless insects between 1.0 to 5.0 mm in length. They have laterally compressed bodies, and their mouthparts are structured for puncturing the skin to suck blood. Because of a superelastic protein (resilin) located in the thorax above the hind legs, the flea can jump 150 times its own length (about 2.5 feet). This is equivalent to a man jumping the length of three football fields! Its acceleration of 140 g's is 50 times the acceleration of the space shuttle after liftoff. The flea then cartwheels end over end until it reaches its host.

Of the more than 2000 species and subspecies of fleas worldwide, only a few actually parasitize dogs and cats. It is therefore not rational to extrapolate facts about different flea species to the ones that affect pets. The predominant flea affecting dogs and cats varies geographically. In most of North America *Ctenocephalides felis* is the most common flea of both dogs and cats. In some areas, however, *Pulex irritans* or *Echidnophaga gallinacea* are more commonly reported. In Great Britain *Ctenocephalides canis* appears to be the most common flea recovered from dogs.

Fleas are not only pests; they also transmit a number of important diseases to dogs and cats, including the following:

- Tapeworm infection
- Plague
- *Pasteurella* infection
- Typhus
- Tularemia

Life Cycle (see Figures 2-2 to 2-4)

The life span of fleas is quite variable, and they can live up to 6 to 12 months as adults. However, most adult fleas only live for 1 to 2 weeks; during this time their main goals are to feed and lay eggs. The life cycle may be completed in as little as 3 weeks, but this time is quite variable, depending on environmental factors. Optimal conditions include temperatures of 18° to 27° C (65° to 80° F) and relative humidities above 70%. Fleas can survive but do not thrive at extreme temperatures, low humidity, or high altitudes. This accounts for the geographic diversity of the flea problem.

A female flea is capable of laying up to 2000 eggs during a lifetime. Eggs are laid on the pet, not in the environment. The first eggs are produced within 48 hours of the first blood meal. For various reasons, these eggs may fall off the animal and into the environment where they continue their development. When eggs are deposited in areas where the pet spends a great deal of time, development is more likely. This is because flea feces will also be present in these areas, which will serve as a future food source.

	TABLE 2-1	
SOME IMPORTANT EXTERNAL PARASITES OF DOGS AND CATS		
PARASITE	IMPORTANT SPECIES	COMMON NAME
Fleas	*Ctenocephalides felis*	Cat flea
	Ctenocephalides canis	Dog flea
	Pulex irritans	Human flea
	Pulex simulans	Small mammal flea
	Echidnophaga gallinacea	Sticktight flea
	Ceratophyllus spp.	Bird and hedgehog flea
	Xenopsylla cheopis	Rat flea
Ticks	*Rhipicephalus sanguineus*	Brown dog tick
	Dermacentor variabilis	American dog tick
	Dermacentor andersoni	American wood tick
	Otobius megnini	Spinose ear tick
	Ixodes dammini	Deer tick
	Ixodes scapularis	Black-legged tick
	Amblyomma americanum	Lone Star tick
Lice	*Trichodectes canis*	Biting louse (dog)
	Heterodoxus spiniger	Biting louse (dog)
	Felicola subrostrata	Biting louse (cat)
	Linognathus setosus	Sucking louse (dog)
Mites	*Demodex canis*	Demodex mite
	Demodex felis	Demodex mite
	Sarcoptes scabiei	Scabies mite
	Notedres cati	Scabies mite
	Otodectes cynotis	Ear mite
	Cheyletiella spp.	*Cheyletiella* mite
	Trombicula alfreddugèsi	North American chigger
	Lynxacarus radovsky	Cat fur mite
	Pneumonyssoides caninum	Sinus mite
	Dermanyssus gallinae	Red poultry mite
Nematodes	*Pelodera strongyloides*	*Pelodera*
	Dirofilaria immitis	Heartworm
	Uncinaria	Hookworm
	Ancylostoma	Hookworm
	Necator	Hookworm
	Gnathostoma	Hookworm
	Dracunculus insignis	Guinea worm

The energy expenditures of the cat flea are incredible when it comes to reproduction. During the first week, the female flea can lay 40 to 50 eggs per day. Because of the size of the flea egg, the female has to consume 15 times its body weight in blood to accomplish this.

Flea eggs typically hatch in 4 to 7 days. First stage larvae feed on organic material and fecal pellets. Second stage larvae emerge after a week and molt to the third larval stage within another week. The pupal stage then follows in response to a decrease in endogenous juvenile major growth hormone. (If artificially high levels of juvenile growth hormone are maintained in the environment by application of an insect growth regulator, larvae never pupate and eventually die.) The adult flea emerges from the pupal stage in several days to 2 weeks. An emerging adult flea may survive as long as a year before its first blood meal, but after this time it must feed on a regular basis.

Newly emerged adult fleas are attracted to pets by the warmth of the pet's body, its move-

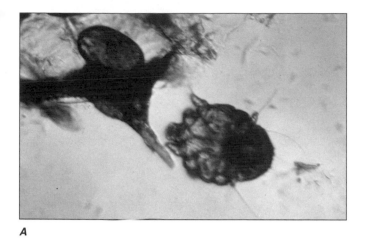

A

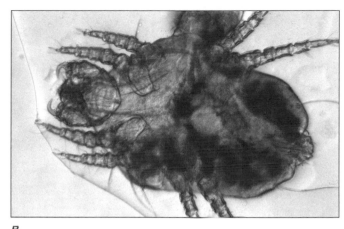

B

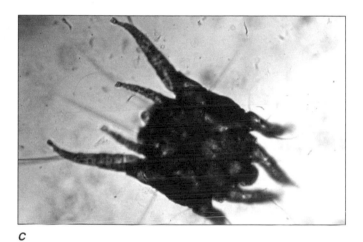

C

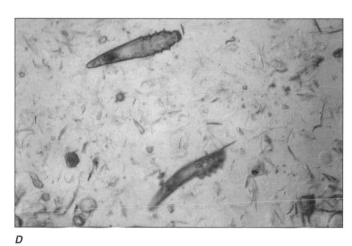

D

ments, and exhaled carbon dioxide. These young adults are the ones that bite humans in the infested environment. Once the fleas have become accustomed to their preferred dog or cat host, they are unlikely to feed on humans.

There are many misconceptions about the activities of the adult flea. Contrary to much of the published information, the cat flea *(C. felis)*, the primary flea parasite of dogs and cats, does not spend most of its time in the environment. Some literature suggests that this flea spends 90% of its time in the environment rather than on the pet. This statistic likely reflects studies done on the rodent flea rather than the cat flea. The rodent flea, the carrier of plague, tends to jump on, take a blood meal, and then jump off to digest the meal and lay eggs. This is *not* the case with *C. felis*.

C. felis is considered a permanent parasite unless it falls off or is physically removed. This flea is metabolically dependent on a constant food source and does not jump off willingly. Once it has emerged from its pupa and has had a blood meal,

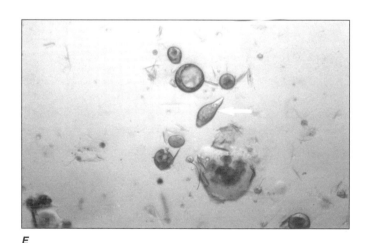

E

Figure 2-1. *Ectoparasites.* **A**, Sarcoptes scabiei *adult and egg;* **B**, Cheyletiella yasguri *(courtesy of G.S. Kedan);* **C**, Otodectes cynotis; **D**, Demodex canis *adults;* **E**, Demodex canis *egg in scraping* (arrow); **F**, *trombiculid mite (courtesy of W.H. Miller, Jr., New York State College of Veterinary Medicine, Cornell University);* **G**, *unengorged and engorged female* Rhipicephalus *ticks;* **H**, Pelodera *larva evident on skin scraping;* **I**, *cutaneous dirofilariasis—microscopic section from a dog with dirofilariasis. Note microfilaria in capillary* (arrow).

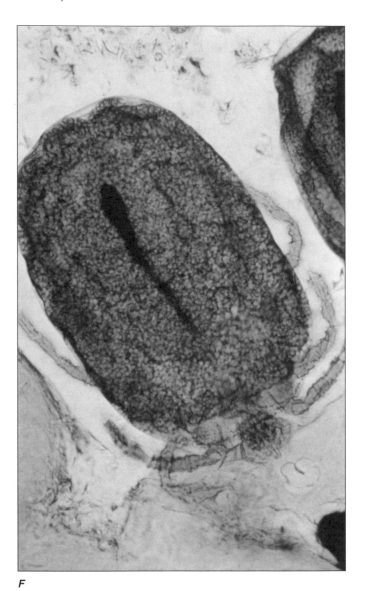

F

Figure 2-1. Cont'd.

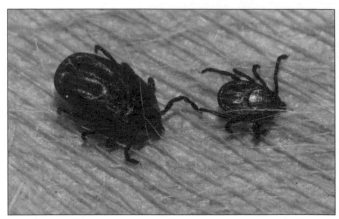

G

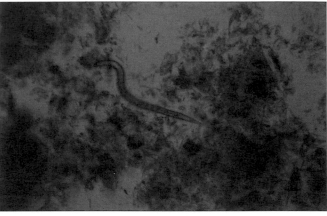

H

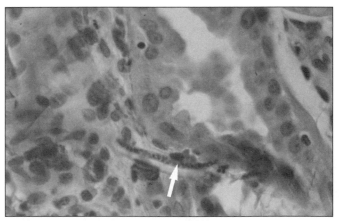

I

it must feed almost continuously. Fleas are deposited in the environment as pets move around or groom themselves or when eggs fall off the fur and develop off the host. This may also contribute to some of the confusion regarding flea statistics. Adult fleas are the only stage that actively feeds on dogs and cats; the eggs, larvae, and pupae do not. In a typical flea population the adults only account for 5% to 10% of the overall number of all life stages (50% of the total population exists as eggs, 35% as larvae, and the balance as pupae). This might be interpreted to mean that the flea only spends 5% to 10% of its time actually feeding, but this does not reflect the situation as it truly exists.

Clinical Signs

Not all animals appear sensitive to flea bites, and cats especially may be asymptomatic carriers.

An animal's flea population is also quite variable; some may have large numbers of fleas without consequence, whereas others are bothered intensely by the bite of only one flea. Animals in the same household may vary considerably in the number of fleas they accommodate. Just as some people tend to attract insects such as mosquitoes while others appear immune, some pets are "flea bags"

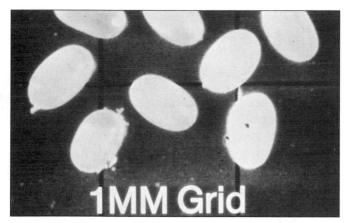

Figure 2-2. Flea eggs. (Courtesy of VetKem.)

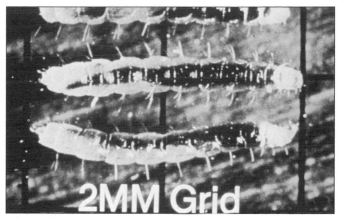

Figure 2-3. Flea larvae. (Courtesy of VetKem.)

and always seem to be plagued by fleas while others never seem to be affected. Therefore flea infestations are a consequence not only of environmental contamination but of individual tendencies as well.

There is a difference between flea infestation, flea bite dermatitis, and flea bite hypersensitivity (flea allergy dermatitis). In a truly flea-allergic animal, the bite of only one flea is sufficient to cause clinical problems for up to 5 days. This is a complex immune reaction involving immediate hypersensitivity reactions (type I), cell-mediated responses (type IV), late onset hypersensitivity, and cutaneous basophil hypersensitivity reactions.

Animals can have flea bite hypersensitivity even if one never finds a flea on that animal. The allergic reaction to flea bites is centered on material present in the flea saliva. Flea saliva contains a low-molecular-weight hapten (4,000 to 10,000 daltons) that binds to dermal collagen to form a complete antigen. Flea saliva also contains histamine-like compounds and enzymes that cause nonimmunologic reactions.

The tendency to become allergic to flea bites is not strictly a chance occurrence. Most cases are seen in:

- Animals with other allergies
- Animals intermittently exposed to fleas
- Animals that have not been exposed to fleas until later in life

Perhaps as a result of some evolutionary strategy, dogs and cats exposed to fleas early in life, and continuously, rarely develop clinical allergies to flea bites. By far, the highest incidence of clinical flea allergies is seen in dogs exposed to fleas on an intermittent basis.

Most infested dogs and cats develop a maculopapular crusting eruption in the area of flea

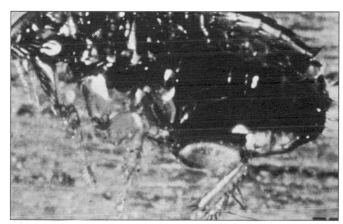

Figure 2-4. Adult flea. (Courtesy of VetKem.)

bites (usually around the base of the tail) with associated hair loss. Pruritus may or may not be present. Some dogs and cats can accommodate fleas while showing no outward signs of discomfort. Other animals show varied responses to the irritating and potentially allergenic nature of the flea bites (see Plates II-1 and II-2). Cats especially may have diverse manifestations of flea dermatitis, including pruritic papular dermatitis (miliary dermatitis), eosinophilic plaque, collagenolytic granuloma (linear granuloma), and symmetrical alopecia (see box on p. 38).

Diagnosis

A flea infestation involving a flea population explosion is usually not difficult to diagnose because at some point the fleas become obvious. Fleas or their fecal debris may be seen on the animal, or owners may have evidence of being bitten themselves. Fleas tend to bite humans mostly around the ankles, but if an infested pet sleeps with its owner, the bites may occur anywhere.

A flea comb is a very handy device for recov-

MANIFESTATIONS OF FLEA BITE HYPERSENSITIVITY IN THE CAT

Miliary dermatitis
Eosinophilic plaque
Collagenolytic granuloma
Symmetrical alopecia

---

ering fleas from pets. Animals suspected of being infested should be combed for several minutes. The areas of the pet offering the best chance to recover fleas are the dorsal midline, the back of the neck, the tailhead, the axillae, and the groin region. The material collected should be examined with a hand lens and then placed on some moistened white paper. The magnified sample may reveal eggs, larvae, or flea feces. Flea eggs are rarely found on dogs and cats as they do not have a sticky coating and tend to drop off into the environment. Flea feces (flea dirt) appears as reddish-black, comma-shaped casts found on the skin surface or in the haircoat. If the material collected turns the moistened white paper a reddish-brown color, it implies that some of the material was digested blood, further evidence of flea infestation.

As a minimum data base, a fecal evaluation and complete blood count are always useful. The stool can be visually assessed for evidence of tapeworm segments, which would be further proof of flea infestation. (Fleas are carriers of tapeworms; dogs can acquire tapeworm infection by ingesting fleas.) The blood counts might reveal evidence of anemia or a peripheral eosinophilia, both of which can be interpreted in light of the suspected diagnosis. Biopsies of skin for histopathologic analysis are sometimes warranted but are unlikely to confirm suspicions. Changes consistent with parasite hypersensitivity are also consistent with many other immunologic processes.

Flea bite hypersensitivity is a complicated phenomenon involving several different immune mechanisms, but a fairly large percentage of hypersensitive animals can be documented with an intradermal allergy test using flea extract. This flea extract is prepared from whole flea parts, not just flea saliva, so it is only an indirect test of flea bite hypersensitivity. The test is performed by shaving a small patch of fur and intradermally injecting 0.05 to 0.1 ml each of the flea allergen (diluted to 1:1000 w/v), a positive control (histamine), and a negative control (saline). Most flea-allergic dogs react positively within 15 minutes, but some may have delayed reactions over the next 24 to 48 hours. Flea-allergic cats tend to react within 30 minutes. It must be noted that up to 40% of normal healthy dogs and 70% of normal healthy cats may react to the intradermal injection of flea extract. This test is therefore only part of the criteria used to diagnose a flea-allergic pet.

If necessary, a therapeutic trial may also be helpful in documenting flea involvement in a pet's dermatologic problems. Various dips, sprays, and pour-ons can be used to dissuade fleas from jumping on and biting. This approach is not foolproof either, because many flea control products only kill fleas after they have bitten the animals. The result is a pruritic skin problem for the next several days whether or not the product eventually kills that particular flea.

It is often important to determine the significance of fleas and flea bite hypersensitivity because the presence of fleas does not necessarily explain the complete dermatologic picture. In many cases dogs or cats may have other skin diseases that are merely "complicated" by fleas. Unless the flea involvement can be determined quickly, proper diagnosis of the true problem may be overlooked.

Treatment

Proper management of flea infestation requires treating the animals and the premises. The most common reasons for flea control failure by owners are poor understanding of the dynamics of the flea population and poor compliance in treatment and preventive protocols. The goal is to:

1. Remove the fleas from the pets
2. Remove the fleas from the house
3. Remove the fleas from the premises
4. Keep the fleas away

Insecticides vary greatly in their ability to kill fleas, remain in the environment, and cause toxicity in pets:

- Pyrethrins (derived from chrysanthemums) are the safest products.
- Pyrethroids are less safe than pyrethrins.
- Carbamates are less safe than pyrethroids.
- Organophosphates are the least safe products.

As always in medicine, there is a tradeoff; the safest products do not persist in the environment and therefore must be frequently applied; the insecticides that are convenient to apply because they last are often the most toxic.

All of the insecticides listed (pyrethrins, pyrethroids, carbamates, organophosphates) share one important disadvantage. They only kill adult fleas. Even repeated applications do not kill the eggs, larvae, and pupae, which account for over 90% of the flea problem in a household. Therefore, if these products are used alone, they must be reapplied every 2 to 4 weeks to kill newly emerged adults. In the last several years, a new class of flea control pharmaceuticals, the insect growth regulators (IGRs), has become available. These products (e.g., methoprene, fenoxycarb) cannot kill adult fleas, but they do kill eggs and larvae in the environment. The combination of IGRs and insecticides has contributed greatly to the ability to sensibly control fleas. Even when these types of products are used together, however, flea control is not absolute because pupae or "pre-emerged" adult fleas may escape relatively unscathed. Repeated treatment with insecticide is needed every 2 to 3 weeks to control this segment of the flea population.

To repeat, there are three stages of flea control:

1. The first stage involves treating all pets to remove fleas and eggs from their bodies.
2. The second stage is to control the flea population in the house.
3. The final stage includes treatment of the outdoor environment.

When these stages have been successfully completed, prevention of recurrence is the next goal.

Treating the Dog and Cat

A flea comb is a very handy device for recovering fleas from pets and is a very worthwhile investment. Animals suspected of being infested should be combed for several minutes over their entire body, and the material collected should be examined with a hand lens. All animals in the household should be bathed with a cleansing shampoo or flea shampoo to remove dirt and fleas. A flea shampoo effectively kills fleas on contact, but once it is rinsed off it offers little residual protection. Because of the lack of residual insecticide, pets are immediately susceptible to infestation after shampooing. Fleas might be found on pets within minutes of bathing. Dips provide the most complete flea kill and last the longest

because the active ingredients are not rinsed off. Dips are more toxic than shampoos, however, because ingredients are allowed to air-dry on the pet and are not removed by rinsing. It is critical that all animals in the household be safely and effectively treated, including other dogs, cats, rabbits, and ferrets.

The best approach, if the owner allows it, is to use safer products such as pyrethrins and pyrethroids in combination with an insect growth regulator. The insect growth regulator stops the further development of eggs that are laid on the pet, even if they drop into the environment. The pyrethrins/pyrethroids kill adults safely but need to be reapplied at regular intervals (usually weekly). Also, the pyrethrins are inactivated by sunlight, which complicates matters somewhat.

When selecting insecticides to use on dogs and cats, safety should be a primary concern. Cats are particularly sensitive to a number of insecticides (including chlorpyrifos and fenvalerate combined with N,N-diethyl-m-toluamide [DEET]). Stronger insecticides used in flea control include the following:

- Carbaryl
- Propoxur
- Dichlorvos
- Phosmet
- Cythioate
- Fenthion
- Chlorpyrifos

For those animals with flea bite hypersensitivity, additional treatment will be needed. Occasionally, low doses of corticosteroids are used to reduce the inflammation of the skin caused by flea bites. Full control can only be achieved when there is 100% control of the flea problem. Hyposensitization (allergy shots) with flea extract has never been regarded as effective, probably as a consequence of the use of whole body flea extracts rather than the allergenic (actually haptenic) component, the flea saliva, as discussed earlier. Effective flea vaccines will likely follow refinement of the hapten into a more specific product.

Inside Flea Control

To be effective, inside flea control must cope with the population dynamics of the fleas. This area requires the most owner education; failure to comply with instructions is likely to result in failure of flea control.

All household programs should do the following:

- Mechanically remove fleas, larvae, pupae, and eggs
- Kill the adults
- Prevent the immature forms from developing to the stage at which they are problematic

Vacuuming should be done before the application of any insecticides and may remove as many as 50% of the flea eggs. Optimally, vacuuming should be done every other day in high traffic areas (for the pets) and every 7 to 10 days elsewhere. Vacuuming not only mechanically removes fleas in different stages of development, but the motion causes pre-emerged adults to hatch so they are susceptible to insecticides. Steam cleaning can also be effective at killing eggs and larvae. Adding chopped up pieces of flea collar, flea powder, or moth balls to the vacuum bag, although not an approved use for these substances, kills developing fleas within this closed environment. Alternatively, the bag should be immediately disposed of or the eggs and larvae trapped inside will continue to develop and new adults can emerge in the home environment. To remove eggs, larvae, and cocoons, pet bedding and other materials with which the pet has contact should be washed weekly.

The next step is to apply a commercial insecticide or borax compound inside the house to kill adult fleas. A pyrethrin-based product is safest, and the microencapsulated forms last about 2 weeks. These insecticides need to be reapplied every 2 weeks (every 3 weeks when the temperature is less than 70° F), even when an insect growth regulator is used. This is important because the IGRs work best on eggs and larvae, and "pre-emerged" adults or pupae can still escape destruction by these products as well as by the insecticides. Recently, borax-based (i.e., sodium polyborate) products have become available that are nontoxic, environmentally safe, and highly effective at controlling flea larvae in the indoor environment. The products are added to the carpeting (1 lb/120 square feet), where they inhibit the development of larval fleas, reduce the emergence of adult fleas, and drastically reduce the number of existing adult fleas. As a bonus, sodium borate also appears to adversely affect cockroaches. At present, this system works best in households that have at least 40% of their surfaces carpeted. Borax definitely has a place in flea control, but, at present, IGRs are easier and less expensive to apply and are less toxic.

The next—and probably most important—step is to use an insect growth regulator to prevent eggs and larvae in the household environment from developing into adults. IGRs are virtually nontoxic, making them an important weapon in the quest for a flea-free environment. It must be remembered, however, that IGRs are not insecticides, and they cannot kill adult fleas. They must be combined with an environmental insecticide or borax-based product to accomplish the whole task. Professional exterminators occasionally are required to treat extensively infested premises.

Outside Flea Control

There are only certain insecticides that are licensed for outdoor use. Most products need to be applied once or twice at 10 day intervals and then on a monthly basis for maintenance. A good strategy is to alternate products because resistance is becoming a recognized problem in flea control. The newer IGRs such as fenoxycarb are not inactivated by sunlight and offer some hope of egg and larval control in the outdoor environment.

Outside flea control is not as big a job as might be expected. Not every inch of yard needs to be treated. Because fleas require warm, moist, and shady areas for development, these regions and those in which the pets spend most of their time should be treated. It is important to concentrate on areas where the pets are usually found and where there is shade and organic debris (e.g., around gardens, patios, porches, dog houses).

Prevention of Recurrence

It is much easier to prevent flea infestation than to treat it. Most owners are unwilling to do what it takes for effective prevention, however. The best way to prevent fleas is to keep all dogs and cats in a flea-free environment. It is hopeless to try to keep fleas off the family dog if the family cat is allowed to wander through the neighborhood and then come indoors. Similarly, it is foolish to treat one pet with fleas and assume the others are not carriers even if they do not seem to be affected.

The best flea repellent to date seems to be a chemical called N,N-diethyl-m-toluamide, more commonly called "DEET." This compound has been incorporated into most human insect repellents. Because poisonings have been reported in dogs, cats, and humans, this product should not be used indiscriminately. The pet product Blockade (Hartz Mountain) should only be used following the manufacturer's directions exactly. The most common repellent used in pet products is 2,3,4,5-bis(2 butylene) tetrahydro-2 furaldehyde (MGK 11) which is found in dips, sprays, and shampoos.

In addition to being mild repellents, pyrethrin sprays and powders are the safest insecticides. Periodic use in dogs and cats is a rational approach to prevention. It is also worthwhile to treat the household with a safe pyrethrin-based product coupled with an insect growth regulator. A borax-based product may also be sufficient. In most cases this represents a safe and effective method of preventing flea infestation.

On the other hand, flea collars, which often contain much stronger insecticides (carbamates, organophosphates), do not come close to meeting their claims as flea repellents. They work best when pets do not have fleas and may be sufficient control when contact with fleas is only intermittent. "Electronic" flea collars promise "high-tech" flea control but reliable scientific studies have never shown them to be effective. Also, since the buzz of electronic flea collars can be heard by pets (though not by humans), the sound may bother dogs and cats more than fleas.

There are often many questions about "natural" flea control, and a basic knowledge is useful when discussing options with clients. Most importantly, pyrethrins and insect growth regulators are both "natural" and safe. Pyrethrins are derived from chrysanthemums, and IGRs are natural insect hormones that do not affect people. These should be the cornerstone of any flea control program. Other natural flea powders are typically made from the following:

- Rosemary
- Wormwood
- Pennyroyal
- Eucalyptus
- Citronella

These ingredients can be made into natural flea collars by adding the oils of these herbs or the herbs themselves (in a pouch) to appropriately sized collars made from cotton or nylon. These remedies should not be dismissed lightly. They may be just as effective as insecticide-impregnated flea collars, and they are certainly far safer. More studies are needed to determine just how well they work.

Products derived from citrus pulp such as d-limonene and linalool have been marketed for flea control. A simple preparation can be made at home by adding sliced lemons to a pot and steeping the concoction for at least 12 hours and then sponging the solution on the pet on a daily basis as needed. Skin-So-Soft (Avon) has also been used as a flea repellent and is applied as a rinse using 1 to 3 tablespoons (15 to 45 ml) per gallon of water. Using too much product leaves the coat very greasy, so moderation is recommended.

Brewer's yeast, thiamine, and garlic have long been regarded by breeders as good flea deterrents, but clinical trials have shown no such merit. This does not mean that they never work but that they could not be shown to consistently deter fleas in any predictable fashion.

The natural approach to flea control is to be commended, but these products should not be used indiscriminately. Poisonings have been reported with the citrus-based products as well as pennyroyal, and virtually any product is capable of causing problems.

TICKS

Ticks are members of the spider family (arachnids) and are blood-sucking parasites capable of transmitting a variety of diseases, including the following:

- Protozoal diseases—e.g., babesiosis, anaplasmosis, cytauxzoonosis, hemobartonellosis
- Rickettsial diseases—e.g., Rocky Mountain spotted fever, ehrlichiosis
- Viral diseases—e.g., St. Louis encephalitis
- Bacterial diseases—e.g., tularemia, borreliosis, coxiellosis

In addition, they produce toxic reactions, dermatologic disorders, paralysis, and anemia.

There are two major families of ticks:

- Soft (argasid) ticks (e.g., *Otobius megnini, Ornithodorus talaje*) have no shield, and the larvae and nymphs are parasitic. *Otobius megnini* parasitizes the external ear canal of small animals, whereas *Ornithodurus talaje* is the cause of Mexican-American relapsing fever.
- Hard (ixodid) ticks (e.g., *Rhipicephalus sanguineus, Dermacentor, Ixodes, Amblyomma, Boophilus, Haemaphysalis*) are the most common ticks affecting dogs. *Rhipicephalus sanguineus, Dermacentor*, and *Ixodes* are also

TABLE 2-2

DISEASES AND ORGANISMS TRANSMITTED BY IXODID TICKS

DISEASE OR ORGANISM	*Rhipicephalus sanguineus*	*Dermacentor andersoni*	*Dermacentor variabilis*	*Amblyomma americanum*	*Amblyomma maculatum*	*Ixodes dammini*
Babesia gibsoni	X					
Babesia canis		X				
Hepatozoon canis	X					
Coxiella burnetii	X	X				
Ehrlichia canis	X					
Pasteurella tularensis	X		X			
Rocky Mountain spotted fever		X	X	X		
Western equine encephalitis		X				
St. Louis equine encephalitis			X			
Leptospira pomona					X	
Borrelia burgdorferi				X		X

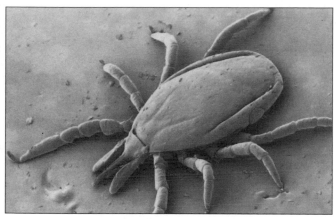

Figure 2-5. An electron micrograph (approximately 250× actual size) of a deer tick nymph. Lyme disease is most often transmitted by a deer tick during this stage of life. Its barbed mouthpart makes removal difficult. (M. Fergione photo/Provided by Boehringer Ingelheim Animal Health, Inc.)

common parasites of cats. The larvae, nymph, and adult stages of hard ticks are all parasitic. Most species require three hosts to complete the four-stage, relatively slow life cycle. (See Table 2-2 for a list of diseaes and organisms transmitted by ixodid ticks.)

Life Cycle

Ticks lay eggs that hatch into larvae and develop into nymphs before becoming adults. After the eggs hatch, each maturation event (called molting) must be preceded by a blood meal. The adult female must also feed on blood prior to laying its eggs. The female drops off the animal to lay its eggs (up to 6000, depending on the species); after they hatch, the larvae climb onto a blade of grass or other object and wait for the presence of a suitable host on which to attach. After feeding on a blood meal (see Plate II-3), some species of ticks stay attached to the host during molting, whereas other species drop back to the ground to molt. Depending on the life cycle, a hard tick is classified as either a one-, two-, or three-host tick (depending on how many hosts the tick feeds on during its development). As a general rule, the more hosts that a tick utilizes, the greater the potential for disease transmission (because of the increased number of animals at risk for infestation).

Clinical Signs

As mentioned previously, ticks can cause a variety of problems. The bites of ticks are irritating, and animals can develop hypersensitivity reactions to tick bites. In fact, the tick is the most potent inducer of cutaneous basophil hypersensitivity, which shares features with both immediate and delayed hypersensitivity reactions. Moreover, depending on the number of ticks, the size and age of the animal, and its overall health, ticks can seriously deplete the blood supply of a pet. This blood loss may result in poor haircoat, weight loss, poor performance, or even death.

Tick paralysis is one manifestation of tick-associated disease. It is primarily caused by female American dog ticks, although other species of ticks have also been reported to cause this condition. The tick injects a toxin that interferes with the stimulation of muscles by nerves. The result is an ascending paralysis. Recovery can be complete within 2 days of tick removal.

Lyme disease is caused by the spirochete bacterium *Borrelia burgdorferi,* spread mainly by the northern deer tick (*Ixodes dammini;* Figure 2-5). *Ixodes scapularis* is the most frequent carrier in the southeastern United States, and *Ixodes pacificus* is the most common in the west. It is probable that the Lone Star tick (*Amblyomma americanum*) and the American dog tick (*Dermacentor variabilis*) are also vectors.

In humans Lyme disease often starts as a characteristic red, circular rash, but soon the bacteria spread to the blood and cause various disorders. In some areas over 50% of dogs may be infected with only 10% actually showing signs. In dogs *Borrelia burgdorferi* infection can cause fever, anorexia, and arthritis, but the characteristic rash seen in humans is an unlikely manifestation. Cats rarely show any clinical signs at all. There is much debate as to the accuracy of blood tests used to diagnose Lyme disease in dogs and cats. It is uncertain whether they predict actual disease or only exposure. It is also suspected that the test may not be specific for *Borrelia* organisms alone. Dogs with periodontal disease associated with spirochete bacteria can test falsely positive. In addition, the development of antibodies to the bacteria (which is measured in the test) may not occur until up to 6 months after tick transmission. Because it takes from 24 to 72 hours for the tick to transmit the bacteria, prompt removal of ticks from pets greatly lessens the chances for infection to occur.

Erlichiosis, also known as "tick fever," is caused by the rickettsial organism known as *Ehrlichia canis.* The brown dog tick is mainly responsible for carrying the organism and transmits infection with its bite. In the acute stage signs are usually mild and include a low grade fever, lack of appetite, and, perhaps, weight loss. In the chronic stages pets might also become lethargic, depressed, and anemic and may suffer from bleeding from the nose or mouth or into the urine. Diagnosis involves blood testing for antibodies to the causative organism. Even after successful treatment, dogs are not immune and can develop the disease again if reexposed. Human ehrlichiosis was first reported in 1986, and all evidence suggests that human ehrlichiosis is contracted only from ticks, not from infected dogs.

Rocky Mountain spotted fever is caused by the rickettsial organism *Rickettsia rickettsii.* The American dog tick *(Dermacentor variabilis)* is the main carrier of the disease in the east, whereas the wood tick *(Dermacentor andersoni)* carries the disease more often in the west. The Lone Star tick *(Amblyomma americanum)* may also be an important carrier of infection. The disease is only infrequently reported in dogs. Although cats have been found with the organism in their system, clinical cases have not yet been reported.

Problems associated with Rocky Mountain Spotted fever include the following:

- Eye problems
- Lethargy
- Anorexia
- Fever
- Seizures
- Discoloration of mucous membranes

Diagnosis can be made with blood testing, but detection is possible only after the animal has been infected for at least 2 to 3 weeks. A good ophthalmic examination can be very suggestive of the disease.

Babesiosis has been uncommonly reported in pets, but many laboratories that are now routinely testing samples are finding positives. The species that infects humans *(Babesia microti)* is not the same as the one that infects dogs *(B. canis)* or cats *(B. felis).* The organism can be transmitted by several species of ticks, including *Dermacentor* spp. and *Rhipicephalus* spp. The condition is diagnosed by finding the organisms parasitizing blood cells or by finding high levels of circulating antibodies in the bloodstream. Clinical babesiosis is characterized primarily by fever and anemia. Dermatologic problems have been reported, usually purpura, petechiae, urticaria/angioedema, and necrosis, and are associated with thrombocytopenia or immune-mediated reactions to infection.

Diagnosis

The diagnosis of tick-related dermatoses first begins with a body search for ticks. The best places to start are the ears, neck, and the region between the toes. The site of tick attachment is often surrounded by a ring of erythema. This area becomes indurated, inflamed, and elevated with continued feeding. The nodule begins to resolve within 4 or 5 days after tick detachment.

If there are any doubts that the erythematous nodules are tick induced, biopsies can be helpful. The findings for tick bites are usually quite specific. There is often a strongly eosinophilic-staining substance over the surface of the epidermis, which appears to correspond to the area of cement substance secreted by the tick. In the dermis there is usually some degree of collagen destruction. Associated hypersensitivity changes can be noticed in some animals.

When ticks are located, they should be carefully removed and then identified. Identification may provide some clue to other diseases the tick might be carrying. For example, parasitization with *Rhipicephalus sanguineus* may warrant blood testing for ehrlichiosis and infestation with *Ixodes dammini* may warrant blood testing for Lyme disease.

Treatment
Control on the Animal

Careful inspection of dogs and humans after walks through wooded areas (where ticks and small host mammals may be found) and careful removal of all ticks can be very important in the prevention of disease. Ticks tend to congregate in the following areas:

- Around the ears
- Between the toes
- Around the head and neck

If only a few ticks are present, they can be plucked out, but it is important to remove the entire head and mouthparts, which may be deeply embedded in the skin. This is best accomplished with forceps designed especially for this purpose; fingers can be used but should be protected with rubber gloves, plastic wrap, or at least a paper towel. The tick should be grasped as closely as possible to the animal's skin and should be pulled upward with steady, even pressure. Do not squeeze, crush, or puncture the body of the tick or you risk exposure to any disease carried by that tick. It is also possible to become infected by hand-to-eye contact after handling the burst tick or a tick contaminated with its own fecal material. Once the tick has been removed, the site should be disinfected. Wash hands with soap and water to minimize risk of contagion. The tick should be disposed of in a container of alcohol or flushed down the toilet. Infection of the site warrants appropriate antibiotic administration.

If several ticks are evident, the entire body should be treated. Most dips designed for this purpose are effective, although engorged female ticks may be difficult to kill. An insecticide must come into contact with the tick directly to be effective. Many of the dips (especially those including permethrin, dioxathion, and chlorfenvinphos) give some residual protection for up to 2 weeks. Perhaps not surprising, flea and tick collars and medallions are usually not effective in treatment. However, flea collars containing appropriate insecticides can aid in tick control for 6 (propoxur) to 16 (chlorfenvinphos) weeks. In most areas of the country, collars should be placed on animals in March (the beginning of the tick season) and changed regularly. Leaving the collar on when the insecticide level is waning invites the development of resistance.

Applying repellents (e.g., DEET, Permanone) prior to and during walks through outdoor areas can also be helpful in preventing tick bites but is not without risk. A better solution is a new type of tick collar that contains amitraz (Preventic®—Allerderm/Virbac), the same product licensed to treat demodectic mange. It prevents the attachment of ticks to the skin and causes ticks already on the skin to detach themselves. One collar performs this function for up to 4 months. If dogs wear this type of collar throughout the tick season, their risk of getting tick-carried diseases (e.g., Lyme disease, tick fever) is greatly reduced. This is because a tick must often be attached for at least 72 hours to spread disease, and amitraz causes ticks to detach within 48 hours. Amitraz is not an insecticide and does not interfere with flea treatment; on the other hand, it does not aid in flea control because it is not effective against fleas.

Environmental Control

Most ticks are found on vegetation and attach to pets and humans as they walk by. Removal of underbrush and leaf litter and thinning of trees in areas where tick control is desired are recommended. These actions remove the cover and food sources for small animals that serve as

hosts for ticks, and continued mowing of grasses in the area further reduces the probability of tick survival. Ticks must have adequate cover that provides high levels of moisture as well as an opportunity of contact with animals.

Tick control in the environment is difficult because most of the ticks are found in grassy and wooded areas. Currently only chlorpyrifos (Dursban®—VetKem) and tetrachlorvinphos (Rabon®—Fermenta) are registered with the EPA for area-wide control of ticks. Application to problem areas in April or May and then again in June or July offers the best options for practical yet effective tick control.

In contrast to most other ticks, the brown dog tick presents a different problem in that it can infest kennels and runs and can hide within houses and the insulation in attics. Most other ticks need to live in vegetation. The brown dog tick has also been found in crevices in walls, bedding, and debris found around kennels. In severe infestations, especially where ticks are located indoors, professional pest control companies should be used. A variety of insecticide ingredients (e.g., resmethrin, carbaryl, permethrin, chlorpyrifos, dioxathion, allethrin) are registered for tick control around the home.

In kennel situations resin-based paints can be used to seal crevices, which prevents ticks from using these crevices while they are developing. Removal of trash in dog runs and the frequent changing of used bedding can also reduce potential problems related to ticks.

MITE INFESTATION (MANGE)

Mange refers to a group of skin disorders caused by different species of mites, including:

- Demodectic mange
- Sarcoptic mange
- Notoedric mange
- Otodectic mange
- Cheyletiellosis
- Trombiculiasis
- Lynxacariasis

Most of the disorders can be diagnosed and treated specifically depending on the type of mite causing the problem (Table 2-3).

DEMODECTIC MANGE

Demodectic mange (demodicosis; see Plates II-4 and II-5) is a condition seen in both dogs and

TABLE 2-3

DISTINGUISHING FEATURES OF SPECIFIC MITES

MITE	SIZE (μm)	FEATURES
Cheyletiella spp.	265 × 500	Larger than *Sarcoptes* Adults have eight legs plus hook-like mouthparts All legs clearly visible
Chiggers	210 × 450	Larvae have six legs and are yellow to red in color Long thin legs Body shape resembles that of ticks
Demodex canis	40 × 250	Cigar shaped Eggs are spindle shaped Adults and nymphs have eight legs; larvae have six legs
Demodex cati	30 × 200	Smaller and slimmer Oval eggs
Demodex (unnamed)	30 × 110	In epidermal scale of affected cats, rather than hair follicles Short, blunted abdomen
Dermanyssus gallinae	150 × 400	Long legs Stocky palps
Lynxacarus radovsky	250 × 550	Large, dorsally flattened body Almost flea-like in appearance Often found clutching hair shaft
Notoedres cati	200 × 250	Similar to *Sarcoptes* Unsegmented pedicles Suckers on several pairs of legs
Otodectes cynotis	300 × 450	Adults and nymphs have eight legs; larvae have six legs Unsegmented pedicles Males have suckers on all pairs of legs, females on two All legs are clearly visible Males may be seen attached caudally to deuteronymphs
Pneumonyssoides caninum	150 × 400	Long legs Small palps Similar to *Dermanyssus*
Sarcoptes scabiei	200 × 400	Adults are globose with four pairs of legs Long, segmented pedicles Suckers on ends of front legs Oval eggs Anus is caudal

cats caused by different species of *Demodex* mites. Demodicid mites of one species or another are present in small numbers on the skin of all normal mammals, including humans, and are considered noncontagious. In small numbers they do not cause any disease but simply feed on debris within the hair follicles. For *D. canis* the complete life cycle lasts 20 to 35 days. *D. cati* and another currently unnamed *Demodex* species are also normal residents of feline skin. They live within the hair follicles or stratum corneum of cats.

Most dogs acquire demodicid mites while being nursed in the first 2 to 3 days of life. Mites can also be transmitted from one pup to another during this time, after which infestation is unlikely. It is supposed that only dogs and cats with either an inherited or acquired immune deficit develop clinical demodicosis. This allows the mite population to grow unchecked. The adult mites, larvae, and eggs crowd out the hair follicles, and chronic deep infections result.

The extent of the immune deficit and its

BREEDS OF DOGS MOST SUSCEPTIBLE TO DEMODICOSIS	
Afghan hound	Dalmatian
Beagle	Doberman pinscher
Boston terrier	English bulldog
Boxer	German shepherd
Bull terrier	Great Dane
Chinese Shar pei	Old English sheepdog
Collie	Staffordshire terrier
Dachshund	

reversibility determine the course of the disease. Localized disease tends to result in a spontaneous cure, whereas generalized demodicosis often requires significant therapeutic intervention. Though stress may trigger clinical episodes, large numbers of mites produce substances that further suppress the immune system. This secondary immunosuppression can be reversed once the mite population is eliminated, but any underlying primary immune defect cannot be corrected. Most cases in young animals are presumed to be stress-related or associated with an inherited immune deficit. When older animals are affected, the underlying problem is often a concurrent illness or other impairment of the immune system by drugs (e.g., corticosteroids). For example, feline demodicosis has been associated with diabetes mellitus, feline leukemia virus infection, feline immunodeficiency virus infection, systemic lupus erythematosus, toxoplasmosis, upper respiratory infections, and hyperadrenocorticism. Although the Burmese and Siamese breeds of cats may be affected more often than other breeds, strong breed predispositions are much more common in dogs than in cats (see box above).

Clinical Signs

Animals with demodicosis may have a variety of dermatologic lesions depending on the degree of immunologic impairment. Classically, this has been described as localized and generalized demodicosis, but these designations are not really important. What is important is whether or not the condition spontaneously resolves with supportive therapy only.

The skin disease itself is caused by the mites crowding out the hairs within the hair follicles, eventually destroying these follicles. Release of the follicle contents (hair, debris, bacteria, mites) into the dermis causes infection, with associated erythema and alopecia.

In dogs demodicosis can mimic many other disorders, including bacterial pyoderma, dermatophytosis (ringworm), and even allergies. In dogs signs usually include:

- Patches of hair loss
- Variable erythema
- Secondary bacterial complications

The first areas affected are often the head and limbs, but individual tendencies are the rule, not the exception.

In cats demodicosis most often causes localized nonpruritic hair loss on the face, external ear canals, bridge of the nose, eyelids, and skin around the eyes. There is no apparent sex or breed predilection. Generalized feline demodicosis is very rare.

Diagnosis

The diagnosis of demodicosis can be made by finding evidence of demodicid mites, eggs, or larvae on skin scraping:

- On dogs mites are located in the hair follicles. The skin should first be squeezed to help express the mites. Scrapings should be deep enough to draw blood, as evidence that the scrapings actually reached the dermis.
- On cats mites may be in the surface scale or the hair follicles. Both superficial and deep scrapings are indicated.

Occasionally, even deep scrapings do not reveal mites. This is especially true with some breeds (e.g., Chinese Shar pei) or in certain locations (e.g., in cases of interdigital pyoderma). Biopsies are helpful in confirming the diagnosis in these situations.

Once a diagnosis has been made, it is important, whenever possible, to determine the underlying cause of the condition. In the young dog it is important to evaluate family history and to test for stressors such as internal parasites (including heartworm). Additional testing for immunoglobulin levels, T cell reactivity, and metabolic disorders should also be considered. An adult dog that suddenly develops demodicosis should be evaluated for:

- Underlying metabolic diseases (e.g., hypothyroidism, hyperadrenocorticism, diabetes mellitus, liver disease)

- Cancers
- Other prospective causes of immunosuppression

All cats with demodicosis should be evaluated for:

- Viral diseases (e.g., feline immunodeficiency virus, feline leukemia virus)
- Diabetes mellitus
- Hyperadrenocorticism

Additional screening for toxoplasmosis and lupus erythematosus may also be indicated.

Treatment

About 90% of cases of demodicosis in dogs and cats are localized and resolve without treatment in a few months. In these cases management should consist of mild (2.5% to 3.0%) benzoyl peroxide gels or 1% rotenone ointment. In the remaining 10% of localized cases that fail to resolve, animals develop the generalized form of disease, characterized by large areas of hair loss, redness, scaling, and infection.

All dogs and cats with demodicosis should be maintained on an excellent plane of nutrition and kept free of internal parasites, and their skin should be conditioned with appropriate topical therapy. Initially, benzoyl peroxide is often a good choice of shampoo because it tends to flush the hair follicles, removing mites, scale, and debris. Once the underlying immune deficit has been addressed, the majority of cases resolve within several months.

For young dogs conservative therapy alone usually results in resolution by 18 months of age (perhaps not until 3 years of age in some large breeds). Dogs in which the condition does not resolve spontaneously by that time likely have major immunologic defects that may be passed on to future generations. Their symptoms can be alleviated with the use of insecticides to kill the mite population, but their immune defect cannot be corrected.

The best supportive treatments involve the use of:

- Shampoos
- Periodic antibiotic therapy
- Immune stimulants (selected cases only)

The antibiotic selected should be bactericidal in effect (e.g., potentiated penicillins, cephalosporins, fluoroquinolones, or trimethoprim-potentiated sulfonamides) because the animal's immune status is presumably impaired. Immune system stimulants can be natural (e.g., vitamin E, selenium, germanium, coenzyme Q) or injectable (e.g., bacterins), or they can stimulate the immune system as a secondary phenomenon (e.g., levamisole). Although previous studies suggested that vitamin E supplementation (200 mg five times daily) was beneficial, recent studies did not find this to be the case. A recent suggestion that dogs with demodicosis have lower blood levels of selenium than do normal dogs has not been conclusively demonstrated.

Miticidal treatment is not usually recommended until the animal reaches immunologic maturity unless the condition gets progressively worse. The decision to use insecticides in a young animal should be based on the assumption that the animal is immunologically handicapped and would not get better on its own. In a dog with a normal immune system, the mite would not cause problems. The pet should be neutered to make sure it does not pass on its immune deficit to future generations. This should help eliminate the inherited immunoincompetence that allows generalized demodicosis to occur.

Specific treatment for generalized demodicosis in dogs is usually accomplished with amitraz (Mitaban®—Upjohn). Treatment with amitraz (see box on p. 49) is successful in 60% to 80% of cases. Many veterinary dermatologists have found that frequently the dosage must be doubled or the treatment interval halved to eradicate the mites in problem cases; this extralabel drug use must be done at the practitioner's risk, because it is not the manufacturer's recommended use.

More potent forms of amitraz are sometimes used by veterinarians. One ml of a 12.5% solution (e.g., Taktic®—Hoechst-Roussel AgriVet) can be diluted in 100 ml of water to yield a 0.125% amitraz solution. This solution can be sponged onto half the body surface daily, alternating front and back halves. This method of application is useful in particularly resistant cases. Animals should be hospitalized during the first week of therapy and monitored for evidence of side effects such as:

- Drowsiness
- Depression
- Bradycardia
- Anorexia
- Gastrointestinal upset

PROTOCOL FOR USE OF AMITRAZ FOR GENERALIZED CANINE DEMODICOSIS

1. Clip the hair to facilitate penetration of the drug.
2. Use an antiseborrheic shampoo to remove crust and scales. Ideally, this should be done the night before the amitraz dip.
3. Empty the contents of the amitraz vial (10.6 ml) into 7.5 L (2 gallons) of water. This amount may need to be doubled for very large dogs or in chronic cases.
4. Slowly sponge on the entire amount of solution prepared, concentrating on problem areas.
5. Allow the animal to air dry; do not rinse or blow dry.
6. Do not allow the animal to get wet between treatments, or the dip must be repeated.
7. Repeat the dip every 2 weeks (or weekly) until the condition has been adequately controlled. The dog should not be stressed after dipping.
8. Do skin scrapings before each dip. When scrapings are negative on two successive occasions, no further treatment is indicated.
9. For demodectic pododermatitis, apply a mixture of 0.5 ml amitraz in 30 ml of propylene glycol or mineral oil every 3 to 4 days. For dogs with demodectic otitis, a solution of 1 ml amitraz in 10 to 20 ml mineral oil can be instilled into the ear canals.
10. Outdated or opened bottles of amitraz should not be used in treatment. The breakdown products of amitraz are more toxic than the drug itself.

The drowsiness may be minimized by feeding prior to dipping, and there is some anecdotal evidence that yohimbine (Yobine®—Lloyd Laboratories; 0.1 mg/kg IV) may minimize or prevent side effects, although it is not licensed for this use.

Several different options are available for managing refractory cases of canine demodicosis. Recently, milbemycin oxime (Interceptor®—Ciba-Geigy) has been shown in limited clinical trials to be beneficial for dogs with generalized demodicosis. It is not licensed for this use but has been administered experimentally at 0.5 mg/kg once or twice daily. (In practical terms, one 11.5 mg tablet is administered per 22.7 kg body weight once or twice daily.) Treatment is continued 30 days following complete resolution. A related compound, ivermectin, has been disappointing in numerous clinical trials, although it is often very effective for internal parasites. Recently, it has been proposed that ivermectin may actually be useful if it is administered weekly (0.3 mg/kg) together with weekly amitraz dips. Finally, ronnel and trichlorfon are potent organophosphates used in the treatment of demodectic mange. Ronnel (Ectoral—Pitman-Moore) can be used as a 4% solution with propylene glycol (60 ml of Ectoral in 330 ml propylene glycol) or, alternatively, trichlorfon (Neguvon®—Miles) can be diluted to a 3% solution with water. The mix is applied to a third of the body daily and not rinsed off. Solutions must be made up fresh each time. Neither trichlorfon nor ronnel has been approved for use in dogs.

The generalized form of feline demodicosis can be treated with lime-sulfur dips or local application of rotenone. Amitraz, the preferred treatment for canine generalized demodicosis, is harmful to cats even in reduced concentration and is not licensed for use in cats. Amitraz is only indicated in cases of feline demodicosis not responsive to safer forms of therapy.

In general, progress is measured by performing skin scrapings prior to each dip. When scrapings are negative on two successive occasions, the dips are discontinued. Dips must be repeated until no mites are left or the mites will eventually repopulate. This may involve a few dips or many, and some animals require life-long treatment.

SARCOPTIC MANGE

Sarcoptic mange (see Plate II-6) is caused by the scabies mite *Sarcoptes scabiei* var *canis,* a burrowing mite that causes intense pruritus. Recently, infestation with scabies mites has been shown to cause transient decreases in serum levels of immunoglobulin A (IgA). Serum levels tend to return to normal once the condition has been successfully treated.

The mite that affects dogs is a different species of mite than that affecting humans. Nevertheless, canine scabies mites can and do bite humans, although they cannot reproduce on them. Sarcoptid mites can only survive a few days away from their preferred host. Scabies in cats is caused by a related mite, *Notoedres,* although occasionally *Sarcoptes scabiei* can produce mange in this species.

Clinical Signs

Sarcoptic mange arguably causes more itchiness than any other condition in dogs. It is frequently misdiagnosed as other pruritic conditions, including flea bite hypersensitivity, food allergy, inhalant allergy, and contact eruption. The intense pruritus is due to allergenic substances, irritating by-products, and mechanical irritation. Preferred locations for parasitism are:

- Ear margins
- Elbows
- Hocks
- Sternum
- Inguinal area

Lesions noted include papules, erythema, and, frequently, excoriations.

Diagnosis

The diagnosis of sarcoptic mange is complicated by the fact that recovery of the mites is difficult. Skin scrapings recover adults or eggs only about a third of the time. The best areas to scrape are the ear margins and the elbows. Crusted or heavily inflamed areas are poor choices for scrapings because the mites do not thrive in areas of intense inflammation. It is therefore best to scrape areas adjacent to inflamed sites. Because the scabies mites do not burrow beyond the stratum corneum, deep skin scrapings are not necessary and lessen the chances for recovery. Multiple superficial scrapings should be done and the scale evaluated for evidence of parasitism.

Because mites are so difficult to recover, a therapeutic trial is a valid diagnostic approach. Although a diagnosis of sarcoptic mange may be difficult to confirm, cure is relatively easy and straightforward.

Treatment

In general, sarcoptic mange is easy to treat; reinfestation is common, however, if the source is not identified and treated. All animals in the household should be treated. Humans do not usually require therapy because the mites cannot reproduce on people and are eliminated once the animals have been effectively treated.

The treatment of dogs with sarcoptic mange is not difficult but resistance to insecticides is a decidedly geographic variable. Whereas organophosphate dips such as phoxim (Paramite®—Vet-Kem) work in some parts of the country, they cannot be relied upon to be effective everywhere. Use of these products must be repeated weekly for 6 weeks to be effective. Amitraz (Mitaban®—Upjohn) can be successfully used in the treatment of sarcoptic mange and is licensed for this purpose in Canada. Two dips with an interval of 2 weeks are usually sufficient. Ivermectin (0.3 mg/kg SC given twice with a 2 week interval) is also highly successful but is not licensed for this use. Ivermectin is licensed only for the prevention of heartworm disease. The dose of ivermectin needed to kill scabies or *Cheyletiella* mites is approximately 50 times that needed to prevent heartworm. Ivermectin should not be used in collies because it appears to be quite toxic in this particular breed. For young pups (less than 4 months) that are affected, 2.5% lime sulfur used weekly for a minimum of six treatments is the treatment of choice.

NOTOEDRIC MANGE

Notoedric mange (see Plate II-7) is caused by the scabies mite *Notoedres cati*, a burrowing mite that produces intense pruritus. This form of mange generally has a geographic distribution, with enzootic pockets of infestation being recognized. The condition is quite contagious, and humans can acquire the mites through contact with infested cats. *Notoedres* has difficulty reproducing on humans, however. Foxes, rabbits, and, rarely, dogs can also be infested.

Clinical Signs

Infested cats often have intense facial pruritus. Thus the condition is often referred to as "head mange." Other signs include:

- Pronounced erythema
- Scaling
- Crusting
- Hair loss

With chronic infestation cats can become debilitated.

Diagnosis

Notoedric mange is diagnosed by skin scrapings. The mites are relatively easy to recover, unlike the canine variant of scabies. The mites are slightly smaller than canine scabies mites and often plentiful in skin scraping samples.

Treatment

Treatment of cats with notoedric mange requires topical therapies to remove the prominent scale and crust and specific antiparasitic therapy. Treatment can be safely accomplished with 2.5% lime-sulfur dips performed weekly for 4 to 6 weeks. All cats in the household must be treated. Products such as ivermectin and amitraz can clear notoedric mange, but there is little or no indication for their use nor are they licensed for this purpose. The risk involved in their use must be borne by the veterinarian prescribing the products.

CHEYLETIELLOSIS

Cheyletiellosis (see Plate II-8) is caused by several different species of *Cheyletiella* mites (*Cheyletiella yasguri*, *C. blakei*, and *C. parasitovorax*) that affect dogs, cats, rabbits, and, transiently, humans. This disorder has been nicknamed "walking dandruff." *Cheyletiella* mites do not burrow but rather feed on the scales present on the skin surface. These mites are obligate parasites, completing their entire life cycle on the host. They are not strictly host specific, however, and can move between host animals and between animals and humans. The entire life cycle is completed in 35 days. This mite, unlike *Sarcoptes* or *Demodex*, is capable of living in the environment for an extended time, perhaps up to 10 days. Pets acquired from kennels, pet stores, or any other place where large numbers of pets are housed in close proximity to one another are most likely to acquire this important parasite.

Clinical Signs

Cheyletiellosis is highly variable in its presentation. Some animals may be asymptomatic, others may have dandruff, and yet others may be intensely pruritic. The most common presentation in both dogs and cats is a moderately pruritic skin disorder, most common along the topline and head. Scale (dandruff) can be prominent, but this is highly variable.

Diagnosis

Cheyletiella mites are just large enough to be seen with a hand lens, so careful examination of the skin and haircoat may reveal the mites. Otherwise, skin scrapings and acetate tape impressions are the preferred methods of mite recovery. The skin scrapings should be very superficial as these are not bur-

rowing mites. Acetate (Scotch) tape can be used to collect dandruff from all over the body; the tape is then applied to a microscope slide for evaluation. Although many texts suggest that these mites are easy to recover, this is not usually the case. Other techniques that can be used include:

- Raking the coat with a fine-toothed comb or toothbrush
- Fecal evaluation for ova and parasites
- Special vacuuming procedures

In the vacuuming procedure a piece of white tissue paper is secured over the opening of a hand-held vacuum cleaner with a rubber band. The vacuum is then run over the entire coat for several minutes, and the collected debris is added to microscope slides (with mineral oil) for evaluation.

Treatment

The treatment options for cheyletiellosis are the same as for sarcoptic mange. Environmental control may be needed in addition to topical antiparasitic therapy. *Cheyletiella* mite infestation is sometimes quite difficult to treat successfully. All animals in the household must be treated. First, an antiseborrheic shampoo is used to remove prominent scales that may interfere with treatment. In dogs amitraz and ivermectin effectively kill *Cheyletiella* mites when used 2 weeks apart. The products are currently not licensed for this purpose and should be used with appropriate caution. For cats weekly dipping for about 6 weeks with either lime sulfur or phoxim, as well as environmental control measures, usually solves the problem; occasionally, exterminators must be called in.

OTODECTIC MANGE (EAR MITES)

Otodectes cynotis, the common ear mite, is highly contagious among pets. Infection is especially likely when animals are housed in close proximity to one another such as in pet stores, boarding facilities, and breeding establishments. These mites have a 3 week life cycle and 2 month life span. Ear mites feed on epidermal debris and tissue fluids and are capable of causing intense irritation and inflammation.

Clinical Signs

The most common manifestation of ear mites is otitis externa. The mites are capable of irritating the ear canal and causing a hypersensitivity reaction. Problems that can develop include:

- Intense pruritus
- Head shaking
- Heavy, dark, waxy discharge

These problems are not seen in all animals, however. Many animals can be carriers of ear mites and demonstrate no particular problems. Because they appear normal, these animals can be a real threat in the spread of mites and they often go unsuspected when a problem occurs.

Diagnosis

Otodectic mange can be diagnosed by locating the mites by otoscopy or by visualizing them in debris removed from the ear canal. Contrary to popular opinion, it is not always easy to diagnose ear mites. The diagnosis may be suspected in animals with heavy discharge in the ears, especially young puppies or kittens that have been housed close to other animals, which would allow contagion to occur.

Treatment

The treatment of ear mites involves more than just putting parasiticidal drops into the ear canal. The mites are quite mobile and can simply crawl out of the ears and far away from the insecticide (usually to around the tailhead). When the effect of the insecticide wears off and it is safe for them to return, the mites can once again infest the ear canals. Reinfestation is most often the result of incomplete treatment rather than insecticide resistance.

Appropriate treatment consists of the following:

- Flushing the ear canals to remove debris (mineral oil or squalene works best)
- Instilling appropriate parasiticidal products into the ear canal
- Using a whole body antiparasitic spray, powder, or dip

It is important to treat the entire body surface, not just the ears. All animals in the household must be treated; otherwise, they may be harboring the mites, even if they seem to remain unaffected. Suitable ear drops for use include those that contain thiabendazole, rotenone, or methylcarbaryl; diluted amitraz is also effective but is not licensed for this use. The use of ivermectin by injection, orally, or in a topical suspension has been found to be highly effective against ear mites but is also not licensed for this purpose. It is sometimes used for stubborn infestations in kennels or catteries.

CHIGGERS

Trombiculiasis is caused by the larvae of chiggers (e.g., *Trombicula alfreddugèsi*) rather than by adults. Chiggers spend most of their time off the host, and the adults do not feed on animals at all. The larvae may feed on dogs, cats, and other hosts for 3 to 15 days before dropping to the ground to molt. The nymphs and adults then feed on decayed vegetation and no longer bother animals. Transmission occurs when dogs and cats wander through larvae-infested ground, especially in heavily wooded areas. This problem is more prevalent in the late summer and fall.

Clinical Signs

The bites of chigger mites are quite irritating and itchy, and most bites are likely to occur on the head and feet. Occasionally, the larvae may be seen as orange dots on the skin surface. While feeding, the larvae produce intense irritation, inflammation, and pruritus as a result of their salivary secretions. A secondary bacterial pyoderma is a common sequela of infestation.

Diagnosis

The diagnosis may be suspected when pets roam through infested forests in late summer or fall and can be confirmed by finding the mite larvae. Occasionally, the larvae may be seen as orange dots on the skin surface, but skin scrapings are often more helpful. Because the larvae only feed for 3 to 15 days, they may no longer be on the animal by the time it is brought in for examination.

Treatment

Treatment is not difficult because infestation is naturally short-lived and because the larvae are susceptible to most common insecticides. Good choices include carbaryl, amitraz, and pyrethrins; amitraz is not licensed for this use, however.

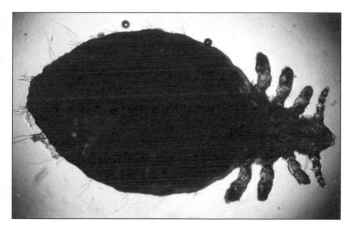

Figure 2-6. Linognathus setosus *(sucking louse) of dogs.*

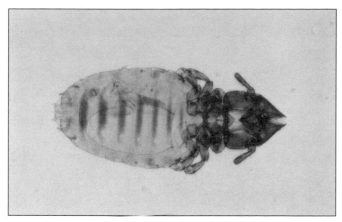

Figure 2-7. Felicola subrostratus *(biting louse) of cats.*

NASAL MITES

Pneumonyssoides caninum is the nasal or sinus mite of dogs. Signs of infestation include:

- Runny nose (rhinitis)
- Itchiness (especially of the face)
- Sneezing
- Respiratory problems

The mite is just large enough to be seen without a microscope and may be found around the nose and muzzle area. Alternatively, it is sometimes seen in preparations of nasal discharge or by careful visualization of the nasal passages with an appropriate instrument (rhinoscope). Ivermectin, the treatment of choice, is quite effective, but it is currently not licensed for this use.

FUR MITES

The fur mite *Lynxacarus radovsky* is a large, fur-grasping parasite of cats. It is more commonly reported in Hawaii, Puerto Rico, Australia, and Fiji and is now becoming more frequently recognized in the continental United States, especially Florida. Fur mites cause a form of miliary dermatitis that is often associated with pronounced scaling as well. When many mites are present, the fur feels almost granular and is described as resembling "salt and pepper." The topline and hindquarters are affected most often. Pruritus may or may not be present. The mite can be transmitted between cats or to humans.

Diagnosis is based on visualization of the mites with a hand lens or by microscopic examination of skin scrapings or plucked hairs. Microscopically, the mite has as a cylindric, sac-like body with eight legs. Treatment may be attempted with 2.5% lime sulfur dips, pyrethrin-based flea products, or 5% carbaryl powder. Flea collars are ineffective against these mites; ivermectin is effective, but it is not licensed for this use.

POULTRY MITES

Dermanyssus gallinae, the red poultry mite, infests birds but can also cause occasional problems in dogs, cats, and humans. Both the nymph and adult stages are parasitic and can cause itchiness and crusting. The areas most often affected are the back and legs of pets. The mite can usually be found on skin scrapings or by the vacuuming technique described for cheyletiellosis. Treatment is effective with most safe acaricides, including pyrethrins, lime sulfur, and ivermectin.

LICE

Lice are wingless insects that are host specific and live only on certain species. They are transmitted by direct contact or via contaminated objects. The entire life cycle, from egg (nit) to nymph to adult, requires about 3 weeks.

Lice are divided into two categories:

- Biting lice (Figure 2-6)
- Sucking lice (Figure 2-7)

Dogs can be infested with biting lice (e.g., *Trichodectes canis, Heterodoxus spiniger*) and sucking lice (e.g., *Linognathus setosus*). Cats are infested only with biting lice (e.g., *Felicola subrostratus, Trichodectes felis*).

Clinical Signs

Dogs or cats infested with lice often have a dull, dry coat with associated hair loss and crusting.

With careful inspection, adult lice and nits can be seen on the haircoat. Animals infested with sucking lice may also be anemic because of blood loss.

Diagnosis

Diagnosis of louse infestation is not difficult because the adult lice and nits are usually clearly visible. Blood counts are advised as anemia can be profound with chronic louse infestation.

Treatment

Treatment is not difficult, because most lice are sensitive to flea products. Treatment must be given to all animals in the household. Although humans may be bitten by canine or feline lice, they do not require any specific treatment if the lice are completely eradicated from the dogs and cats.

FLY-RELATED DERMATOSES

Flies may cause dermatologic conditions in a number of ways:

- Some inflict irritating bites.
- Some lay eggs within wounds (myiasis).
- Others complete their life cycles under the skin.

The following brief discussion will considers biting flies, cuterebriasis, and myiasis.

Fly Bites

Fly bites, especially those of stable flies (*Stomoxys calcitrans*) or black flies (*Simulium* spp.), can be very irritating. Dogs are affected more than cats and, although flies may attack any area of the body, they prefer the head, ears, and lightly haired skin. Lesions appear as little papulocrustous eruptions, with or without associated bleeding.

Diagnosis is sometimes difficult unless the flies are actually seen annoying the dog or cat. Treatment involves cleansing the affected area and, if necessary, applying a topical preparation (e.g., corticosteroid creams, baking soda and water, cooling lotions). If the bites are very bothersome, oral antihistamines or corticosteroids can be given. Applying insect repellents or a thin layer of petroleum jelly to susceptible areas should lessen the problem.

Cuterebriasis

The botfly *Cuterebra* occasionally parasitizes dogs and cats. It lays its eggs in soil, and the larvae later penetrate the skin of passing rabbits and rodents. They then mature to the pupal stage beneath the skin of these animals. Dogs and cats may be affected accidentally if exposed to the larvae during outdoor excursions.

Clinically, affected animals are presented with a nodular growth, often on the face or feet. If unchecked, a larva creates a breathing pore and eventually enlarges the hole, emerges, and pupates on the ground. Treatment involves surgically removing the subcutaneous larva and treating the remaining pocket as an open wound. The larva must not be crushed during extraction, because it would release material that would be extremely irritating to the animal.

Myiasis

Several species of flies lay eggs in organic matter, which then turn into maggots. A female fly typically lays from 50 to 150 eggs in a single batch. For myiasis (see Plate II-9) to develop, an inciting cause must be present, such as:

- Fecal soiling
- Neglected wound or other traumatized area
- Surgical site
- Area containing ocular or salivary discharge

Most larvae only feed on dead tissue and do not invade living skin. Toxins released from the larvae may damage surrounding healthy tissue, however, which then becomes suitable for continued feeding.

It is important to establish a definitive diagnosis of myiasis by analyzing the larvae involved. The screwworm *Cochliomyia hominivorax* has been virtually eradicated from the United States but is occasionally recovered. This is a reportable disease, and the appropriate authorities need to be contacted if it is recovered.

Treatment of myiasis involves:

- Extensive clipping of the affected area
- Flushing with an appropriate antiseptic
- Removal of all larvae
- Debridement of damaged skin
- Treatment of the open wound

A broad-spectrum antibiotic is indicated, as well as continued fly control. Pyrethroids, such as permethrin, are probably the insecticides of choice. Owners should be cautioned not to allow animals outdoors with open sores.

BEES, WASPS, AND HORNETS

Hymenoptera (bees, wasps, and hornets) can induce severe systemic allergic or toxic reactions by their stings. Hymenoptera venom contains many of the mediators of anaphylaxis including histamine, serotonin, and kinins. With multiple stings or enhanced sensitivity, severe systemic reactions can occur.

Recently, an arthropod etiology has been proposed for the condition referred to as "canine eosinophilic furunculosis of the face." Affected dogs tend to have lesions on the dorsal muzzle, which begin as small hemorrhagic areas that progress to extensive swelling and ulceration. When these areas are biopsied, they display striking similarities to mosquito bite hypersensitivity in cats and *Culicoides* hypersensitivity in horses. Bees and wasps are the suspected culprits. The condition responds rapidly to corticosteroid administration.

In animals adversely affected by hymenoptera stings, medical attention should be immediate. Blood should be collected for a complete blood count and urea, alanine transaminase (ALT), and coagulation profiles. Dogs may experience azotemia, inflammatory leukograms, evidence of liver damage, and even disseminated intravascular coagulopathy (DIC).

Conservative treatment for hymenoptera stings includes administration of antihistamines (e.g., diphenhydramine hydrochloride [1 to 2 mg/kg IV or IM]) and, occasionally, epinephrine (0.15 ml of 1:1000 solution SC at site of sting) and corticosteroids (e.g., prednisolone [2 mg/kg orally starting 12 to 24 hours after sting]). Epinephrine is indicated if the reaction is allergic in origin; it is much less beneficial when the animal is in shock. More severe reactions warrant prompt intravenous administration of fluids and electrolytes.

MOSQUITO BITE DERMATOSIS

Mosquitoes bite dogs and cats as well as humans. In cats mosquito bite hypersensitivity has been recognized as one of the causes of the eosinophilic granuloma complex.

The most common clinical signs noted are:

- Papular eruption
- Erosions

- Crusting
- Depigmentation of the skin over the nose
- Papular eruptions of the pinnae
- Footpad hyperkeratosis

Other possible signs include:

- Peripheral lymphadenopathy
- Eosinophilia
- Fever

Biopsies are quite characteristic. The lesions regress when affected cats are isolated from mosquitoes and recur upon reexposure. Response to corticosteroid administration is usually good.

HELMINTH-RELATED DERMATOSES

Nematodes, such as *Pelodera (Rhabditis) strongyloides*, the hookworm *Ancylostoma caninum*, the heartworm *Dirofilaria immitis*, and *Dracunculus insignis*, may also cause skin disorders. Each is discussed briefly because they are a relatively rare cause of dermatitis.

Pelodera Dermatitis

Pelodera (Rhabditis) strongyloides is a free-living nematode often found in organic matter, such as damp hay or straw. Dogs and cats may be affected when this material is used as bedding or through other forms of direct contact. The larvae can actively penetrate a pet's skin. Diagnosis is confirmed by finding the characteristic nematode larvae on skin scrapings. Differential diagnoses should include *Dirofilaria*, *Dipetalonema*, and hookworm infections. Successful treatment includes removing infested bedding and treating with appropriate parasiticidal dips, such as lime sulfur and phoxim.

Hookworm Dermatitis

Hookworms (*Ancylostoma caninum, Ancylostoma braziliense, Uncinaria* spp., *Gnathostoma spinigerum, Necator americanus*) may penetrate a pet's skin, especially the area between the toes, as part of its normal migration. The skin in affected regions becomes pruritic, swollen, spongy, hot, and painful. Once in the skin, the larvae are unable to cross the basement membrane and migrate in the basal cell layer, causing what is known as "creeping eruption." Humans can also become infected. The hookworms can puncture the skin even through a beach towel. In some parts of the world the feline hookworm *Gnathostoma spinigerum* is prevalent and usually infects cats that eat contaminated fish, chicken, frogs, or snakes. The parasite migrates through the body to the subcutaneous tissues.

Confirmation of the diagnosis of hookworm dermatitis is based on finding of hookworm eggs on fecal evaluation coupled with resolution of the skin problems with appropriate parasiticidal therapy. Many of the newer heartworm preventives are also effective against hookworms, but specific treatments (e.g., pyrantel pamoate, fenbendazole) can be prescribed if necessary. A second anthelmintic treatment should be repeated 2 to 3 weeks after initial treatment. All animals in the household as well as any with which they have contact should be treated. Environmental control may also be warranted. Borax (10 lb per 100 square feet [0.5 kg/m²] can be used to treat contaminated soil.

Heartworm Dermatitis

The heartworm *Dirofilaria immitis* only occasionally causes skin disorders. Heartworms are usually found in the heart and pulmonary arteries, but sometimes the immature forms (microfilariae) are found in the blood vessels of the skin and can cause itchiness, redness, and even lumps. Most affected dogs show pruritic, erythematous, nonfollicular papules and nodules on the face, neck, and trunk. Diagnosis can be made by finding microfilariae on skin scrapings or with biopsies. Positive blood tests are supportive. Treatment with Caparsolate® (Sanofi Animal Health), levamisole, or ivermectin should result in remission of the skin disorder.

Dracunculiasis

Infection with *Dracunculus insignis* is uncommon in dogs and cats. Typically, these slender nematodes cause a large fluid-filled subcutaneous swelling. This cystic cavity is often located on the legs or head. Microscopically, the parasites resemble heartworms. Surgical removal is the treatment of choice.

LEISHMANIASIS

Leishmaniasis is a rare protozoal disease caused by five species of the nonmotile flagellated protozoa *Leishmania*. Most cases in dogs and cats result from infection with either *L. donovani* or *L. chagasi*. Cats are affected much less often than are dogs. Sandflies *(Phlebotomus, Lutzomyia, Sergentomyia, Psychodopygus)* are the insect vectors most responsible for the spread of these organisms. Although infection is more common in the Mediterranean region of Europe, enzootic areas are now recognized in the southwestern United States (i.e., Oklahoma, Texas). The organism parasitizes and multiplies within macrophages.

Clinical Signs

Clinically, leishmaniasis can occur as a strictly cutaneous, mucocutaneous, and or visceral form. The clinical presentation is less variable in cats than in dogs and is usually limited to cutaneous changes involving crusting ulcerated lesions of the lips, nose, eyelids, ears, and, occasionally, the trunk.

Diagnosis

A diagnosis of leishmaniasis is made on the basis of clinical findings, cytologic, serologic and histopathologic examination, and culture. Biopsy specimens should be split into two—half is used for impression cytology and histopathology and the other half is used for culture. The portion for culture is wrapped in sterile gauze moistened with sterile saline and transferred to appropriate media. Touch impressions of tissue on microscope slides are placed in methyl alcohol for fixation 3 minutes and then into Wright's stain for 45 minutes. The leishmanial organisms, best highlighted with Giemsa stains, have a rod-like kinetoplast, and are most often found within macrophages. An indirect fluorescent antibody test using *L. donovani* promastigotes and rabbit–anticanine IgG conjugates has been described but is not commonly available to practitioners.

Treatment

Host immunity plays an important role in clinical expression, and resolution of cutaneous leishmaniasis usually results in permanent immunity. Treatment of leishmaniasis may involve the use of ketoconazole in the same dosages used for systemic mycoses or pentavalent antimony compounds. Because of the public health significance of leishmaniasis, owner counseling should be done before treatment is started.

GUIDE TO SAFE INSECTICIDE USE
(see Appendix on pp. 60–70)

Examples of commonly used insecticides, repellents, and insect growth regulators are provided in the box at right. Technicians and hospital staff are frequently exposed to these compounds without understanding the potential risks involved. It is also clear that many owners receive insecticides for home use without appropriate counseling regarding safety.

Pyrethrins

The safest products to use in parasite control are always pyrethrin-based insecticides and insect growth regulators. Pyrethrins are derived from the chrysanthemum flower. They can still cause side effects in animals, and humans can also develop a rash if they are sensitive to the products. The pyrethrins do not persist in the environment for long unless they are microencapsulated; they are also biodegradable and inactivated by sunlight.

Pyrethroids

The pyrethroids are synthetic formulations of the pyrethrins. Their effects last longer than their natural cousins, but they also may be slightly more toxic. Synergists used in flea preparations that inhibit various enzymes of insects (e.g., piperonyl butoxide, MGK 264, sesamin) may also increase the toxicity of pyrethroids in mammals. In addition, carbamates and organophosphates are esterase inhibitors and can potentiate the toxicity of pyrethroids if used concurrently. The regular pyrethroids are classified as type I compounds, but those that contain a specific chemical moiety (alpha-cyano-3-phenoxybenzyl group) are classified as type II compounds. These type II compounds are exceptionally potent but also can result in several side effects.

Organophosphates/Carbamates

The organophosphates and carbamates have a long-lasting effect but are potentially much more toxic than the pyrethrins. They are commonly incorporated into sprays, flea collars, and dips and are fairly stable in the environment, lasting for many weeks. The toxic effects of organophosphates and carbamates can be potentiated by other drugs, including antibiotics (e.g., gentamicin, lincomycin), inhalant anesthetics, some tranquilizers, and some antihistamines (e.g., cimetidine). Most poisonings

INSECTICIDES, REPELLENTS, AND INSECT GROWTH REGULATORS	
Class	**Examples**
Pyrethrins	Pyrethrin
Pyrethroids	Allethrin, d-trans allethrin, deltamethrin, fenvalerate, d-phenothrin, resmethrin, tetramethrin
Carbamates	Carbaryl, bendiocarb, propoxur
Organophosphates	Chlorfenvinphos, chlorpyrifos, cythioate, diazinon, dichlorvos, dioxathion, fenthion, malathion, phosmet, propetamphos, temephos, tetrachlorvinphos
Repellents	N,N-diethyl-m-toluamide (DEET)
Insect growth regulators	Methoprene, fenoxycarb
Formamidines	Amitraz
Avermectins	Ivermectin, milbemycin oxime

result when owners apply an organophosphate or carbamate dip to the pet, then apply an organophosphate or carbamate flea collar, and then use an organophosphate or carbamate spray or "bomb" in the house. Within the veterinary hospital, poisoning can result when individuals do several dips in a row, without proper protection.

Signs and symptoms of organophosphate and carbamate toxicity include:

- Pinpoint pupils
- Blurred vision
- Tightness in the chest
- Wheezing
- Sweating
- Nausea
- Vomiting
- Diarrhea
- Cramps

Possible long-term side effects may involve the immune system, the reproductive system, and the nervous system (decreased alertness, sleep disorders, memory loss, paranoia). The carbamates and organophosphates block the enzyme acetylcholinesterase and can result in toxicities if not carefully handled. These products should only be used in well-ventilated areas, and extreme care should be used to avoid any skin contact. Do not apply insecticides more frequently or at higher concentrations than recommended by label instructions. If you are dipping dogs or cats, choose the safest product, wear protective clothing, and apply the product in well-ventilated areas only. Do not attempt to do several animals in a row; share the duties, and decrease your risks.

Insect Growth Regulators

The insect growth regulators are not insecticides and are safe to use in all flea control programs. Most last in the environment for about 2 months. These products stop immature forms of fleas from developing into adults, thereby breaking the life cycle. They are extremely safe and unlikely to cause poisonings. Because these products do not kill adult fleas (they are insect hormones, *not* insecticides), they may be combined with insecticides for a more comprehensive effect.

Boric Acid

Boric acid (e.g., borax, sodium polysorbate) is becoming increasingly popular as an environmental flea control product. In humans repeated small doses of boric acid tend to be more toxic than a single acute dose. Poisoning may result in vomiting or diarrhea; the preparations are not caustic, however, and serious damage is rarely seen. Boric acid is rapidly absorbed through mucous membranes, abraded skin, and the gastrointestinal tract but not through intact skin. Young animals are more susceptible than adults. Borax preparations should be applied by trained professionals wearing gloves and face gear. Exposure to boric acid dust can cause irritation of the eyes and respiratory tract.

Citrus Acid–Based Products

The citrus acid–based flea products are generally regarded as safe, but some real concerns involving their use need to be addressed. At least one product made from crude citrus oil extract was found to be potentially fatal to cats. This is one example in which a "natural" product can be much more dangerous than the refined and stan-

dardized products. The most immediate sign of d-limonene toxicosis in cats is mild to severe hypersalivation, which last 15 minutes to 1 hour. Most signs abate without consequence within 6 hours. The toxic effects of d-limonene are increased if an animal is exposed concurrently to the synergist piperonyl butoxide, which is commonly found in most insect sprays and powders.

DEET

DEET is not a common component in flea products, but it is found in many insect repellents used by humans. It is combined with fenvalerate in the pet product Blockade (Hartz Mountain). Despite the overall safety of DEET, it has frequently been implicated in poisonings of children, dogs, and cats. In pets (especially cats) side effects include:

- Tremors
- Vomiting
- Excitation
- Ataxia
- Seizures

In severe cases death may occur. The main threat to humans is from repeated exposure, because up to 48% of the product can be absorbed directly through the skin. This chronic exposure has resulted in progressive brain damage in children. The risks are worse in areas where Lyme disease is prevalent as DEET is a common tick repellent.

Amitraz

Amitraz is licensed for the treatment of demodectic mange. Many veterinary dermatologists have found that the dosage often must be increased (doubled) or the treatment interval shortened (halved) from the manufacturer's recommendations to eradicate the mites in problem cases. This extralabel use is at the veterinarian's and owner's risk. Since it first appeared in the marketplace with almost miraculous claims, amitraz has now been accepted as a useful product but not one that can cure all cases. Side effects are rare but may include:

- Sedation
- Low blood pressure
- Bloat
- Vomiting

Ivermectin and Milbemycin

Ivermectin is licensed as a heartworm preventive but has also been found to be effective in the treatment of many other parasites, albeit at higher doses. It paralyzes nematodes and arthropods by its stimulatory effect on the neurotransmitter gamma-aminobutyric acid (GABA). The product is generally regarded as quite safe but, for some reason, collies and their crossbreeds are very prone to being poisoned by this product. In all dogs heartworm testing should precede treatment as ivermectin also kills heartworm microfilariae, causing serious complications. It is generally administered by subcutaneous injection or orally for the treatment of mites, although it is not licensed for this use.

A cousin of ivermectin, milbemycin oxime, has recently been introduced as a heartworm preventive. Milbemycin has experimentally been given orally as a treatment for demodectic mange. It is not currently licensed for this use, however.

APPENDIX: CLASSIFICATION BY TYPE OF PRODUCT[a]

This listing is arranged according to product classes defined as follows:

Class 1: aerosol spray and mist products for use on pets
Class 2: nonaerosol spray and mist products for use on pets
Class 3: shampoo products
Class 4: collars
Class 5: dip or sponge-on products
Class 6: dust and powder products

Class 7: any topical liquid preparation that is not a dip, sponge-on, spray, mist, or shampoo
Class 8: cream rinse preparations
Class 9: foggers for environmental use
Class 10: liquid sprays for environmental use
Class 11: systemic preparations

CLASS	COMPANY	PRODUCT NAME[b]	PRINCIPAL ACTIVE INGREDIENTS	ACTION[c]	SPECIES[d]	FREQUENCY OF ADMINISTRATION	PRECAUTIONS[e]	MISCELLANEOUS COMMENTS
Class 1: Aerosol Spray	Vet-Kem	Pet Spray	o-Isopropoxyphenyl methylcarbamate	1	D, C	See product label	See product label	Pleasant smell; excellent coverage; long-lasting killing power; 14 oz
	Veterinary Products Laboratories	VIP™ Flea Repel™	Pyrethrins, permethrin	1, 3	D, C	As needed	Avoid contact with eyes, skin, clothing	On-animal or premise use
		VIP™ Flea Spray	d-Limonene	1	D, C	As needed, every 2 days	Avoid contact with eyes, skin, clothing	Do *not* use more than once every 2 days
		VIP™ Flys-Off Aerosol	Butoxypolypropylene glycol	3	D	As needed	Avoid contact with eyes, food, skin, clothing; see product label	Protects against flies, gnats, and mosquitoes; can be used as a surface repellent
Class 2: Nonaerosol Spray	Bio-Ceutic Animal Health	14-Day Flea & Tick Spray	Pyrethrins, permethrin	1, 2	D, C	14 days for fleas, 7 days for ticks	See product label	
		Buzz Off™	Pyrethrin, methoxychlor	1, 2, 3	H	3–4 times weekly	See product label	Water base
		Buzz Off™ II	Permethrin	1, 2, 3	H	As needed	See product label	Effective against flies, lice, ticks (including deer ticks), mites, mosquitoes, cockroaches, and spiders
		Permectrim™ II Horse & Stable Spray	Permethrin	1, 2	H	See product label	See product label	
		Permectrin™ Pet, Yard & Kennel Spray	Permethrin	1, 2	D, C	See product label	See product label	Effective against fleas, lice, ticks (including deer ticks), and mange mites

CLASS	COMPANY	PRODUCT NAME[b]	PRINCIPAL ACTIVE INGREDIENTS	ACTION[c]	SPECIES[d]	FREQUENCY OF ADMINISTRATION	PRECAUTIONS[a]	MISCELLANEOUS COMMENTS
	CIBA-GEIGY Animal Health Coopers Animal Health (A Pitman-Moore Company)	Sustain™ Flea & Tick Spray for Dogs	Fenoxycarb, permethrin, pyrethrins	1	D	See product label	See product label	Controls and repels gnats, mosquitoes, biting flies, houseflies, cockroaches, silverfish, and spiders; can also be used as a premise spray
		Expar® Insecticide/Repellent	Permethrin	1, 3	D, H	See product label; as needed	Do *not* use on cats	Controls lice; repels gnats, mosquitoes, biting flies
		Mistaway® Extra	Pyrethrins, piperonyl butoxide	1, 3	D, C, H	As needed	See product label	
	DVM Pharmaceuticals	DuraKyl™ Pet Spray	Resmethrin	1, 3	D, C	Weekly	See product label	Kills fleas, ticks, lice; coat and skin conditioner; 16 oz plastic bottle
		SynerKyl™ Pet Spray	Pyrethrins, permethrin	1, 3	D, C	As needed	Do not use on nursing puppies or kittens under 3 mo of age	
	Fermenta Animal Health	Dermatological Mist Plus (TechAmerica)	Pyrethrins, permethrin	1	D, C	See product label	See product label	Contains aloe vera; safe for use on weaned puppies and kittens over 12 wk of age
		EctoGard™ Pet Spray (TechAmerica)	Fenoxycarb, permethrin, s-bioallethrin, synergists	1, 2, 3	D, C	See product label; as needed	See product label	Use with environmental products
		Feline & Puppy Mist (TechAmerica)	Pyrethrins, synergists	1	D, C	See product label	See product label	Ideal for cats, kittens, puppies; convenient fingertip sprayer
		Flea-Kill Mist (TechAmerica)	Pyrethrins, synergists	1, 3	D, C	See product label	See product label	Fast-acting; convenient trigger sprayer
	Fort Dodge Laboratories	Nolvacide® Mist II with Nolvasan®	Pyrethrins, permethrin	1	D, C	Every 14 days or as needed	See product label; do *not* use on nursing kittens or puppies	Available as 16 oz pump spray or in gal quantities
	HAVER, Miles Animal Health Products	PARA™ Mist	Pyrethrins	1, 2, 3	D, C	Daily if needed	See product label	Alcohol base; available in 16 and 32 oz bottles with/without sprayers and in gal refills
		PARA™ Mist W.B.	Pyrethrins	1, 2, 3	D, C	Daily if needed	See product label	Water base; available in 16 and 32 oz bottles with/without sprayers and in gal refills
	Merck AgVet Division	Sectrol® Pet and Household Flea Spray	Microencapsulated pyrethrins	1, 2	D, C	As needed	See product label	Kills fleas on pets for 8 days; also a premise spray; odorless
		Sectrol® Pet Spray	Microencapsulated pyrethrins	1, 2	C, C	Repeat as needed	See product label	Kills fleas on pets for 8 days; excellent knockdown; pleasant scent; kills ticks, including deer ticks
	Pitman-Moore	DEFEND™ Just-for-Cats	Pyrethrins, piperonyl butoxide	1, 3	C	See product label	See product label	Quick kill of fleas; contains grooming agent

Cont'd.

APPENDIX—Cont'd

CLASS	COMPANY	PRODUCT NAME[b]	PRINCIPAL ACTIVE INGREDIENTS	ACTION[c]	SPECIES[d]	FREQUENCY OF ADMINISTRATION	PRECAUTIONS[e]	MISCELLANEOUS COMMENTS
Class 2: Nonaerosol Spray—Cont'd.	Schering-Plough Animal Health	Escort® Flea & Tick Pet Spray	Pyrethrins, piperonyl butoxide	1, 3	D, C	As needed	Do not spray pet's eyes, face, genitalia; avoid treatment of nursing puppies and kittens	Keep away from open flame
	SmithKline Beecham Animal Health	Adams™ Flea & Tick 14-Day Residual Mist	Pyrethrins	1, 3	D, C	As needed	See product label; avoid treatment of nursing puppies, kittens	Use as often as necessary on dogs, cats, nonnursing puppies and kittens; do not oversaturate
		Adams™ Flea & Tick Mist	Pyrethrins with synergists and repellent	1, 3	D, C, H	As needed	See product label; avoid treatment of nursing puppies, kittens	
		Adams™ Flea & Tick Spray for Dogs with Dursban	Chlorpyrifos, pyrethrins	1	D	As needed	Dogs only; do *not* use on cats	
		Adams™ Tick Killer	Permethrin, pyrethrins	1, 3	D	Daily for 2–3 days; repeat every 5–10 days	Avoid contact with eyes and mucous membranes	Avoid treatment of nursing puppies under 6 wk of age unless prescribed by veterinarian
		MYCODEX® '14' Spray	Permethrin, 0.25%; pyrethrins, 0.10%	1	D	As needed	See product label	Controls fleas up to 14 days; aqueous vehicle, no alcohol; dogs only
		MYCODEX® Aqua-Spray	Pyrethrins, 0.20%	1	D, C	As needed	See product label	Aqueous base, no alcohol
	Vet-Kem	Ovitrol™ Plus Flea Spray	Pyrethrins, Precor	1, 2	D, C, H	See product label	See product label	Kills fleas and flea eggs on animal before they fall into the environment; breaks the flea life cycle; 16 and 32 oz
		Vet-Kem® Flea & Tick Pump Spray	Pyrethrins, piperonyl butoxide	1	D, C	See product label	See product label	Kills fleas, ticks, lice; alcohol or water base; 16 oz
		Vet-Kem® Water-Based Flea & Tick Pump Spray	Pyrethrins, piperonyl butoxide	1	D, C	See product label	See product label	Kills fleas, lice, and ticks; contains lanolin; 16 oz
	Veterinary Products Laboratories	VIP™ Dermatological Flea & Tick Spray	Pyrethrins	1	D, C	As needed	See product label	Contains special skin and coat conditioners (coconut and aloe vera); noncholinesterase inhibitor
		VIP™ Flys-Off Lotion Spray	Butoxypolypropylene glycol	1	D, C	As needed	Avoid contact with eyes, food, skin, clothing; see product label	Spray on directly or apply with cloth sprayed with repellent
		VIP™ Ovi-Cide™ Plus Pet Spray	Linalool, d-limonene	1, 2	D, C	As needed	See product label	Kills adult fleas, eggs, larvae, pupae
		VIP™ Pet Spray	d-Limonene, linalool	1, 2	D, C	As needed, every 2 days	Avoid contact with eyes, skin, clothing	Kills all four stages of flea life cycle; pleasant citrus scent; do *not* use more than once every 2 days

CLASS	COMPANY	PRODUCT NAME[b]	PRINCIPAL ACTIVE INGREDIENTS	ACTION[c]	SPECIES[d]	FREQUENCY OF ADMINISTRATION	PRECAUTIONS[e]	MISCELLANEOUS COMMENTS
	Virbac Laboratories	DuoCide® Long Acting Spray	Pyrethrins, permethrin	1, 3	D, C	Twice weekly	See product label	In an Aqua-soothe™ water base vehicle; woodlands fresh fragrance
		D-F-T	Carbaryl, 2.5%	1, 3	D	Weekly	Cholinesterase inhibitor	
		D-F-T Plus	Pyrethrins, 0.06%; carbaryl, 2.5%	1, 3	D	Weekly	Cholinesterase inhibitor	
		Supra-Quick Mist™	Pyrethrins, 0.10%	1, 3	D, C	Daily or as needed	See product label	Will not irritate skin with dermatologic problems
		Ultra-Sect R Mist™	Pyrethrins, 0.15%	1, 3	D, C	Daily or as needed	See product label	"Tamed alcohol" base has low odor; reduces sting to sensitive skin
Class 3: Shampoo	Bio-Ceutic Animal Health	Sectilin™ Flea & Tick Mousse	Pyrethrins	1, 2	D, C	As needed	See product label	Cleanses without using water
		Sectilin™ Shampoo	Pyrethrins, 0.06%; piperonyl butoxide, 0.12%	1, 2	D, C, H	As needed	See product label	Contains protein-base surfactant
	Coopers Animal Health (A Pitman-Moore Company)	Expar® Shampoo	Permethrin	1	D, C	As needed	See product label	Also kills lice
		Thionium® Shampoo with Expar®	Permethrin	1	D, C	As needed	See product label	Controls lice
	DVM Pharmaceuticals	DuraKyl™ Shampoo	Resmethrin	1, 3	D, C	As needed	See product label	Kills fleas, ticks, lice; skin and coat conditioner; 8 oz plastic bottle or gallon size
		SynerKyl™ Shampoo	Pyrethrins, permethrin	1, 3	D, C	As needed	Do *not* use on nursing puppies or kittens under 3 mo of age	
	EVSCO Pharmaceuticals	Theradex/D-Flea™	Pyrethrins, piperonyl butoxide	1	D, C	1–2 times weekly	See product label	
	Fermenta Animal Health	Flea and Tick Shampoo Plus (TechAmerica)	Pyrethrins	1, 3	D, C	See product label	See product label	Concentrate (can be diluted); leaves coat clean and glossy
	Fort Dodge Laboratories	Novalcide® Shampoo with Nolvasan®	Pyrethrins	1, 3	D, C	Repeat as needed	See product label	Available in 8 oz or gallon volumes
	HAVER, Miles Animal Health Products	FLEATOL™ Shampoo	Pyrethrins	1, 2, 3	D, C	As needed	See product label	Available in 8 oz or gallon containers
	Merck AgVet Division	Q-Sect™ Flea Mousse Shampoo	Pyrethrins	1, 2	D, C	As needed	See product label	Lathering mousse shampoo with good flea kill
	Pitman-Moore	KFL® Insecticide Shampoo	Pyrethrin, 0.5%	1	D, C	As needed	See product label	Natural pyrethrins
	SmithKline Beecham Animal Health	Adams™ Flea & Tick Shampoo	Pyrethrins	1	E, C	Every 7–10 days	See product label	Natural pyrethrins
		MYCODEX® Pet Shampoo with 3X Pyrethrins	Pyrethrins, 0.15%; piperonyl butoxide, 1.5%	1	D, C	As needed semiweekly	See product label	Triple strength for severe problems
		MYCODEX® Pet Shampoo with Allethrin	Allethrin, 0.12%	1	D, C	Semiweekly	See product label	Gentle flea shampoo

Cont'd.

APPENDIX—Cont'd

CLASS	COMPANY	PRODUCT NAME[b]	PRINCIPAL ACTIVE INGREDIENTS	ACTION[c]	SPECIES[d]	FREQUENCY OF ADMINISTRATION	PRECAUTIONS[e]	MISCELLANEOUS COMMENTS
Class 3: Shampoo—Cont'd.		MYCODEX® Pet Shampoo with Carbaryl	Carbaryl, 0.5%	1	D, C, H	Weekly	See product label	Strong defense against fleas and ticks
	Vet-Kem	Vet-Kem® Flea & Tick Shampoo	Pyrethrins, piperonyl butoxide	1	D, C	See product label	See product label	Kills fleas, ticks, lice; 8 oz, 1 gal
		Vet-Kem® Flea & Tick Shampoo Plus	Pyrethrins, piperonyl butoxide	1	D, C	See product label	See product label	Contains 0.15% natural pyrethrins; kills fleas, ticks, lice; 12 oz, 1 gal
		Vet-Kem® Flea & Tick Super Concentrate Shampoo	Pyrethrins, piperonyl butoxide	1	D, C	See product label	See product label	Kills fleas, ticks, and lice; contains coconut conditioners; 8 and 64 oz
	Veterinary Products Laboratories	VIP™ Flea Control Shampoo	d-Limonene	1	D, C	As needed	May cause eye irritation; harmful if swallowed	Pleasant citrus scent
		VIP™ Ovi-Cide™ Plus Citrus Scent Shampoo	Linalool	1, 2	D, C	As needed	See product label	Kills adult fleas, eggs, larvae, pupae; pleasant citrus scent; noncholinesterase inhibitor
		VIP™ 26% Pyrethrins Concentrated Flea Shampoo	0.26% pyrethrins	1	D, C	As needed	May cause eye irritation; harmful if swallowed; see product label	Kills fleas; contains lanolin and silicones; 1:6 dilution
	Virbac Laboratories	DuoCide® Shampoo	d-trans® allethrin, sumithrin	1	D, C	As needed	See product label	Kills fleas on dogs and cats and brown dog ticks on dogs
		Parid-X™ Shampoo	Pyrethrins, 0.075%	1	D, C	As needed	See product label	Concentrated (12 oz makes ½ gal)
		Pesticidal Shampoo	Pyrethrins, 0.05%	1	D, C	As needed	See product label	
Class 4: Collar	Fermenta Animal Health	Pet Insecticide Collar	DDVP	1	D, C	Every 3 mo	See product label	Available in two strengths (one for cats, one for dogs)
	Schering-Plough Animal Health	Duration® 6	Chlorpyrifos	1	C	Change 11 mo for fleas, 6 mo for ticks	See product label	Do *not* use on sick or debilitated cats or kittens younger than 12 wk of age; maximum effectiveness within 2–3 days
		Duration® 11	Chlorpyrifos	1	D	Change 12 mo for fleas, 7 mo for ticks	See product label	Do *not* use on sick or debilitated dogs or puppies younger than 12 wk of age; maximum effectiveness within 2–3 days
		Escort® Flea & Tick Collar for Cats	Diazinon	1	C	Change 5 mo for fleas and ticks	See product label	Do *not* use on sick or convalescing animals or on kittens younger than 12 wk of age; maximum effectiveness within 3–4 days

CLASS	COMPANY	PRODUCT NAME[b]	PRINCIPAL ACTIVE INGREDIENTS	ACTION[c]	SPECIES[d]	FREQUENCY OF ADMINISTRATION	PRECAUTIONS[e]	MISCELLANEOUS COMMENTS
		Escort® Flea & Tick Collar for Dogs	Diazinon	1	D	Change 5 mo for fleas and ticks	See product label	Do *not* use on sick or debilitated dogs or on puppies younger than 12 wk of age; maximum effectiveness within 3–4 days
		Escort® Plus Flea & Tick Collar for Cats	Diazinon	1	C	Change 5 mo for fleas and ticks	See product label	Do *not* use on sick or convalescing animals or on kittens younger than 12 wk of age; maximum effectiveness within 3–4 days
		Escort® Plus Flea & Tick Collar for Dogs	Diazinon, fatty acids	1	D	Change 5 mo for fleas and ticks	See product label	Do *not* use on sick or debilitated dogs or on puppies younger than 12 wk of age; maximum effectiveness within 3–4 days
		Escort® Signal Flea & Tick Collar for Cats	Diazinon	1	C	Change 5 mo for fleas and ticks	See product label	Do *not* use on sick or convalescing animals or on kittens younger than 12 wk of age; maximum effectiveness within 3–4 days; includes reflective strip
		Escort® Signal Flea & Tick Collar for Dogs	Diazinon	1	D	Change 5 mo for fleas and ticks	See product label	Do *not* use on sick or debilitated dogs or on puppies younger than 12 wk of age; maximum effectiveness within 3–4 days; includes reflective strip
	Solvay Animal Health	Dirodan® Flea & Tick Collar for Dogs	Dursban, 8%; chlorpyrifos	1	D	12 mo for fleas, 7 mo for ticks	See product label; cholinesterase inhibitor	Do *not* use on sick or debilitated dogs or on puppies younger than 12 wk of age; also helps prevent sarcoptic mange for 5 mo; 24 in. collar
		Dirodan® Saf-T-Stretch Flea & Tick Collars for Cats	Dursban, 3%; chlorpyrifos	1	C	11 mo for fleas, 6 mo for ticks	See product label; cholinesterase inhibitor	Do *not* use on sick or debilitated cats or on kittens younger than 12 wk of age; collar gives if caught on fixed object; 13 in. collar
	Vet-Kem	Breakaway™ Flea & Tick Collar for Cats	o-Isopropoxyphenyl methylcarbamate	1	C	Change every 5 mo	See product label	Unique breakaway feature

Cont'd.

APPENDIX—Cont'd

CLASS	COMPANY	PRODUCT NAME[b]	PRINCIPAL ACTIVE INGREDIENTS	ACTION[c]	SPECIES[d]	FREQUENCY OF ADMINISTRATION	PRECAUTIONS[e]	MISCELLANEOUS COMMENTS
Class 4: Collar—Cont'd.		Dursban Flea & Tick Collar for Dogs	Chlorpyrifos	1	D	Change 11 mo for fleas, 7 mo for ticks	See product label	Helps prevent sarcoptic mange for up to 5 mo
		Flea & Tick Collar for Dogs	o-Isopropoxyphenyl methylcarbamate	1	D	Change every 5 mo	See product label	Kills fleas and ticks for up to 5 mo
		Tick & Flea Collar for Cats	o-Isopropoxyphenyl methylcarbamate	1	C	Change every 5 mo	See product label	Kills fleas and ticks for up to 5 mo
	Veterinary Products Laboratories	VIP™ Flea & Tick Collar for Dogs & Cats	2-Phenol methylcarbamate	1	D, C	Every 5 mo	Avoid contact with eyes, skin, clothing; see product label	Metered release technology; heavy metal O-ring
	Virbac Laboratories	DuoCide® Flea and Tick Collar for Cats	Chlorpyrifos, 3%	1	C	Up to 11 mo	See product label	Safety stretch feature
		DuoCide® Flea and Tick Collar for Large Dogs	Chlorpyrifos, 8%	1	D	Up to 12 mo	See product label	
		DuoCide® Flea and Tick Collar for Small and Medium Dogs	Chlorpyrifos, 8%	1	D	Up to 12 mo	See product label	
		Preventic®	Amitraz 9%	1, 3	D	Every 4 mo	See product label	Prevents attachment of ticks; no activity against fleas
Class 5: Dip/Sponge-on	Coopers Animal Health (A Pitman-Moore Company)	Expar® 3.2% EC	Permethrin	1, 3	D	Every 3 wk	Do *not* use on cats	Controls lice
	DVM Pharmaceuticals	DuraKyl™ Pet Dip	Pyrethrins, rotenone	1, 3	D, C	Weekly	See product label	
	Fermenta Animal Health	Flea and Tick Dip for Dogs (TechAmerica)	Chlorpyrifos	1	D	See product label	See product label	Kills fleas for 28 days; effective on ticks and mange mites
	Fort Dodge Laboratories	Dermethrin™ Pet Dip	Permethrins	1	D, C	Every 2 wk	Do *not* use on sick, debilitated, or old animals; toxic to fish	Pleasant smelling
	Merck AgVet Division	Duratrol® Flea & Tick Dip for Dogs	Microencapsulated chlorpyrifos	1, 2	D	Not more than every 21 days	See product label	Kills fleas on dogs for 28 days; no knockdown; kills ticks, including deer ticks
	Pitman-Moore	Sprecto®-D Flea/Tick Dip	Permethrin, pyrethrins	1, 3	D, C	Four weeks	See product label	Nonoffensive odor
	SmithKline Beecham Animal Health	Adams™ 14 Day Flea Dip	Permethrin, pyrethrins	1, 3	D, C	Every 7–14 days	See product label	Use on dogs over 12 wk old; do *not* use on cats
		Adams™ Flea & Tick Dip	Malathion	1, 3	D	Repeat as needed	See product label	Dogs only; do *not* use on cats
		Adams™ Flea & Tick Dip with Dursban	Chlorpyrifos	1, 3	D	28 days for fleas; 21 days for ticks	See product label	
		Adams™ Pyrethrin Dip	Pyrethrins	1, 3	D, C, H	As needed	See product label	Do *not* use on puppies, kittens, foals less than 6 wk of age

CLASS	COMPANY	PRODUCT NAME[b]	PRINCIPAL ACTIVE INGREDIENTS	ACTION[c]	SPECIES[d]	FREQUENCY OF ADMINISTRATION	PRECAUTIONS[e]	MISCELLANEOUS COMMENTS
	Vet-Kem	Paramite® Sponge-on or Dip	Phosmet	1	D	See product label	See product label	16 day control of fleas and brown dog ticks; 4 oz, 1 and 5 gal
		Vet-Kem® Pyrethrin Dip for Dogs & Cats	Pyrethrins	1	D, C	See product label	See product label	Kills fleas, ticks, lice, mites; 8 oz and 1 gal
	Veterinary Products Laboratories	VIP™ Flea & Tick Dip for Dogs	Chlorpyrifos	1	D	Every 4 wk	Avoid contact with skin, eyes, clothing	Do *not* repeat treatment more than once every 4 weeks
		VIP™ Flea Dip	d-Limonene	1	D C	Every other day	Do *not* get into the eyes or on clothing or skin	Pleasant citrus scent; conditions and deodorizes coat; safe for use on cats
		VIP™ Pyrethrin Flea & Tick Dip	Pyrethrins	1	D, C	As needed	Harmful if swallowed; avoid contamination of feed and utensils	
	Virbac Laboratories	Ban-Guard® Dip	Dursban, 3.84%	1	D	Monthly	Cholinesterase inhibitor; do *not* use on cats	Controls sarcoptic mange mites
		DuoCide® Dip	Permethrin, 2.3%	1, 3	D, C	Every 2 wk	See product label	Kills fleas, ticks, lice
Class 6: Dust/Powder	Fermenta Animal Health	Flea and Tick Dust Plus (TechAmerica)	Carbaryl, pyrethrins, rotenone	1, 3	D, C	See product label	See product label	Combines three effective insecticides; no offensive odor
	SmithKline Beecham Animal Health	Adams™ Flea & Tick Dust II	Pyrethrins with synergist and carbaryl	1	D, C	As needed	See product label	Can use on cats, dogs, puppies, and kittens over 4 wk of age
	Vet-Kem	Flea & Tick Powder	Carbaryl	1	D, C	See product label	See product label	Kills fleas and ticks; can be used on puppies and kittens older than 4 wk of age; 5 oz
		Paramite® Insecticidal Dust for Dogs	Phosmet	1	D	See product abel	See product label	Aids in prevention of sarcoptic mange; 8 oz
	Veterinary Products Laboratories	VIP™ Flea & Tick Powder	Carbaryl, pyrethrins with amorphous silica gel	1	D, C	Once weekly	Do not breathe dust; avoid contact with skin	Quick knockdown with residual
Class 7: Topical Liquid	Coopers Animal Health (A Pitman-Moore Company)	EXspot™	Permethrin	1	D	Every 28 days, as needed (no more than every 7 days)	Do *not* use on cats; see product label	Kills and repels fleas, ticks, and deer ticks up to 28 days
	Fort Dodge Laboratories	Foam Control™	1% propoxur (gendran)	1	D, C	2 wk for fleas, 1 wk for ticks	See product label	A fast-breaking topical foam product (not a shampoo) that is applied along top line of animal's back; also kills lice
	Merck AgVet Division	Sectrol® Flea Foam	Microencapsulated pyrethrins	1, 2	D, C	As needed	See product label	Kills fleas on pets for 8 days; excellent knockdown; kills ticks, including deer ticks

Cont'd.

APPENDIX—Cont'd

CLASS	COMPANY	PRODUCT NAME[b]	PRINCIPAL ACTIVE INGREDIENTS	ACTION[c]	SPECIES[d]	FREQUENCY OF ADMINISTRATION	PRECAUTIONS[e]	MISCELLANEOUS COMMENTS
Class 7: Topical Liquid—Cont'd.	Pitman-Moore	DEFEND™ EXSPOT® Insecticide for Dogs	Permethrin	1, 3	D	See product label	See product label	Up to 4 wk residual control with one application
	Virbac Laboratories	Supra-Quick Roll-on™	Pyrethrins, 0.10%	1, 3	D, C	Daily or as needed	See product label	Roll-on application; does not frighten pets
Class 8: Cream Rinse	Coopers Animal Health (A Pitman-Moore Company)	Expar® Cream Rinse	Permethrin	1, 3	D, C	Every 2–3 wk	See product label	Controls lice
Class 9: Fogger	CIBA-GEIGY Animal Health	Sustain™ Household Fogger	Fenoxycarb, bioallethrin	1		See product label	See product label	
	Coopers Animal Health (A Pitman-Moore Company)	Impass™ Plus Fogger	Fenoxycarb, permethrin, pyrethrin	1, 2		Every 6 mo	Do *not* apply to pets	Quick knockdown plus residual control of adult fleas; prevents flea reinfestation for up to 6 mo
	Fermenta Animal Health	EctoGard™ Fogger (TechAmerica)	Fenoxycarb, pyrethrins, permethrin	1, 2		See product label	See product label	New; stops flea development for 32 wk; ovicidal after recommended application
	Pitman-Moore	DEFEND™ CFII Fogger	Permethrin, tetramethrin	1		See product label	See product label	
		Professional Home Treatment Kit	2 Sprecto-CF (4 oz); 1 Sprecto-CF (8 oz); 1 Sprecto-CCR	1, 2		Every 4 wk	See product label	
		Sprecto® Foggers	Permethrin, tetramethrin	1, 2		Every 4 wk	See product label	
	SmithKline Beecham Animal Health	Adams™ Automatic Room Fogger with Dursban	Chlorpyrifos, pyrethrins	1, 2		Every 30 days for adults, 42 days for larvae	See product label; harmful if swallowed	Covers up to 5000 sq ft of unobstructed space
	Vet-Kem	Siphotrol® Plus Fogger	Precor, permethrin	1, 2		See product label	See product label	Kills preadult fleas for 30 wk; 6 and 11½ oz, three 6-oz in a pack
		Vet-Fog®	Permethrin	1		See product label	See product label	Kills fleas, ticks, roaches, flying moths, spiders, ants; 6 and 11½ oz
	Veterinary Products Laboratories	VIP™ Fogger	Fenvalerate	1, 2		See product label	See product label	Kills fleas, roaches, ants, spiders, flying moths, mosquitoes, flies, crickets; 4 oz size covers 4000 cu ft
Class 10: Liquid Spray	Bio-Ceutic Animal Health	Permectrin™ II Horse & Stable Spray	Permethrin	1, 2	H	See product label	See product label	Effective against flies, lice, ticks (including deer tick), mites, mosquitoes, cockroaches, and spiders; can be used as premise spray
		Permectrin™ Pet, Yard & Kennel Spray	Permethrin	1, 2	D, C	See product label	See product label	Effective against fleas, lice, ticks (including deer ticks), and mange mites; can be used as premise spray

Cont'd.

CLASS	COMPANY	PRODUCT NAME[b]	PRINCIPAL ACTIVE INGREDIENTS	ACTION[c]	SPECIES[d]	FREQUENCY OF ADMINISTRATION	PRECAUTIONS[e]	MISCELLANEOUS COMMENTS
	CIBA-GEIGY Animal Health	Yard & Kennel Spray	Chlorpyrifos	1, 2		See product label	See product label	Hose-end spray
		Sustain™ Flea & Tick Household Spray	Fenoxycarb, permethrin, pyrethrins	1	D	See product label	See product label	
		Sustain™ House & Kennel Aerosol	Fenoxycarb, chlorpyrifos	1	D	See product label	See product label	
	Coopers Animal Health (A Pitman-Moore Company)	Expar® Home & Carpet Spray	Permethrin	1, 3		Every 10 wk	See product label; do *not* use on cats	Available as spray; for use on dogs and premises; also controls cockroaches, silverfish, spiders
		Impass® Complete Premise Spray	Fenoxycarb, chlorpyrifos	1, 2		Every 6 mo	See product label	Inverted aerosol delivery system treats up to 1500 sq ft
		Impass® Home & Carpet Spray	Fenoxycarb, 1.0% permethrin, pyrethrin	1, 2		Every 6 mo	See product label	Quick knockdown plus residual control of adult fleas; prevents reinfestation for up to 6 mo
	Fermenta Animal Health	EctoGard™ House and Carpet Spray (TechAmerica)	Fenoxycarb, permethrin	1, 2		See product label	See product label	New; stops flea development for 32 wk; ovicidal after recommended application
	Merck AgVet Division	Duratrol® Household Flea Spray	Microencapsulated chlorpyrifos	1, 2		As needed	See product label	Kills adult fleas for 90 days and flea larvae for 90 days; odorles, nonstaining; available with pump-up sprayer
		Duratrol® Yard Spray	Microencapsulated chlorpyrifos	1, 2		As needed	See product label	Kills fleas outdoors for 30 days; comes with hose sprayer; also kills deer ticks
		Sectrol® Pet and Household Flea Spray	Microencapsulated pyrethrins	1, 2		As needed	See product label	Also a pet spray for direct application to dogs or cats; kills fleas indoors for 30 days; odorless
	Pitman-Moore	Sprecto® Complete Carpet & Room Spray	Chlorpyrifos, d-trans allethrin	1, 2		As needed	See product label	
	Schering-Plough Animal Health	Escort® Flea & Tick Home & Carpet Spray	d-trans allethrin, chlorpyrifos	1		As needed	Do not allow children or pets to contact treated surface until spray dries	Chlorpyrifos is a cholinesterase inhibitor
	SmithKline Beecham Animal Health	Adams™ Surface Spray	Allethrin, chlorpyrifos	1, 2		As needed	Do *not* apply to animals; do *not* apply to finished wood surfaces	
		MYCODEX® Lawn Spray Concentrate	Cyano (3-phenoxyphenyl) methyl 4-chloro-alpha-(1-methylethyl) benzeneacetate	1		As needed every 7–14 days	See product label	Hose-end sprayer

APPENDIX—Cont'd

CLASS	COMPANY	PRODUCT NAME[b]	PRINCIPAL ACTIVE INGREDIENTS	ACTION[c]	SPECIES[d]	FREQUENCY OF ADMINISTRATION	PRECAUTIONS[e]	MISCELLANEOUS COMMENTS
Class 10: Liquid Spray—Cont'd.	Vet-Kem	Siphotrol Plus® II House Treatment	Precor, chlorpyrifos, pyrethrin	1, 2		See product label	See product label	Kills fleas, ticks, roaches; kills preadult fleas for 30 wk; 32 and 64 oz; also available in kit that contains pump-up sprayer
		Vet-Kem® Siphotrol Premise Spray	Precor, pyrethrins	1, 2		See product label	See product label	Kills fleas; kills preadult fleas for 30 wk; can be used on dogs or premises; 12 oz
		Vet-Kem® Yard & Kennel Spray	Chlorpyrifos	1		See product label	See product label	Kills fleas and ticks in yards, kennels, and doghouses; 16 oz; hose-end sprayer or refill
	Veterinary Products Laboratories	VIP™ Concentrated Yard Spray	Fenvalerate	1		7–14 days	Do not get into eyes or on skin or clothing	A noncholinesterase inhibitor
		VPL Lawn Spray Concentrate	Fenvalerate	1		7–14 days	Do not get into eyes or on skin or clothing	A noncholinesterase inhibitor; 8 oz size covers 3000 sq ft
Class 11: Systemic	HAVER, Mobay Animal Health	PROBAN® Tablets & Liquid	Cythioate	1	D	Twice weekly or every third day	Cholinesterase inhibitor; do *not* use for greyhounds or for pregnant, sick, stressed, postsurgical dogs	Safe for heartworm-positive dogs and adults or puppies of all ages
		PROSPOT® Solution	Fenthion	1	D	Every 2 wk	Cholinesterase inhibitor; do *not* use on puppies younger than 10 wk of age, or for sick, stressed, convalescing dogs	Safe for heartworm-positive dogs; safe during all stages of female reproduction; safe use on breeding males not established; five sizes for dogs weighing between 5 lb and 160 lb; cleared by FDA

Reprinted from *Vet Tech* 13(4):256–264, 1992.
[a]Product labels should be reviewed carefully before any product is used. In all cases, keep insecticide products out of the reach of children and pets. Inclusion of a product in this guide does not represent endorsement by the publisher or author.
[b]Proprietary names are listed.
[c]Action key: 1 = adulticidal; 2 = larvicidal; 3 = repellent.
[d]Species key: D = dog; C = cat; H = horse. If no species is indicated, the product is for environmental use.
[e]Any product specified as a cholinesterase inhibitor should *not* be used in conjunction with other pesticides.

RECOMMENDED READINGS

Ackerman LJ: Demodicosis in cats. *Mod Vet Pract* 65:751–753, 1984.

Bukowski J: Real and potential occupational health risks associated with insecticide use. *Compend Contin Educ Pract Vet* 12(11):1617–1626, 1990.

Bussieras J, Chermette R: Amitraz and canine demodicosis. *JAAHA* 22:779–782, 1986.

Cowell AK, Cowell RL, Tyler RD, Nieves MA: Severe systemic reactions to Hymenoptera stings in three dogs. *JAVMA* 198(6):1014–1016, 1991.

Dorman DC: Pyrethrin poisoning in dogs and cats. *Companion Anim Pract* 2(8):12–13, 1988.

Dorman DC: Diethyltoluamide (DEET) insect repellent toxicosis. *Vet Clin North Am [Small Anim Pract]* 20(2):387–389, 1990.

Dryden MW, Long GR, Gaafar SM: Effects of ultrasonic flea collars on *Ctenocephalides felis* on cats. *JAVMA* 195(12):1717–1718, 1989.

Ferrer L, Rabanal R, Rondevila D, et al: Skin lesions in canine leishmaniasis. *J Small Anim Pract* 29:381–388, 1988.

Fischer K: Cuterebra larvae in domestic cats. *Vet Med* 78:1231–1233, 1983.

Foley RH: Parasitic mites of dogs and cats. *Compend Contin Educ Pract Vet* 13(5):783–800, 1991.

Folz SD: Canine scabies (*Sarcoptes scabiei* infestation). *Compend Contin Educ Pract Vet* 6:176–180, 1984.

Garris GI: Control of ticks. *Vet Clin North Am [Small Anim Pract]* 21(1):173–183, 1991.

Gilbert PA, Griffin CE, Rosenkrantz WS: Serum vitamin E levels in dogs with pyoderma and generalized demodicosis. *JAAHA* 28:407–410, 1992.

Greene RT et al: Trombiculiasis in a cat. *JAVMA* 188:1054–1055, 1986.

Hendrix CM: Facultative myiasis in dogs and cats. *Compend Contin Educ Pract Vet* 13(1):86–93, 1991.

Hooser SB: D-limonene, linalool, and crude citrus oil extracts. *Vet Clin North Am [Small Anim Pract]* 20(2):383–385, 1990.

Horton ML: Rhabditic dermatitis in dogs. *Mod Vet Pract* 61:158–159, 1980.

Hoskins JD, Cupp EW: Ticks of veterinary importance. *Compend Contin Educ Pract Vet* 10:564–580, 1988.

Merchant SR, Taboada J: Dermatologic aspects of tick bites and tick-transmitted diseases. *Vet Clin North Am [Small Anim Pract]* 21(1):145–155, 1991.

Moriello KA: Dermatologic manifestations of internal and external parasitism. *Companion Anim Pract* 2(3):12–17, 1988.

Panciera DL, Stockham SL: *Dracunculus insignis* infection in a dog. *JAVMA* 192:76–78, 1988.

Paradis M, Villeneuve A: Efficacy of ivermectin against *Cheyletiella yasguri* infestation in dogs. *Can Vet J* 29:633–635, 1988.

Scheidt VJ: Common feline ectoparasites. Part 1: Clinical syndromes. *Companion Anim Pract* 1(1):6–11, 1987.

Scheidt VJ: Common feline ectoparasites. Part 2: *Notoedres cati, Demodex cati, Cheyletiella* spp and *Otodectes cynotis. Feline Pract* 17(3):13–23, 1987.

Scheidt VJ: Common feline ectoparasites. Part 3: Chigger mites, cat fur mites, ticks, lice, bot fly larvae and fleas. *Companion Anim Pract* 1(2):5–15, 1987.

Schick MP, Schick RO: Understanding and implementing safe and effective flea control. *JAAHA* 22:421–434, 1986.

Scott DW, Vaughn TC: Papulonodular dermatitis in a dog with occult filariasis. *Companion Anim Pract* 1(1):31–35, 1987.

Sosna CB, Medleau L: External parasites: Life cycles, transmission, and the pathogenesis of disease. *Vet Med*, pp 538–547, June 1992.

Sosna CB, Medleau L: The clinical signs and diagnosis of external parasite infestation. *Vet Med*, pp 549–564, June 1992.

Sosna CB, Medleau L: Treating parasitic skin conditions. *Vet Med*, pp 573–586, June 1992.

CHAPTER THREE
Diagnosis and Management of Bacterial Skin Diseases

*U*nder normal circumstances, there are hundreds or even thousands of microbes on every square centimeter of skin surface. These bacteria are normally confined to the skin surface and the immediate openings of the hair follicles, with the hair roots and glandular structures being virtually sterile.

Microbes that have evolved to live on dog or cat skin are referred to as "resident" bacteria. In the dog and cat normal resident microbes include:

- *Staphylococcus epidermidis*
- *Staphylococcus simulans*
- *Corynebacterium* spp.
- *Clostridium (Micrococcus)* spp.
- *Malassezia* yeasts (formerly *Pityrosporum* spp.)
- *Demodex* mites

Transient cutaneous bacteria of dogs and cats include:

- *Proteus* spp.
- *Pseudomonas* spp.
- Coagulase-positive staphylococci (e.g., *Staphylococcus intermedius* in dogs, *Staphylococcus aureus* in cats)

Bacterial skin diseases are commonly encountered and are frequently referred to as "pyodermas" (derived from the Latin words for pus [pyo] and skin [derm]). This term is not always accurate (pus is not a feature of all bacterial skin diseases), but it likely will continue to be used in the veterinary nomenclature.

Although bacteria are often identified as the cause of pyoderma, only a relatively small percentage of cases are truly caused by highly pathogenic microbes. Most infections in dogs and cats are actually opportunistic, with infection only occurring under a specific set of conditions. Because even healthy dogs and cats typically have many microbes on their skin, it is rare that resident or transient flora represent the root cause of the pyoderma. The key issue with most pyodermas is to determine the reason that the infection is occurring. Is the organism sufficiently pathogenic

to overwhelm an animal's defense mechanisms, or are these mechanisms somehow impaired? In the vast majority of cases, there is an underlying problem that allows the skin to be preyed upon by opportunistic microbes. Possible causes for a decreased resistance to infection might include some immune deficit, allergies, hormonal problems (e.g., hypothyroidism), and parasitism.

The concept of underlying problems in pyoderma is important with respect to diagnosis and treatment. A diagnosis of cutaneous bacterial infection, or pyoderma, is rarely helpful. In most cases, antibiotic therapy improves the situation only temporarily. Because the skin is never sterile, recurrence of the pyoderma should be anticipated if the underlying problem is not addressed. The deeper the infection, the more immune compromise of the animal is likely.

In dogs *Staphylococcus intermedius* is a common pathogen, implicated in over 95% of canine pyodermas. Puppies acquire this microbe from their mothers during birth and the first few days of life. Bacterial counts of the organism are higher at the vaginal opening of pregnant bitches than at any other site. After this time the bacteria does not appear to be transferable between dogs. Because *Staphylococcus intermedius* is not contagious, a critical question is whether the pyoderma is a result of the potency of the bacteria or reduced host defenses. As already discussed, some inciting factor usually allows the bacteria to colonize the skin in larger than normal numbers. The staphylococci then secrete a number of important enzymes and toxins, which serve to complicate the situation.

Some bacterial skin diseases cause considerable pruritus, which is often treated as a separate entity. This is often referred to as bacterial or staphylococcal hypersensitivity (obviously, not hypersensitivity in the traditional sense). These conditions are probably best labeled pruritic pyodermas or pruritic staphylococcal disease, because therapy with antibiotics eliminates not only the infection but the pruritus as well.

TYPES OF BACTERIAL SKIN DISEASES

Bacterial skin diseases are often grouped into four categories:

- Superficial pyoderma
- Intermediate pyoderma
- Deep pyoderma
- Atypical pyoderma

Superficial Pyoderma

Superficial (or surface) pyodermas are cutaneous bacterial infections that involve only the very top layers of the epidermis. They tend not to extend into the hair follicles and certainly do not damage the dermis extensively.

In dogs this category includes:

- Pyotraumatic dermatitis
- Skin fold pyodermas
- Juvenile pustular dermatitis

In cats this category includes:

- Impetigo
- Ecthyma

Pyotraumatic Dermatitis (Hot Spots)
(see Plate III-1)

Pyotraumatic dermatitis (hot spots) is a common cutaneous eruption, especially in long-coated breeds. This acute superficial infection evolves over a period of hours as a result of self-inflicted trauma. The underlying causes include, but are not limited to, the following:

- Allergies
- Ear infections
- Irritated anal sacs
- Buildup of humidity within a dense haircoat
- Borreliosis

Clinically, an animal with pyotraumatic dermatitis has a well-delineated patch of oozing and erythema. The redness makes the infection appear to be very deep, but actually only the very superficial layers of the skin are involved. The diagnosis can often be made by history and clinical evaluation. Touch impressions of skin exudates usually reveal a mixed cell inflammatory infiltrate of nonspecific etiology. Biopsies can confirm the diagnosis, if necessary, and reveal the superficial nature of the condition.

Management is rather routine and straightforward. Hot spots can be prevented if the underlying cause is corrected. For treatment of acute cases, however, the area should be clipped to the skin surface, leaving a wide margin of normal skin. This helps prevent the extension of infection, as well as matting of the haircoat. The area should then be gently but thoroughly cleansed with an antiseptic (e.g., chlorhexidine) and gently patted dry. No ointments, creams, or occlusive dressings should be applied to the area; this tends to seal in infection and drive the process deeper. A water-based astringent can be dispensed; most contain *Hamamelis* (witch hazel) or Burow's solution and aqueous hydrocortisone. Depending on the depth of the process, a short course of antibiotics (e.g., 7 to 14 days) may be prescribed, as well as anti-inflammatory doses of corticosteroids.

Skin Fold Pyodermas

Skin fold pyodermas are the result of bacterial proliferation in folds of skin that tend to be continually traumatized by friction and that do not have adequate ventilation. Different parts of the body are affected in different animals, including:

- Whole body folds (e.g., Shar peis)

- Facial folds (e.g., pugs)
- Lip folds (e.g., spaniels; see Plate III-2)
- Vulvar folds (e.g., older bitches)
- Tail folds (e.g., Boston terriers)

Clinically, the conditions involve erythema and often exudation in problem areas. Biopsies are rarely necessary for confirmation, but impression smears of the exudate may provide useful information about the extent of bacterial involvement.

In most cases, management involves life-long care unless the owners elect to have the folds surgically altered. Because long-term antibiotics are a poor treatment option, topical therapy on a daily or every other day basis is indicated. The area between the folds needs to be routinely cleansed with a gentle antiseptic (e.g., chlorhexidine) and carefully dried.

Juvenile Pustular Dermatitis (Impetigo)

Juvenile pustular dermatitis (also known as impetigo and puppy pyoderma) is a benign process in which pustules (pimples) are noted on the ventral and inguinal area. Affected puppies are otherwise completely healthy and are not bothered much by the condition.

Diagnosis is made by history and clinical signs but can be confirmed by biopsy if necessary. Impression smears can be made by puncturing a pustule and collecting the contents on a microscope slide. Routine blood stains are adequate for evaluation. Cytologic examination reveals neutrophils and, occasionally, evidence of phagocytized cocci. Staphylococci are commonly cultured from intact pustules, but other pustules may be sterile.

Treatment includes therapy with antibacterial products (e.g., benzoyl peroxide, chlorhexidine) and, rarely, a 7 to 10 day course of antibiotics. Although impetigo is very contagious in humans, this is not at all the case in dogs. There is no problem of contagion or zoonotic potential for juvenile pustular dermatitis in the dog.

Impetigo and Ecthyma

Superficial pyodermas in the cat are often referred to as impetigo and ecthyma, but neither are particularly good terms for these conditions. These superficial bacterial eruptions are seen most often in kittens.

Clinically, oozing sores appear on the back of the neck and may expand to involve the head,

chest, and ventral area. These lesions may stem from overzealous mouthing by the queen as she carries the kittens. The most common organisms recovered, *Pasteurella multocida* and beta-hemolytic streptococci, usually are controlled with amoxicillin or ampicillin and topical antiseptics or astringents. Affected areas should first be clipped before topical preparations are applied. Occlusive ointments and creams should not be used.

Intermediate Pyodermas

Intermediate pyodermas refer to cutaneous bacterial infections of the hair follicles (folliculitis; see Plate III-3) and the surrounding tissues (perifolliculitis). These conditions involve more than just the superficial aspects of the epidermis but not the deeper dermis or subcutaneous tissue. Most cases of intermediate pyoderma are not primary events. There are usually underlying problems (e.g., allergy, hypothyroidism) that allow the infection to become established and proliferate.

Clinically, folliculitis and perifolliculitis are characterized by pinpoint papular or pustular eruptions with associated scaling and hair loss. The hair loss usually occurs in a round patch and may be confused with dermatophytosis (ringworm). The extent of the process is easiest to visualize on the sparsely haired regions on the abdomen. In these areas, it is common to find papules, pustules, focal hyperpigmentation, and round, peeling rims of scale (epidermal collarettes). The round lesions are sometimes referred to as "target lesions."

Diagnosis is normally made on the basis of clinical signs, cytology, histopathologic examination of biopsies, and bacterial culture. Biopsies of pustules usually demonstrate perifolliculitis and folliculitis, which are histopathologic findings only and not clinical diagnoses. Cytologic examination is also useful. A pustule can be pricked with a needle, with the pus expressed onto a microscope slide and highlighted by a variety of stains. Usually, there are abundant neutrophils, many of which contain engulfed microorganisms. *Staphylococcus intermedius,* a gram-positive coccoid bacteria, is associated with folliculitis in the vast majority of canine cases. In cats staphylococci are also frequently recovered from superficial and intermediate pyodermas; *Staphylococcus aureus* is the most common of the coagulase-positive staphylococci, followed by *S. intermedius* and *S. hyicus.* Of the coagulase-negative staphylococci *S. similans* is the most commonly recovered, followed by *S. epider-*

midis and *S. xylosus. Pasteurella multocida* and beta-hemolytic streptococci are also important pathogens in feline pyodermas. Culture of an aspirate from an intact pustule can be used if the problem is a chronic or recurrent one. Samples collected from old, excoriated, or chronic lesions are likely to provide numerous contaminant organisms. If biopsies are taken, the tissue can be aseptically sectioned and submitted for histopathologic evaluation.

Management of intermediate pyodermas involves correcting any underlying problems (e.g., allergy, endocrine disorders) and treating the bacterial component with topical and oral antibacterial agents. Intermediate pyodermas usually require antibiotics for at least 10 days and often 3 to 4 weeks. Bacteriostatic antibiotics such as lincomycin, chloramphenicol, and erythromycin are good first choices for cases of folliculitis in dogs. The more potent antibacterial agents should be reserved for chronic or recurrent cases, in which an underlying cause cannot be identified and corrected. In cats more potent antibacterial agents such as potentiated penicillins and cephalosporins may be needed as empirical first treatments. Bathing with an antiseptic wash (e.g., benzoyl peroxide, chlorhexidine, cetrimide) also helps decrease bacterial population on the skin surface. Once the underlying cause is identified and corrected, the folliculitis should disappear in response to systemic and topical therapy.

Deep Pyoderma

Deep pyodermas usually result from the extension of an intermediate pyoderma but may also be introduced by skin trauma. The two most common types of deep pyodermas are:

- Furunculosis
- Cellulitis

Furunculosis (see Plate III-4) refers to a folliculitis in which the affected hair follicles have ruptured. Fistulous tracts may appear at the skin surface, providing an outlet for trapped pus and debris.

Cellulitis (see Plate III-5) is an infection of the deeper tissues that spreads between tissue planes. If the infection is well circumscribed and a cavity of pus forms, it is referred to as an abscess. Abscesses usually result from traumatic inoculation of microorganisms into the dermis or panniculus. They may appear as firm to fluctuant subcutaneous nodules that exude pus and are painful to the touch. The most common cause of abscesses in cats is bite wound infection.

Deep pyodermas are serious medical problems that usually imply a significant immune deficit or inoculation of harmful bacteria by bite wounds or trauma. Inoculation can occur by many routes, including needle tracks and foreign objects (e.g., thorns, plant awns, wire). A deep cellulitis documented in the German shepherd appears to be the result of a serious cell-mediated immune deficit.

Diagnosis of deep pyoderma can usually be made by clinical evaluation and impression smear cytology of exudates, but histopathologic examination of biopsies and bacterial cultures are advocated in most cases. The latter approach is worthwhile because underlying problems are to be anticipated and antibiotic therapy may be needed for weeks or months. Ultimately, successful treatment depends on identifying and eliminating the underlying cause. If this cannot be accomplished, long-term antibacterial therapy is unavoidable. This treatment is expensive and may lead to resistance to multiple antibacterial agents and increase the possibility of drug reactions. In cats with chronic abscesses, underlying causes (e.g., feline leukemia virus, feline immunodeficiency virus, atypical pyodermas, mycoplasmal infection, fungal infection, neoplasia) should be investigated.

Management of deep pyodermas depends on topical antibacterial therapy and often prolonged administration of antibiotics. Potent antibiotics such as the potentiated penicillins, amoxicillin-clavulanate, and the cephalosporins are often employed to penetrate into the deeper tissues involved. Resistance to other antibacterial agents is common. Antiseptics such as tris(hydroxymethyl)-aminomethane-EDTA (tris-EDTA) can be very useful in flushing fistulous tracts. Bacteria exposed to tris-EDTA are more susceptible to antibiotics.

For patients with abscesses, surgical drainage, flushing with appropriate antiseptic agents, and judicious use of hot compresses should precede antibacterial therapy. This is facilitated by clipping the fur to expose the entire affected area. In cats abscesses usually result from bite wounds from other cats and many different oral microorganisms (e.g., anaerobic streptococci, *Fusobacterium, Bacteroides, Escherichia coli, Pasteurella,* mycoplasmas) may become inoculated into the subcutaneous tissues. Establishing effective drainage is the most important aspect of therapy. For routine abscesses administration of amoxicillin accompanied by surgical drainage is sufficient. For chronic or recurrent abscesses or those associated with devitalized tissues, administration of metronidazole or clindamycin may be indicated. Abscesses resulting from infection with mycoplasma-like organisms often respond to tetracycline therapy. To prevent further episodes of abscess development, cats should be isolated from potential combatants and, when feasible, castrated. Sequelae to abscess development include extension of the infection to pyothorax, bone and joint infection, and nasal and sinus infection.

When no underlying cause for a deep pyoderma is evident, long-term antibiotic therapy is often augmented with the use of immune stimulants. This is attempted because it is assumed that animals with recurrent deep infections likely have some impairment of their immune function. Products used for this purpose include:

- Derivatives of the cell wall of staphylococci—e.g., Staphoid® A-B (Coopers Animal Health), Staphage lysate (SPL)® (Delmont Laboratories), Lysigin (Bio-Ceutic)
- *Propionibacterium*—e.g., ImmunoRegulin® (ImmunoVet)
- Mycobacteria—e.g., Regressin® (Vetrepharm Research)

The anthelmintic levamisole is also used occasionally because it has been shown to augment the immune system, but it has been shown to cause serious side effects in some cases. These immune stimulants cannot be expected to restore a defective immune system, but they appear to be successful in about 65% to 70% of cases. Because each product has different mechanisms, an animal that does not respond to one type may respond to another. At present, the only other alternative is long-term antibacterial use, which has its own disadvantages.

Atypical Pyodermas

Some conditions do not fit neatly into any of the categories described above. Many of these conditions are not even caused directly by bacteria.

Acne

Acne is common in both dogs and cats, but these conditions are not identical in these two species nor are they analogous to acne in humans.

In many ways acne is better characterized as a defect in the keratinization process, in which accumulation of scale and debris in hair follicles results in inflammation. Chronic antibiotic therapy is unlikely to significantly improve the situation.

In dogs certain breeds such as the Great Dane, Doberman pinscher, bulldog, and bull terrier are particularly at risk, but any animal may be affected. Development of inflammatory papules and nodules is seen on the chin and often around the lips. The cause of feline acne is unknown. Comedones and papules may progress to abscesses and draining tracts.

Diagnosis can be made following clinical evaluation, but biopsies can confirm suspicions if necessary. Treatment must consist of frequent cleansing with antiseptics (e.g., alcohol, benzoyl peroxide, chlorhexidine, povidone-iodine) and the use of astringents. The condition improves spontaneously in some dogs as they grow older. In severe conditions topical benzoyl peroxide gels and vitamin A derivatives (e.g., Retin-A® 0.05% cream—Ortho Pharmaceutical) may help clear clogged hair follicles. These preparations may cause irritation, however, especially in cats. In severe or refractory cases, oral isotretinoin (Accutane®—Roche Dermatologics) can be tried at a dosage of 1 to 2 mg/kg/day, but side effects may occur. Application of topical antibacterial agents (e.g., clindamycin, tetracycline, erythromycin) may have some benefit for cats and dogs with acne, as has been seen in humans. Supplementation with omega-3 and omega-6 fatty acid supplements can help resolve the situation in cats, an indication that fatty acid metabolism is an important factor in the development of this disease.

Actinomycotic Mycetoma (see Plate III-6)

Actinomycotic mycetomas are bacterial granulomas caused by the gram-positive filamentous bacteria *Nocardia*, *Actinomyces*, and *Streptomyces griseus*. They are relatively rare in dogs as well as cats. The term mycetoma, also used to refer to a family of fungal disorders, implies the presence of swelling (tumefaction), draining tracts, and tissue "grains" of microbes. The adjective "actinomycotic" indicates that the microbes causing the mycetoma are from the Actinomycete family. *Actinomyces* is the organism most commonly responsible in dogs, whereas *Nocardia* is more common in cats. Infections are most often caused by contamination of existing wounds.

Clinically, actinomycotic mycetoma consists of localized or generalized nodules, ulcers, and abscesses that often discharge material. The exudate often include "grains," which are gritty colonies of microbes.

Diagnosis is confirmed by cytologic examination, aerobic and anaerobic bacterial culture, and histopathologic examination of biopsies employing special stains to highlight the organisms. Fine needle aspirates of lesions may reveal the characteristic gram-positive filamentous branching bacteria in about two-thirds of cases. The samples are often highly cellular and include numerous mature, nondegenerative neutrophils. *Actinomyces* is anaerobic or microaerophilic, whereas *Nocardia* is aerobic.

Therapy with the penicillins is usually attempted for *Actinomyces* infection, and trimethoprim-sulfa regimens (trimethoprim fraction at 2.2 mg/kg bid) are used for *Nocardia* and *Streptomyces* infections. Treatment is often required for 3 months or more. The combination of surgical excision and antibiotic administration is superior to antibiotic use alone. These organisms pose no threat to humans or other animals.

Bacterial Hypersensitivity

Bacterial hypersensitivity, a commonly used but somewhat controversial term, refers to a bacterial folliculitis of dogs that is particularly pruritic. Other terms used for this condition include:

- Pruritic pyoderma
- Pruritic superficial folliculitis
- Staphylococcal hypersensitivity

It is possible that hypersensitivity reactions are involved, though documentation has been incomplete. It is presumed that most affected animals have underlying disorders, such as hypothyroidism, allergies, keratinization disorders, or immune dysfunction.

Clinical signs include:

- Folliculitis
- Erythematous pustules
- Seborrheic plaques
- Hemorrhagic bullae

The diagnosis of true "bacterial hypersensitivity" requires biopsy because evidence of vasculitis (inflammatory reaction around the blood vessels) is needed. Also, a modified intradermal allergy test can be performed using diluted staphylococcal cell wall extracts such as Staphoid® A-B (Coopers Animal Health) and Staphage lysate

(SPL)® (Delmont Laboratories). The extract is diluted 50:50 with sterile saline, and 0.1 ml is injected intradermally, along with histamine and saline controls. All sites are evaluated in 15 minutes and again in 24 to 48 hours. The specificity of this test is relatively poor because many normal dogs react within the first 15 minute period. Recent research has also shown that some dogs with recurrent pruritic pyodermas have high serum concentration of IgE directed against staphylococcal antigens.

Management includes treatment with antibiotics and elimination of any underlying problems. The diagnosis is confirmed when both the folliculitis and pruritus are resolved following antibiotic therapy alone. Use of corticosteroids is not indicated in these cases as it only serves to confuse the issue. If underlying problems are not identified, long-term maintenance involving daily administration of antibiotics or immune stimulants may be needed. For long-term antibacterial use, bactericidal drugs (e.g., oxacillin, cephalosporins, trimethoprim-sulfas, amoxicillin-clavulanate) given once daily are usually satisfactory, but the possibility of adverse reactions should be anticipated.

Bacterial Granuloma (Botryomycosis)
(see Plate III-7)

Bacterial granuloma is a rare microbial infection of dogs and cats in which the microorganisms have been effectively walled off but not eliminated. The walled off bacteria are protected from the body's immune system. Antibacterial agents usually cannot readily penetrate the granuloma.

Diagnosis of this condition relies on histopathologic examination of biopsies and culture and sensitivity tests. The name botryomycosis (from the Greek words for bunch of grapes [botrys] and fungus [mykes]) was coined because early pathologists thought that the histopathologic arrangement resembled bunches of grapes. Since that time, it has been documented that the cause is not fungal, so the term "mycosis" is also inaccurate.

Treatment can be curative if the granuloma can be surgically removed. Because granulomas have a poor blood supply, most antibiotics cannot penetrate the area where the bacteria are located. Although culture and sensitivity testing is useful, it may erroneously indicate that some antibacterial agents would be effective that in reality could not penetrate the walls of the granuloma. Bactericidal antibiotics such as potentiated penicillins or cephalosporins may be combined with rifampin, an antibiotic that is able to penetrate the granuloma. Rifampin cannot be used on its own because of rapid development of resistance. Some side effects (e.g., increased liver function enzymes, bilirubinuria) have been recognized, and complete blood counts (CBCs) and organ profiles should be periodically evaluated. The response is only complete when the underlying problem (e.g., allergy, hypothyroidism) is identified.

Callus Pyoderma

Callus pyoderma is an infection of traumatized calluses. The calluses form on areas of recurrent impact, and repeated trauma drives hairs and debris into the callus, resulting in infection. Calluses are commonly found on the elbows and hocks of large breeds (e.g., Great Dane, St. Bernard) and on the sternum of other breeds (e.g., dachshund, Doberman pinscher). They are only rarely encountered in cats.

The diagnosis is not difficult as the calluses are thick, dry, and cauliflower-like and limited to the areas of the elbows, hocks, and sternum. Management is complicated by the fact that treatment must also be directed at environmental aspects contributing to the condition. For instance, dogs sleeping on a concrete patio have nothing to insulate their skin from the hard surface when they first drop down on their elbows or hocks. Antibiotic therapy does not improve this situation. Therapy is often only symptomatic and includes weight reduction, keeping the animal on a padded surface, or having it fitted with protective pads (e.g., hockey elbow pads or a padded vest for sternal calluses). Owners should apply emollient lotions (e.g., Vaseline Intensive Care), gels (e.g., Kerasolv Gel—DVM Pharmaceuticals) or creams (urea or lactic acid) to affected areas on a daily basis. Surgical alternatives may be considered but they are often more hazardous and less effective than they are worth.

Interdigital Pyoderma

Interdigital pyoderma is a complex of disorders that cause inflammatory lesions between the toes. It does not appear that all of these disorders are bacterial in origin, but the literature has been confusing to date. The condition is most common in Great Danes, bulldogs, German shepherds, boxers, and dachshunds, but it may occur in any breed.

Clinical signs include:

- Inflammatory papules and nodules between the toes
- Accompanying draining tracts

Diagnostic testing might include cytologic examination of direct smears, skin scrapings, bacterial and fungal cultures, fecal evaluation for parasites, biopsies, immune panels (e.g., antinuclear antibody [ANA] assay, IgA analysis), thyroid profiles, and allergy testing. Many of these disorders are presumed to be immunologic, rather than bacterial, in origin.

Successful management requires identification and correction of the disorder(s) and antibiotic therapy for up to 6 to 8 weeks. The antibacterial agent should be selected on the basis of culture and sensitivity tests. The feet should also be soaked daily with an appropriate antiseptic such as chlorhexidine or povidone-iodine. In advanced cases surgical drainage may be required to expose sites of infection.

Mycobacteriosis

Mycobacterial infections are quite variable in animals, but they are relatively rare. Types of these infections include:

- Tuberculosis
- Leprosy
- Atypical mycobacterial infections

Cutaneous Tuberculosis

Cutaneous tuberculosis has been documented in both dogs and cats. These infections are transmissible to humans, and appropriate preventive care should be taken. Most infections are caused by *Mycobacterium bovis*, but *M. avium* and *M. tuberculosis* also have been implicated. The diagnosis of cutaneous tuberculosis requires histopathologic examination of biopsies, microbial culture, and biochemical tests of frozen tissues. Treatment is usually not attempted because of the public health significance of the disorder.

Leprosy

Feline leprosy has been recognized as a disease entity distinct from cutaneous tuberculosis and atypical mycobacteriosis. The agent responsible for the condition is thought to be *Mycobacteri-*

um lepraemurium, which causes rat leprosy, rather than *M. leprae*, which causes human leprosy. Because the identity of the microbe has not been confirmed and the public health significance remains uncertain, care should be taken when handling infected felines. The disease is thought to be transmitted by the bites of infected rats. Diagnosis involves cytologic examination and histopathologic examination of biopsies. The bacterium responsible for feline leprosy cannot be cultured; cultures are negative even when mycobacteria are identified on cytologic or histopathologic examination. The treatment of choice is complete excision of the lesions. An alternative is clofazimine (Lamprene®—Geigy Pharmaceuticals) given orally at 8 mg/kg sid for 6 to 8 weeks and then twice weekly at that dosage for another 6 to 8 weeks.

Atypical Mycobacteriosis (see Plate III-8)

Atypical mycobacteriosis is more common than either tuberculosis or leprosy and is caused by several opportunistic genera of mycobacteria that are found in the environment. Species implicated include:

- *Mycobacterium fortuitum*
- *M. phlei*
- *M. chelonei*
- *M. smegmatis*
- *M. xenopi*

These mycobacteria are mainly common soil and water inhabitants that may contaminate existing wounds. Infection is also more common in immunocompromised animals. Affected animals develop localized nodules that may ulcerate and drain.

The diagnosis of atypical mycobacteriosis can be confirmed with cytologic examination, culture, or histopathologic evaluation. Samples collected for histopathology usually require staining with Ziehl-Neelsen, Fite, Kinyoun carbolfulschin, or Auramine-O fluorescent staining to highlight the microbes. Routine cytologic preparations prepared with routine blood stains or acid-fast stains often reveal the large, acid-fast rods in direct smears of exudate. Culture for atypical mycobacteria requires Löwenstein-Jensen agar. Transport media are often sufficient to preserve samples during shipment to special laboratories capable of culturing the organisms. Most cultures are positive in less than 4 days; other mycobacteria may require 8 weeks. Laboratories must be informed that atypical mycobacteria are suspected, or they will not hold the cultures long enough. Overgrowth by other bacteria in the first 48 to 72 hours may confuse the picture if the laboratory personnel are not prepared. Also, the laboratory should be notified to incubate the cultures at both 30° C and 37° C as different mycobacteria require different temperatures for culture.

Management of these cases is complicated by the fact that only complete surgical excision is likely to be curative. Spontaneous remission may also occur, but it is uncommon. The use of the aminoglycosides kanamycin, gentamicin, and amikacin may be suggested by sensitivity testing, but cats are quite prone to the ototoxicity and nephrotoxicity of these agents, especially amikacin. Amikacin (5 to 7 mg/kg SC or IM bid for 2 to 4 weeks) may be used initially before converting to safer long-term antimicrobial agents. Kidney function must be carefully monitored during treatment. Safer alternatives include enrofloxacin and doxycycline. The initial treatment of choice is probably enrofloxacin at 5 mg/kg every 24 hours, but the selection is best made on the basis of sensitivity testing. Recently, combination topical and systemic enrofloxacin was used to treat atypical mycobacteriosis. An oral dosage (2.5 mg/kg bid) was combined with a topical preparation (combination of enrofloxacin with dimethyl sulfoxide in a 1:1 solution; 2.5 mg/kg bid) to provide a total dosage of 5 mg/kg bid. The solution was applied to the affected areas twice daily. Resolution of lesions was reported after 2 months of therapy.

Clofazimine (Lamprene®—Geigy Pharmaceuticals) can be used in recurrent or resistant cases. For solitary lesions, controlled localized heating may offer yet another alternative. The area can be desensitized with local anesthesia and the surface temperature heated to 50° C for 30 seconds with a radiofrequency heat generator. The treatment should be repeated in 1 week. This treatment was recently reported to be successful against human *M. chelonei* infection.

Nasal Pyoderma

Nasal pyoderma is a deep pyoderma confined to the dorsal aspects of the nose and muzzle. It is most common in long-nosed breeds (e.g., collie, German shepherd) and may or may not be the result of rooting in the dirt. Probably many conditions originally described as nasal pyoderma were in reality immune-mediated disorders such as cutaneous lupus erythematosus.

Diagnosis can be confirmed with skin scrapings, cytologic examination, and biopsies; bacterial and fungal cultures should also be performed. Therapy includes antibiotic treatment (often for 3 to 8 weeks), gentle cleansing with an antiseptic wash (e.g., chlorhexidine, benzoyl peroxide, povidone-iodine), and protection against further trauma. Appropriate therapy often leads to a complete recovery, but scarring may result if the area is not protected.

Perianal Pyoderma (see Plate III-9)

Perianal pyoderma (also referred to as perianal fistulae and anal furunculosis) is a perplexing problem of uncertain cause. There is very little evidence to support the contention that this is a true bacterial disease. It is most common in the German shepherd and Irish setter breeds. The condition affects twice as many males as females. Researchers have explored many possible etiologies (e.g., overproduction by local secretory glands, poor ventilation associated with low tail carriage, anal sac disease, hip dysplasia). To date, nothing conclusive has been demonstrated.

The diagnosis can often be made on clinical grounds. Confirmation requires histopathologic assessment of biopsies. Cultures are beneficial if antibiotic therapy is being contemplated; the most common organisms recovered on culture include:

- *E. coli*
- *Staphylococcus aureus*
- beta-Hemolytic streptococci
- *Proteus mirabilis*

Management of these cases is often disappointing because response to antibiotics, corticosteroids, or surgery is inconsistent. The best therapy option to date has been cryosurgery, with multiple freezes; removing part of the tail musculature, neutering, and extirpation of the anal sacs may also be indicated. In addition, chemical cauterization may be successful. After removal of the anal sacs the fistulous tracts are debrided; the remaining tissue is cauterized with 75% silver nitrate, 80% liquefied phenol, or 10% Lugol's solution. Preliminary successes with isotretinoin (Accutane®—Roche Laboratories) at 1.0 mg/kg daily suggest that this disorder may share some similarities with acne. Isotretinoin is not licensed for use in dogs.

Plague

Plague, a rare disease in cats, is caused by the organism *Yersinia (Pasteurella) pestis*. Cats normally acquire the infection by eating contaminated rats or rabbits and can transmit the disease to humans through bite wounds or scratches. Lesions include subcutaneous abscesses and lymph node enlargement (buboes). Only perhaps 10% of cases are pneumonic with lung involvement. Most of the cases in North America are in the Southwest, principally New Mexico.

Diagnostic studies should include microscopic and bacteriologic examinations of lymph node aspirates and blood. In most cases the lymphadenomegaly is submandibular. Blood should be drawn for culture, serologic examination, CBC, and cytologic examination. Evaluation of the blood smear or lymph node aspirate for bipolar-staining, gram-negative coccobacilli is best accomplished with Wayson or Giemsa stain. Confirmation can be made by fluorescent antibody testing, which is quick but not positive in all cases. Public health officials should be notified of any suspected cases. Necropsy or handling of animals suspected of having the disease should only be performed by experienced and properly garbed individuals. Every effort must be made to contain possible extension of the infection.

Treatment may be undertaken with tetracycline or chloramphenicol, but affected animals pose a public health danger. Flea control is also of paramount importance as fleas are the sylvatic vector of plague.

Streptococcal Lymphadenitis

Streptococcal lymphadenitis is a contagious disease of cats caused by a Lancefield Group G beta-hemolytic streptococcus. The disease causes an acute inflammatory reaction of the lymph nodes, especially in the region of the head and neck. There is usually evidence of systemic infection. The organism first colonizes the tonsils, then spreads in the lymphatic system of the head and neck. Diagnostic testing includes biopsies of the tonsils and microbial culture. Treatment with potentiated penicillins or erythromycin is usually curative.

DIAGNOSING BACTERIAL INFECTIONS IN DOGS AND CATS

A list of bacterial sampling techniques is presented in Table 3-1.

TABLE 3-1

BACTERIAL SAMPLING TECHNIQUES

TYPE OF LESION	TECHNIQUE
Superficial pustule	1. Clip hair around lesion, if necessary, avoiding trauma to surface of pustule. 2. Gently wipe surface of pustule with alcohol and let dry. 3a. Open pustule with No. 10 or No. 11 sterile scalpel blade. **OR** 3a. Aspirate exudate from pustule using a fine needle and syringe. b. Force exudate to surface by carefully squeezing open pustule. b. Place exudate from syringe and needle onto sterile swab. c. Touch sterile swab to the exudate, avoiding contact with surrounding skin or hair. 4. Streak directly onto agar plate or place in transport medium.
Crusty lesion	1. Clip hair around lesion, if necessary, leaving crust intact. 2. Gently wipe surface of crust and surrounding area with alcohol and let dry. 3. Remove crust with forceps using as aseptic a technique as possible. 4. Rub sterile swab over the moist surface directly beneath the crust, avoiding contact with surrounding area. 5. Streak directly onto agar plate or place in transport medium.
Deep pyoderma with tract but no pustule	1. Clip hair from site of lesion. 2. Wipe surface of lesion with alcohol and let dry. 3. Apply pressure to deeper layers of skin, forcing the exudate onto the surface. 4. Touch sterile swab to exudate, avoiding contact with surrounding skin or hair. 5. Streak directly onto plate or place in transport medium.
Deep pyoderma with unruptured pustule	1. Clip hair from area, if necessary, avoiding trauma to pustule. 2. Gently wipe surface with alcohol and let dry. 3a. Open pustule with No. 10 or No. 11 sterile scalpel blade. **OR** 3a. Aspirate exudate from pustule using a fine needle and syringe. b. Insert swab into cavity and rub vigorously. b. Place exudate from syringe and needle onto sterile swab. 4. Streak directly onto agar plate or place in transport medium.
Deep pyoderma with ulcerated skin	1. Clean area of lesion with soap and water. 2. Swab area with alcohol. 3. Infiltrate lesion subcutaneously with local anesthetic. 4. Use 6 mm biopsy punch to obtain plug of skin at the site to be cultured. 5. Carefully split the plug longitudinally, cutting from the bottom to the surface with a No. 10 or No. 11 sterile scalpel blade. 6. Place sterile swab into the midsection of the split biopsy and rub vigorously, avoiding contact with the surface. 7. Streak directly onto agar plate or place in transport medium.

Direct Microscopic Examination

Direct microscopic examination of cutaneous lesions is one of the quickest and most helpful diagnostic tests available. Unfortunately, it is also rarely done in clinical practice.

Whenever possible, a pustule should be aspirated and the contents examined microscopically. The hematologic stains (Wright's or Giemsa) are quite suitable, because much of the contents are white blood cells (especially neutrophils and lymphocytes). When pyoderma is suspected but there are no pustules, surface crusts can be removed and touch impressions made. Abscesses can be aspirated and fistulous tracts gently squeezed to express contents.

Direct microscopic examination is valuable because it provides immediate information. If *Demodex* mites are noted, diagnostic efforts should be redirected. Acantholytic keratinocytes (rounded pink epidermal cells) suggest the pustules may have originated as pemphigus blisters. Budding yeasts suggest *Malassezia* rather than bacterial infection.

If bacteria are noted in samples, it is important that they be described (e.g., whether they are cocci, bacilli, coccobacilli, spirilli) and their location (e.g., extracellular, within neutrophils) reported. Much information can be gleaned from this rapid assessment. For example, if cocci are noted in smears but cultures grow *E. coli* or *Pseudomonas*, contamination of the sample is likely.

Additional information can be derived from other stains on fresh samples, even if cultures are also being performed. One of the most useful is Gram staining (see box at right), which should be available in most veterinary facilities. Bacteria that stain purple (e.g., *Staphylococcus, Streptococcus*) are termed gram-positive. Those that lose their purple color and stain red (e.g., *E. coli, Pseudomonas*) are classified as gram-negative.

Culture and Sensitivity Testing

Bacterial culture and sensitivity testing are commonly done, but even more commonly the information they provide is misinterpreted. The culture is only as representative as the sample collected, and the sensitivity testing really does not indicate appropriateness of an antibacterial agent.

Bacteria are common residents on the skin surface and mucous membranes and within the ear canals. Swabs taken from these areas are likely to be culture positive, even in animals without bacterial disease. Opportunistic infection is com-

---

GRAM STAINING PROCEDURE

1. Make a smear of presumed bacterial contents on a clean microscope slide.
2. Pour on crystal violet and let stand 30 seconds. Rinse.
3. Pour on iodine solution and let stand 30 seconds. Rinse.
4. Wash with decolorizer for 5–10 seconds until no more purple washes off. Rinse.
5. Pour on safranin or basic fuchsin and let stand 30 seconds. Rinse.
6. Air dry or blot dry, then examine microscopically. Gram-positive bacteria stain purple. Gram-negative bacteria stain red.

---

monplace. For example, any scratch or laceration of a dog's skin results in colonization by staphylococci within 48 hours. Although the bacteria can be cultured readily, that does not mean they are primary pathogens requiring antibiotic therapy.

All normal dogs and cats can resist infection by resident and transient microbes. Without this ability, all dogs and cats would continually have infections; as has been noted, there are hundreds, if not thousands, of microbes on every square centimeter of skin surface. Therefore most opportunistic cutaneous infections in dogs and cats are the result of predisposing causes, including trauma to the skin or any process that interferes with immune competence, even temporarily.

Bacterial infections are often seen secondarily in animals with:

- Allergies
- Keratinization disorders (seborrhea)
- Endocrine problems
- Fungal infections
- Immunologic diseases

Any process that alters the body's defense mechanisms predisposes an animal to bacterial infection and decreases its resistance to infection.

The diagnosis of bacterial infections entails more than just growing bacteria on a culture medium. Cultures must always be interpreted in light of the clinical picture.

The culture is accomplished by sampling the skin tissue as aseptically as possible and placing the material on appropriate growth media. Suitable samples cannot be harvested by swabbing the skin surface. Appropriate samples must be collected by surgical biopsy or by sterile aspiration of an intact pustule. In either case the skin surface is first swabbed with alcohol or other antiseptic (e.g., chlorhexidine, povidone-iodine) to reduce numbers of contaminant bacteria. Bacteria in the deeper aspects of the dermis or subcutis rather than surface microbes are usually the source of the infection.

Blood agar is used as an initial culture medium for bacteria. After 18 to 24 hours of incubation, the presence of numerous colonies of bacteria indicate an infection. The bacteria are then identified. The first step is Gram staining, as described above.

Gram-positive bacteria should then be tested for catalase:

- Staphylococci are catalase-positive (most of the staphylococcal pyodermas in dogs are also coagulase-positive).
- Streptococci are catalase-negative.

Gram-negative bacteria should be tested for oxidase:

- Bacteria such as *Pseudomonas* and *Pasteurella* are oxidase-positive.
- Coliforms (e.g., *E. coli)* are oxidase-negative.

More information on bacterial identification can be found in textbooks on microbiology.

It is not valid to transfer bacterial growth to sensitivity testing media without identification. If many different types of bacteria are present, contamination must be considered. In dogs most cases yield coagulase-positive *Staphylococcus intermedius;* in cats staphylococci, streptococci, and *Pasteurella multocida* are all common isolates.

Sensitivity testing, the term used for the next part of the procedure, is really a misnomer. Once the bacterial species have been identified, samples from four to five well-isolated colonies of the same type are inoculated into 4 to 5 ml of trypticase soy broth and incubated at 35° C for 2 to 8 hours until the medium becomes slightly turbid. The sample's turbidity is adjusted to that of a standard (McFarland 0.5) through dilution with normal saline. If a standard is not available, an approximation can be made by adding three to seven well-spaced colonies in about 2 ml of sterile saline or by using the Prompt System (BBL). A sterile cotton swab is used to streak some of the sample onto a Mueller-Hinton agar plate. Inoculated plates should be allowed to dry for 15 to 30

minutes at room temperature. Small paper discs saturated with different antibacterial agents are placed on the agar plate. The agar plates should be incubated at 37° C within 15 minutes of applying the discs.

The antibacterial agent in each disc diffuses into the agar (the heaviest concentration of antibacterial agent being closest to the disc), inhibiting the growth of susceptible bacteria surrounding each disc. Colonies of bacteria growing close to an antibacterial disc over the next 16 to 18 hours are presumed to be resistant to that drug. A region of no growth (zone of inhibition) surrounding a disc indicates sensitivity to that antibacterial agent. These zones are measured and interpreted, and bacteria are classified according to a standard table as sensitive, intermediate, or resistant (Table 3-2).

In some laboratories antimicrobial susceptibility is predicted based on the breakpoint minimum inhibitory concentration (MIC) agar dilution technique. With MIC testing the antimicrobial agents to be tested are incorporated into agar and plated bacteria are observed for the presence or absence of growth. Several different concentrations of each drug are used, providing a conditional recommendation of sensitive or resistant status relative to the antimicrobial agents tested.

The problem with sensitivity testing is that it does not accurately predict whether an antibiotic will successfully treat the infection. In many ways the term "resistance testing" would be more appropriate. If the test suggests that the microbe is resistant to a particular antibiotic, it is probably valid. The most appropriate antibiotic can then be selected on this basis coupled with information such as the site of infection, presence or absence of a granuloma or abscess, and the time frame needed for treatment. For example, sensitivity information is probably invalid in most cases when the sample comes from a swab of the ear canal. Only when an oral antibiotic is being considered for systemic therapy would this information be of any value.

Other problems with sensitivity testing include the following:

- Abscesses and granulomas tend to wall off infection, making them inaccessible to most antibiotics, regardless of the results of sensitivity testing.
- Some drugs are inactivated by contact with blood, pus, or damaged tissue and may not exert any antibacterial effect.

TABLE 3-2
ZONES OF INHIBITION FOR VARIOUS ANTIBACTERIAL AGENTS

ANTIBACTERIAL ON DISK	REPRESENTATIVE ANTIBIOTIC	DISC CONTENT (µg)	ZONE OF INHIBITION (mm)		
			RESISTANT	INTERMEDIATE	SENSITIVE
Amoxicillin-clavulanate	Clavamox®[a]	30	<20	—	>20
Ampicillin	Ampicillin	10	<21	21–28	>28
Carbenicillin	Carbenicillin	100	<18	18–22	>22
Cephalothin	Keflex®[b]	30	<15	15–17	>17
Chloramphenicol	Chloramphenicol	30	<15	15–17	>17
Clindamycin	Lincocin®[c]	2	<15	15–20	>20
Cloxacillin	Orbenin-DC®[a]	1	<10	10–13	>13
Enrofloxacin	Baytril®[d]	46	<16	16–20	>20
Erythromycin	Erythromycin	15	<14	14–17	>17
Gentamicin	Gentocin®[e]	10	<13	—	>13
Kanamycin	Kantrim®[f]	30	<14	14–17	>17
Methicillin	Staphcillin[g]	5	<10	10–13	>13
Nitrofurantoin	Furacin®[a]	300	<15	15–16	>16
Rifampin	Rifampin	5	<25	—	>25
Sulfonamides	Sulfas	300	<13	13–16	>16
Tetracyclines	Tetracycline	30	<15	15–18	>18
Trimethoprim-sulfa	Tribrissen®[h]	1.25/23.75	<11	11–15	>15

[a] SmithKline Beecham Animal Health.
[b] Dista Products.
[c] Upjohn.
[d] Miles.
[e] Schering-Plough Animal Health.
[f] Fort Dodge Laboratories.
[g] Apotecon.
[h] Coopers Animal Health.

- Other drugs cannot penetrate the skin surface in an adequate concentration to be effective.
- Many cutaneous infections require weeks or months of antibiotic treatment. Products like aminoglycosides (e.g., gentamicin), which can only be administered safely for days or weeks, are poor choices for treatment, regardless of sensitivity test results.

Therefore information from bacterial culture and sensitivity testing should be regarded as diagnostic clues and not definitive results. Almost any animal with a skin disorder is likely to have secondary bacterial complications. These bacteria may be cultured, but treatment with an appropriate antibacterial agent does not correct the underlying problem. Treatment failures involving therapy indicated by culture and sensitivity testing should prompt the investigator to consider underlying disorders.

The antibacterial agents selected for the discs are a matter of convention (e.g., lincomycin is assessed with a clindamycin disc, cephalexin with a cephalothin disc, and enrofloxacin with a ciprofloxacin disc).

EMPIRICALLY SELECTING AN ANTIBIOTIC

Antibiotics can be selected by evaluating the clinical circumstances as well as by culture and sensitivity testing. In uncomplicated cutaneous pyodermas of dogs, *Staphylococcus intermedius* can be suspected as it is recovered in 95% of cases. Because there is much information about the success of various antibiotics against this microbe, a valid selection can often be made empirically. On the other hand, some antibiotics can be dismissed because there is evidence that they do not work well in practice. Ampicillin, amoxicillin, and tetracycline have poor therapeutic value for canine pyodermas, regardless of sensitivity test results. Moreover, the aminoglycosides (e.g., gentamicin and kanamycin) are too toxic to be used for the long periods required for skin infections.

For first-time canine pyodermas it is valid to suspect that *Staphylococcus intermedius* is responsible and to begin treatment on this assumption. At this time the likely underlying cause must be determined or the infection will likely recur soon after the antibiotic has been discontinued. At this first instance, it is advisable to use a narrow-spectrum, bacteriostatic antibiotic such as lincomycin and erythromycin. Chloramphenicol is also suit-

able. If some degree of immune compromise (e.g., prior corticosteroid administration, demodicosis) is suspected, a bactericidal antibiotic such as oxacillin or dicloxacillin should be selected.

For first-time feline pyodermas the cause is likely to be *Pasteurella multocida*, beta-hemolytic streptococci, *Fusobacterium,* or *Bacteroides.* Penicillins such as amoxicillin should be effective in most cases.

For recurrent or chronic infections, antibiotics should be selected on the basis of culture and sensitivity testing. Samples for culture should not be obtained while animals are receiving antibacterial agents; a minimum withdrawal time of 72 hours is necessary. Potentiated penicillins, cephalosporins, fluoroquinolones, and trimethoprim-potentiated sulfonamides are likely needed in chronic cases. In canine pyodermas most of the staphylococcal isolates produce beta-lactamase (penicillinase), which inactivates simple penicillins. For feline pyodermas more potent antibacterial agents such as potentiated penicillins and cephalosporins are often selected. Doxycycline is the treatment of choice for feline mycoplasmal infections.

GUIDE TO ANTIBIOTICS (Table 3-3)

Antibiotics are divided into two main classes based on their effects on microbes:

- Bactericidal antibiotics kill bacteria outright.
- Bacteriostatic antibiotics inhibit the growth of bacteria so they can be disposed of by the immune system.

Some antibiotics can be both bactericidal and bacteriostatic, depending on the dosage at which they are administered.

Penicillins

Penicillins belong to the beta-lactam group of antibiotics. Clavulanic acid and sulbactam are also part of this group and act by inhibiting certain enzymes (beta-lactamases) produced by bacteria that would normally destroy the beta-lactam antibiotics. Thus clavulanic acid combined with simple penicillins such as amoxicillin is effective against bacteria that produce beta-lactamase. These bacteria would normally be resistant to products like amoxicillin and ampicillin but become susceptible with the inclusion of the clavulanic acid. Sulbactam also works synergistically with penicillins and cephalosporins and has weak antibacterial

TABLE 3-3

SYSTEMIC ANTIBIOTICS

DRUG (GENERIC NAME)	ACTION	TYPE	DOSAGE/ ADMINISTRATION	COMMENT
Oxacillin	Bactericidal	Penicillin	15–20 mg/kg tid PO	β-Lactamase resistant
Cloxacillin	Bactericidal	Penicillin	15 mg/kg tid PO	β-Lactamase susceptible
Penicillin G	Bactericidal	Penicillin	20,000 U/kg qid PO	Cat bite abscess
Ampicillin	Bactericidal	Penicillin	22 mg/kg PO	Bacterial feline dermatoses
Amoxicillin	Bactericidal	Penicillin	12 mg/kg PO	Bacterial feline dermatoses
Nafcillin	Bactericidal	Penicillin	20 mg/kg bid PO	β-lactamase resistant
Amoxicillin-clavulanate	Bactericidal	Penicillin	12–14 mg/kg PO	β-lactamase resistant
Cefadroxil	Bactericidal	Cephalosporin	22 mg/kg bid PO	May be given tid
Cephalexin	Bactericidal	Cephalosporin	22 mg/kg tid or 30 mg/kg bid PO	High efficacy
Cephradine	Bactericidal	Cephalosporin	20–30 mg/kg bid PO	High efficacy
Trimethoprim-sulfa	Bactericidal	Trimethoprim-sulfa	30 mg/kg sid or bid PO	Potential to lead to keratoconjunctivitis sicca
Gentamicin	Bactericidal	Aminocyclitol	4 mg/kg bid SC	Only used in generalized resistant deep pyoderma or septicemia; ototoxic; nephrotoxic
Enrofloxacin	Bactericidal	Fluoroquinolone	5 mg/kg bid PO	Not for use in young animals
Lincomycin	Bacteriostatic	Lincosamide	20 mg/kg bid PO	Good first-line antibiotic
Clindamycin	Bacteriostatic	Lincosamide	5.5 mg/kg bid PO	Abscesses, wounds
Erythromycin	Bacteriostatic	Macrolide	15 mg/kg tid PO	Vomiting common
Chloramphenicol	Bacteriostatic	Chloramphenicol	50 mg/kg tid PO	Good first-line antibiotic

activity against most gram-positive and some gram-negative organisms; it works best against *Neisseria* and *Bacteroides* infections in humans. Most staphylococci affecting dogs produce beta-lactamase. Beta-Lactamase–resistant penicillins (e.g., cloxacillin, oxacillin, dicloxacillin, flucloxacillin, amoxicillin, ticarcillin) combined with clavulanic acid or sulbactam, are effective against cutaneous bacterial infections.

Some of the newer families of penicillins include:

- Carboxypenicillins (e.g., carbenicillin, ticarcillin)
- Ureidopenicillins (e.g., piperacillin, azlocillin)
- Amdinopenicillins (e.g., amdinocillin)
- 6-Methoxypenicillins (e.g., temocillin)

These penicillins are worth mentioning but have few uses in dermatologic therapy. They are most effective against gram-negative microbes, especially *Pseudomonas*.

Cephalosporins

Like penicillins, cephalosporins are part of the beta-lactam family of antibiotics. They include some of the most potent antibacterial agents used in veterinary medicine, such as cephalexin, cefadroxil, and cephradine. New generations of cephalosporins and penicillins are constantly being formulated as organisms develop resistance to existing varieties. Because these products are very important in human medicine, they should only be used when absolutely necessary in animals as indiscriminate use will result in an increased bacterial resistance.

The third-generation cephalosporins include moxalactam, ceftriaxone, cefoperazone, cefotaxime, and cefotaxime. They have marked activity against anaerobic and aerobic gram-negative organisms but minimal effect on aerobic gram-positive organisms. They are therefore of little benefit in the management of canine staphylococcal pyodermas.

Aminocyclitols

Aminocyclitols, also known as aminoglycosides, are potent and potentially toxic antibiotics that are rarely used systemically in canine or feline pyodermas. They include streptomycin, gentamicin, neomycin, kanamycin, amikacin, tobramycin, and spectinomycin. Toxicity is very common with long-term use, especially ototoxicity and kidney damage. Because skin diseases often require antibiotic therapy for weeks or months, these products are poor choices despite their excellent efficacy. Aminocyclitols are usually prescribed for dermatologic use only in the form of topical solutions applied to the surface of the skin, where the risk of toxic side effects is greatly reduced. They are ototoxic, however, and should not be instilled into the ear canal unless it is known that the ear drum is intact.

Macrolides and Lincosamides

Macrolides (e.g., erythromycin) and lincosamides (e.g., lincomycin, clindamycin) are bacteriostatic antibiotics that are effective against about 75% of cutaneous bacterial infections in dogs. Although they do not function in exactly the same manner, it appears that animals resistant to either drug show cross-resistance for the other. The principal side effect of erythromycin is digestive upset, including vomiting and diarrhea, but this is rarely seen with lincomycin. These antibi-

otics are excellent choices for first-time pyodermas in dogs because of their narrow spectrum of activity and overall safety. Clindamycin (e.g., Antirobe®—Upjohn) is used to treat abscesses or deep, infected wounds.

Potentiated Sulfonamides

Combinations of trimethoprim or ormethoprim with sulfonamides (such as sulfamethoxazole, sulfadimethoxine, or sulfadiazine) are bactericidal and often effective in the treatment of canine pyodermas. These combination products are much more effective than administration of the antibiotics individually. Side effects are few but include a slight risk of decreased tear production (keratoconjunctivitis sicca), thrombocytopenia, and a lupus erythematosus–like syndrome in Doberman pinschers. (Whether this is a breed-related susceptibility to sulfa drugs has not been determined, but it is best to avoid use of this product in Dobermans, if possible.) The combination of ormethoprim and sulfadimethoxine (Primor®—Hoffman-La Roche) is less likely to cause reduced tear production than other combinations, but other adverse reactions (e.g., behavioral abnormalities) have been reported with its use.

Fluoroquinolones

Fluoroquinolones are bactericidal antimicrobial agents related structurally to nalidixic acid. Many different fluoroquinolones (e.g., norfloxacin, ciprofloxacin, ofloxacin, enoxacin, pefloxacin, fleroxacin) are available in human medicine, but only enrofloxacin is available for use in dogs. They work uniquely by inhibiting the A subunit DNA gyrase, which appears to be essential for DNA replication. This group of antibacterial agents has efficacy against many gram-negative and gram-positive bacteria as well as mycoplasmas, chlamydiae, and perhaps, atypical mycobacteria. They do not work well against streptococci and anaerobic organisms, making them less useful for feline infections. Fluoroquinolones such as enrofloxacin (e.g., Baytril®—Miles) quickly reach serum levels and kill bacteria rapidly. They have an excellent spectrum of activity but reach lower levels in the skin and subcutis than they do in most other tissues. In general, they are not meant to be used for more than 10 days, although they are commonly dispensed for periods of up to 3 weeks. They should be used cautiously during periods of active growth because they can cause lesions of articular cartilage. A good rule of thumb is to not use these products in pups less than 12 months of age. Enrofloxacin is currently not licensed for use in cats.

Chloramphenicol

Chloramphenicol is a broad-spectrum, bacteriostatic antibiotic that penetrates tissues well. It is usually successful in treatment of simple bacterial infections, but development of resistance by organisms is an ever increasing problem. Liver function enzymes and blood counts should be carefully monitored throughout treatment.

Rifampin

Rifampin has a broad spectrum of activity and has the ability to penetrate septic foci, granulomas, and abscesses. It can also enter phagocytic cells and kill intracellular bacteria. Rifampin is not licensed for use in either dogs or cats. Because of the rapid onset of bacterial resistance to this drug, rifampin is usually administered in combination with another bactericidal antibiotic, such as potentiated penicillin or cephalosporin. Indications for use of rifampin include bacterial granuloma (botryomycosis) and chronic deep-seated abscesses. Side effects are more common in dogs than in people, and liver function enzymes should be carefully monitored.

RECOMMENDED READINGS

Ackerman L: Cutaneous bacterial granuloma (botryomycosis) in 5 dogs: Treatment with rifampin. *Mod Vet Pract* 68:404–409, 1987.

Bahri LE, Blouin A: Fluoroquinolones: A new family of antimicrobials. *Compend Contin Educ Pract Vet* 13(9):1429–1433, 1991.

Bevier DE: Canine staphylococcal pyoderma: Choosing the appropriate antibiotic. *Vet Med Rep* 2:288–291, 1990.

DeBoer DJ: Canine staphylococcal pyoderma: Newer knowledge and therapeutic advances. *Vet Med Rep* 2:254–266, 1990.

DeBoer DJ, Moriello KA, Thomas CB, Schultz KT: Evaluation of a commercial staphylococcal bacterin for management of idiopathic recurrent superficial pyoderma in dogs. *Am J Vet Res* 151(4):636–639, 1990.

Dow SW, Jones RL, Rosychuk RAW: Bacteriologic specimens: Selections, collection, and transport for optimum results. *Compend Contin Educ Pract Vet* 11:686–702, 1989.

Eidson M, Thilsted JP, Rollag OJ: Clinical, clinicopathologic, and pathologic features of plague in cats: 119 cases (1977–1988). *JAVMA* 199(9):1191–1197, 1991.

Ihrke PJ: Therapeutic strategies involving antimicrobial treatment of the skin in small animals. *JAVMA* 185:1165–1168, 1984.

Keane DP: Chronic abscesses in cats associated with an organism resembling mycoplasma. *Can Vet J* 24:289–291, 1983.

Kirpensteijn J, Fingland RB: Cutaneous actinomycosis and nocardiosis in dogs: 48 cases (1980–1990). *JAVMA* 201(6):917–920, 1992.

Kunkle GA et al: Rapidly growing mycobacteria as a cause of cutaneous granulomas: Report of five cases. *JAAHA* 19:513–521, 1985.

Kwochka KW, Kowalski JJ: Prophylactic efficacy of four antibacterial shampoos against *Staphylococcus intermedius* in dogs. *Am J Vet Res* 52(1):115–118, 1991.

Levine N, Rothschild JG: Treatment of *Mycobacterium chelonae* infection with controlled localized heating. *J Am Acad Dermatol* 24:867–870, 1991.

Matushek KJ, Rosin E: Perianal fistulas in dogs. *Compend Contin Educ Pract Vet* 13(4):621–627, 1991.

Miller WH Jr: Deep pyoderma in two German shepherd dogs associated with a cell-mediated immunodeficiency. *JAAHA* 27(5):513–517, 1991.

Monroe WE, August JR, Chickering WR, Sriranganathan N: Atypical mycobacterial infections in cats. *Compend Contin Educ Pract Vet* 10:1044–1048, 1988.

Paradis M, Lemay S, Scott DW, et al: Efficacy of enrofloxacin in the treatment of canine bacterial pyoderma. *Vet Dermatol* 1:123–127, 1990.

Prescott JF, Baggot JD: Antimicrobial susceptibility testing and antimicrobial drug dosage. *JAVMA* 187:363–368, 1985.

Prescott JF, Yielding KM: In vitro susceptibility of selected veterinary bacterial pathogens to ciprofloxacin, enrofloxacin and norfloxacin. *Can J Vet Res* 54:195–197, 1990.

Riviere JE: Calculation of dosage regimens of antimicrobial drugs in animals with renal and hepatic dysfunction. *JAVMA* 185:1094–1097, 1984.

Rosenkrantz WS: The pathogenesis, diagnosis, and management of feline acne. *Vet Med*, pp 504–512, May 1991.

Studdert VP, Hughes KL: Treatment of opportunistic mycobacterial infections with enrofloxin in cats. *JAVMA* 210(9):1388–1390, 1992.

Sullivan PS, Arrington K, West R, McDonald TP: Thrombocytopenia associated with administration of trimethoprim/sulfadiazine in a dog. *JAVMA* 201(11):1741–1744, 1992.

White PD, Kowalski JJ: Presentation at the annual meeting of the American Academy of Veterinary Dermatology, Phoenix, 1991.

White SD: Pyoderma in five cats. *JAAHA* 27(2):141–146, 1991.

CHAPTER FOUR
Diagnosis and Management of Fungal Skin Diseases

*F*ungal skin diseases are relatively common in dogs and cats and are referred to as "mycoses." They are grouped into three main classes (see box on p. 92, top):

- Superficial fungal infections
- Intermediate fungal infections
- Deep (systemic) fungal infections

SUPERFICIAL FUNGAL INFECTIONS

DERMATOPHYTOSIS (RINGWORM)

Dermatophytosis is a contagious fungal disorder seen in dogs and cats that can also be spread to humans (Figure 4-1). In dogs and cats, three species account for over 95% of all cases and each has its own preferred reservoir, as follows:

Species	Reservoir
Microsporum canis	Cat
Microsporum gypseum	Soil
Trichophyton mentagrophytes	Rodent

This information is important when considering how the infection was acquired and where to direct treatment efforts.

Medical doctors often refer to dermatophytosis as tinea, and this term is then modified to reflect the body parts involved. For example:

Generalized dermatophytosis	=	tinea corporis
Scalp infection	=	tinea capitis
Groin infection (jock itch)	=	tinea cruris
Foot problem (athlete's foot)	=	tinea pedis

Another way of describing dermatophytes is by their preferred environments, as follows (see examples in the box on p. 92, bottom):

- Anthropophilic fungi are preferentially adapted to humans.
- Geophilic fungi are preferentially adapted to the soil.
- Zoophilic fungi are preferentially adapted to animals.

All dermatophytes, regardless of their preferences, are capable of causing infections in humans and animals.

Clinically, dermatophytosis is quite variable (see Plates IV-1, IV-2, and IV-3) and only rarely are "rings" evident. In veterinary medicine "rings" are more often indicative of bacterial folliculitis than they are of dermatophytosis. Dermatophytes are "skin lovers," but they only invade dead skin; they do not penetrate living tissue or survive in areas of severe inflammation. Moreover, they only parasitize actively growing hair; once a hair follicle is damaged, dermatophytes migrate outward in search of intact ones.

Animals with dermatophytosis may have no visible problems, or they may display changes that include hairless patches with scal-

FUNGAL DISORDERS OF PETS

Class	Disorder	Genus of Most Common Pathogen
Superficial	Dermatophytosis	*Microsporum* *Trichophyton* *Epidermophyton*
	Yeast infection	*Malassezia* *Candida*
Intermediate	Eumycotic mycetoma	*Acremonium* *Curvularia* *Madurella* *Petriellidium* *Pseudoallescheria*
	Hyalohyphomycosis	*Aspergillus* *Chrysosporium* *Paecilomyces* *Penicillium*
	Phaeohyphomycosis	*Cladosporium* *Drechslera* *Phialophora*
	Phycomycosis	*Absidia* *Mucor* *Rhizopus*
	Protothecosis	*Prototheca*
	Pythiosis	*Pythium*
	Rhinosporidiosis	*Rhinosporidium*
	Sporotrichosis	*Sporothrix*
Systemic (deep)	Blastomycosis	*Blastomyces*
	Coccidioidomycosis	*Coccidioides*
	Cryptococcosis	*Cryptococcus*
	Histoplasmosis	*Histoplasma*

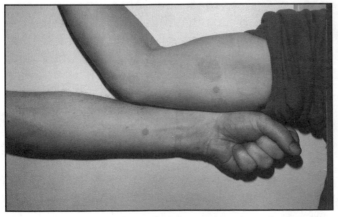

Figure 4-1. Clinical dermatophytosis in an infected veterinarian and staff member.

DERMATOPHYTE CATEGORIES

Dermatophyte Category	Example
Anthropophilic	*Trichophyton rubrum* (athlete's foot fungus)
Geophilic	*Microsporum gypseum*
Zoophilic	*Microsporum canis*

STEPS FOR PROPER USE OF A WOOD'S LAMP

1. Turn lamp on and allow it to warm up for at least 5 to 10 minutes before use.

2. Spend a minimum of 5 minutes examining animal with lamp. Some hairs do not fluoresce immediately.

3. Select hairs that fluoresce with a green color for direct microscopic examination or for dermatophyte culture.

4. Less than half of all cases of dermatophytosis can be expected to fluoresce.

DIRECT MICROSCOPIC EXAMINATION

1. Collect hairs or scales for examination by plucking or scraping.
2. Apply saline, KOH, or chlorazol fungal stain to clean microscope slide.
3. Add collected material to solution on slide. Apply coverslip.
4. Heat fix for several (5 to 30) seconds.
5. Press paper towel over slide and coverslip to remove excess liquid.
6. If KOH or chlorazol fungal stain was used, allow samples to stand before examining, as follows: 5 to 10 minutes for hairs, 5 minutes for skin scrapings, 30 minutes for nail scrapings.
7. Lower condenser on microscope, half-close substage or condenser diaphragm, and scan slide for fungal elements.

ing, an inflamed rash, or actual lumps. These differences reflect the activities of the immune system. Animals with the *fewest* clinical signs likely have the *most* fungi.

Dermatophytes are common in the environment, but not all animals (or humans) are equally susceptible to infection. Animals that are stressed or whose immune status is compromised are likely to be the least resistant to infection.

Diagnosis

Dermatophytosis cannot be reliably diagnosed by visual inspection alone. Confirmation requires finding microscopic evidence of infection or the presence of characteristic spores and hyphae growing on appropriate culture media.

Wood's lamp evaluation (see box above) is a quick and common test for dermatophytosis, but it is not diagnostic. This light source filters ultraviolet light through nickel oxide and causes some dermatophytes to fluoresce green on the hair shafts. Unfortunately, of the three common dermatophytes of dogs and cats, only *Microsporum canis* fluoresces and then only about 40% of the time. *M. adouini*, *M. distortum*, and *Trichophyton schoenleinii* also fluoresce, but they are much more common in humans than they are in animals. Consequently, Wood's lamp evaluation is not a very reliable diagnostic test. Its best use is as a guide to help select hairs for fungal culture and direct microscopic examination. It is important to allow the Wood's lamp to warm up for 5 to 10 minutes before use, or its sensitivity will be even less. All patients should be evaluated in a darkened room to enhance the recognition of any fluorescence. Also, because infected hairs do not necessarily fluoresce immediately, at least 5 minutes

should be spent with this evaluation technique to optimize chances for success. It must be remembered that only the keratin of hairs invaded by the dermatophyte fluoresces, the fungal arthrospores and surface scale do not.

Direct microscopic examination is an important diagnostic test for dermatophytosis but requires careful evaluation and a certain amount of expertise. When viewed by an experienced technician, characteristic spores and hyphae can be detected about 60% to 70% of the time. Suspicious hairs are plucked for examination. Ideally, the selected hairs should appear abnormal visually; sometimes they are described as "fuzzy" or "sick." A Wood's lamp can also be used to aid in the selection process. If no hairs appear abnormal, selection of the hairs from the periphery of lesions is more likely to yield positive results than those from the center. Potassium hydroxide (KOH), commonly used in human preparations, is not usually needed for veterinary samples. Animal dermatophytes are located on the outside of the hair shaft (i.e., ectothrix) and therefore the hair does not need to be digested to see hyphae or spores. The hair samples collected are mixed with mineral oil, saline, or fungal stains on a clean microscope slide, covered with a coverslip, and microscopically evaluated (see box above). The 4× or 10× objective lens is used to scan the slide quickly and identify individual hairs that have evidence of hair shaft damage. Then the high dry or oil immersion lens can be used to confirm the

Figure 4-2. Distorted hair shaft on direct microscopic examination. Numerous fungal spores and hyphal structures are evident on higher magnification.

findings of characteristic hyphae and spores (Figure 4-2).

The proper identification of fungal elements requires practice. The inexperienced technician may find it difficult to distinguish spores from pigment and hyphae from keratin. It is not possible to identify the genus or species of fungus with this test. As an aid to locating fungal elements, chlorazol fungal stain is often helpful because it stains hyphae green against a gray background. This stain can be purchased commercially or formulated as shown in the first box at right.

This solution is applied to a microscope slide. The plucked hairs or scrapings from skin or claws are added to the slide. A coverslip is applied, and the slide is gently heated for several seconds and then allowed to stand. The amount of time that the slide is left to stand before evaluation depends on the sample (hairs for 5 to 10 minutes, skin scrapings for 5 minutes, and nail scrapings for 30 minutes). The slide is not heated to the point of boiling because this can disrupt the fungi and create artifacts. Before viewing, a paper towel should be pressed over the slide and coverslip to spread out the material and remove excess KOH. Microscopic objectives can be permanently etched by contact with KOH.

To view the specimen, the substage or condenser diaphragm should be closed halfway and the condenser lowered almost all the way. Adjustments are made to obtain best contrast with the specimen. The sample is scrutinized for the presence of hyphae, arthrospores, or, occasionally, budding cells. The characteristic macroaleuriospores of the different dermatophyte species are not evident on direct microscopy; they are only seen following fungal culture.

MAKING CHLORAZOL FUNGAL STAIN

1. Dissolve 100 mg chlorazol black E dye in 10 ml DMSO.
2. Add 90 ml saline containing 5 g KOH (10% to 20%).

PROTOCOL FOR CULTURING DERMATOPHYTES

1. Select samples for culture. Wood's lamp can be used to help select contaminated hairs or scales. Use sterile toothbrush for inapparent infections.
2. Inoculate material onto DTM and/or a fungal sporulating medium (Sabouraud dextrose, Mycosel, Mycobiotic).
3. If contagion from large animals is expected, add two to three drops of liquid B vitamins to media.
4. If media are in capped vials, be sure the caps are not tightened.
5. Incubate at 30° C and 30% humidity. Alternatively, keep at room temperature but in darkened environment.
6. Check cultures daily for evidence of fungal growth and color change of DTM from amber to red. Most dermatophytes grow as fluffy white colonies. Ignore any color change that occurs after 2 weeks.
7. Examine microscopically all fungal growth for purposes of identification.

Another stain that can be used immediately for cytologic preparations is chlorphenolac solution. It can be prepared by mixing 50 g of chloral hydrate with 25 ml of liquid phenol and 25 ml of liquid lactic acid. Scales and hair can be dissolved in a few drops of the solution and examined under a microscope with reduced lighting.

Biopsies for histopathologic evaluation sometimes reveal fungal elements in the keratinized layers of the epidermis, claws, or hair follicles. In general, the number of fungal elements present is inversely proportional to the amount of inflammatory reaction. If necessary, these fungal elements can be highlighted with the use of special stains (e.g., periodic acid–Schiff [PAS] or acid orcein Giemsa [AOG]).

Fungal culture (see second box above) is the most reliable method of confirming dermatophytosis, but it may take as long as 3 weeks to identify fungi by this method. Identification of fungi is important in animals because it often provides clues to how the infection was contracted. The culture of dermatophytes can be easily accomplished within a veterinary hospital or at a diagnostic laboratory. If the sample is to be sent elsewhere, the material is placed on black paper (for contrast), and the paper is folded and put in an envelope so that none of the specimen is lost.

To aid in the recovery of specific dermatophytes, special diagnostic media have been formulated. Dermatophyte test medium (DTM) is created by adding a variety of ingredients to Sabouraud agar. An antibacterial agent (usually gentamicin, chlortetracycline, or chloramphenicol) is added to inhibit bacterial growth, and an antifungal agent (usually cycloheximide) is added to inhibit nondermatophyte fungal growth. Finally, a pH indicator (usually phenol red) is often added to the solution so that the medium will change color as the pH increases. Because dermatophytes preferentially use the protein in the medium first, they produce alkaline metabolites that turn the medium from amber to red. This color change is designed as a convenience only and is not diagnostic on its own. An alternative to DTM is Mycosel or Mycobiotic agar, which uses chloramphenicol as the antibacterial agent and cycloheximide as an agent to inhibit saprophytic fungi.

Dermatophyte test medium is not foolproof and has a number of disadvantages. Several other microbes can result in color changes; the overgrowth of nondermatophytes on the medium will also eventually result in a color change. Most commercial dermatophyte test media were formulated for recovery of human pathogens, which are not necessarily those that infect animals. Some ringworm species that infect cattle and horses (e.g., *Trichophyton verrucosum* and *T. equinum)* have additional requirements for B vitamins (inositol and thiamine, and niacin, respectively) than other dermatophytes. If contagion from large animals is suspected, add two to three drops of liquid B vitamins to the medium. Finally, the colony morphology and microscopic features of dermatophytes growing on this medium are frequently not optimal for diagnostic purposes.

Samples are collected for dermatophyte culture in a similar fashion to those used in direct microscopic evaluations. The surface of the skin is first disinfected with 70% isopropyl alcohol. The alcohol is allowed to evaporate before sampling. Suspect hairs or scrapings from claws or skin are

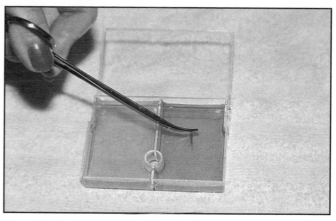

Figure 4-3. Applying hairs to culture media.

collected and are gently placed on, not embedded in, the surface of the agar (Figure 4-3). If the animal is completely asymptomatic, a sterilized toothbrush can be combed through the coat and the bristles touched to the agar surface. Suspect samples should be applied sparingly, or contamination is likely to occur (see Plate IV-4). It must be remembered also that dermatophytes are aerobic and require oxygen for growth. If the DTM is in a capped vial, the cap must not be tightened or inhibition of fungal growth will result. Ideally, fungal cultures should be incubated at 30° C with 30% humidity, but they also can grow if kept at room temperature, preferably in a cupboard or darkened enclosure.

To optimize the chances of growing and identifying dermatophytes in culture, it is advisable to use two different forms of media. DTM is convenient for many cases, but a rapid sporulating medium such as Sabouraud dextrose agar is often valuable because it produces standard colony morphology and provides more structural details for microscopic examination.

Most dermatophytes grow as fluffy white colonies (see Plate IV-5) in 3 to 10 days but some of the large animal varieties may take up to 3 weeks. Color change is usually evident within the first week, and any color change that occurs after 2 weeks should be disregarded. All growth on the fungal culture medium, whether there is a color change or not, must be evaluated microscopically before confirming or rejecting any diagnosis. Collect fluffy fungal growth from the medium with either a moistened swab or a "flag" made of transparent tape. Apply the material to a clean microscope slide moistened with saline or special fungal stains. Lactophenol cotton blue is the most commonly used fungal stain for this purpose and stains the hyphae, macroaleuriospores (macroconidia), and microaleuriospores (microconidia) a blue color (Figure 4-4).

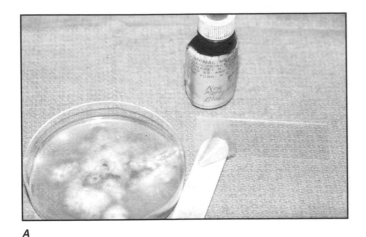

A

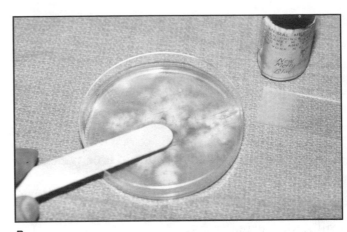

B

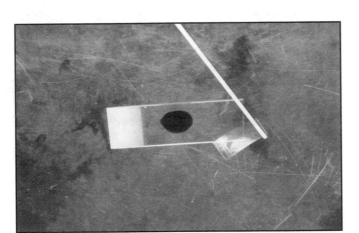

C

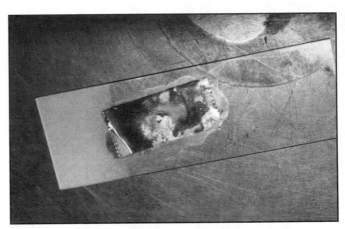

D

Figure 4-4. Acetate tape technique for fungal identification. **A**, *Materials include fungal culture, applicator, acetate tape, microscope slide, lactophenol cotton blue, or new methylene blue.* **B**, *Gently touch tape, which is attached to the end of the applicator with the sticky tape surface outside, to the surface of the culture.* **C**, *Place tape with sticky surface down onto glass slide over drop of stain.* **D**, *Smooth tape on glass slide and examine under microscope.* **E**, *Macroconidia of* Microsporum gypseum *(low power).*

Fungal identification (see box on p. 97) depends on the presence of characteristic macroaleuriospores (macroconidia) and hyphae. To facilitate identification, it may be necessary to transfer growth to Sabouraud dextrose agar or other media designed to enhance sporulation. Some fungal culture kits provide segmented compartments containing different types of media so that identification can be made without additional delays. *Microsporum canis* produces spindle- or canoe-shaped macroconidia with thick walls and, often, a knob on the terminal end. It appears compartmentalized, often having six or more cells (Figure 4-5). One-celled microconidia may also be apparent. *Microsporum gypseum* appears similar to *M. canis* in many respects. However, the macroconidia of *M. gypseum* are often more numerous, lack the knob on the terminal end, and frequently

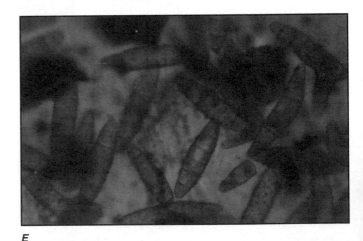

E

have less than six cells (Figure 4-5). One-celled microconidia may be seen as well. *Trichophyton mentagrophytes* may rarely produce elongated, canoe-shaped macroconidia, but it is most often identified by the presence of globose microconidia and/or spiral hyphae (Figure 4-5). Other important dermatophytes as well as contaminants can be identified by searching for characteristic hyphal and spore forms (Figures 4-5 and 4-6).

FEATURES OF DERMATOPHYTES	
Organism	**Features**
M. canis	Spindle-shaped macroconidia; thick walls Knob on terminal end Compartmentalized, often with six or more cells
M. gypseum	Macroconidia often more numerous than *M. canis* Lack of knob on terminal end Compartmentalized, often with less than six cells
T. mentagrophytes	Rarely produce spindle-shaped macroconidia Globose microconidia Spiral hyphae

Treatment

The significance of dermatophytosis may vary from a mild inconvenience to a major skin disease. Treatment depends on many criteria and is tailored to the individual animal. Mild infections are self-limiting and may spontaneously regress (over months to years); other infections are chronic, debilitating, and poorly responsive to therapy. Individual infected hairs may contaminate an environment for up to 18 months, which poses a risk of repeated infection even if the condition clears spontaneously.

The aim of treatment is threefold:

* Clear the infection.
* Prevent spread to other animals and humans.
* Decontaminate the environment to prevent future infections.

For localized infections treatment may only involve trimming the area and applying suitable antifungal creams or ointments (see first box on p. 100). This is rarely satisfactory because most dogs and cats have such dense haircoats that the fungi are likely to be more widespread than suspected. Good products for "spot" treatment include miconazole, clotrimazole, and ketoconazole. Human products abound in the marketplace, and suitable antifungal ingredients include tiocona-

zole, econazole, oxiconazole, isoconazole, sulconazole, naftifine hydrochloride, haloprogin, and ciclopirox olamine. Nystatin, a common prescription item for humans with yeast infections, is not very effective against ringworm fungi. Tolnaftate is also a common human antifungal agent but has limited applications in animals.

Because most dermatophyte infections in animals are actually more generalized than they appear, it is advisable to clip the haircoat as short as possible. It must be remembered that the fungi are located in the hair follicles. Antiseptic cleansers (see second box on p. 100) should be used twice weekly, and they should be worked well into the skin to maximize their antifungal action. Some antifungal products used as weekly or twice weekly dips include:

* Chlorhexidine (e.g., Nolvasan®—Fort Dodge Laboratories)—A very convenient product that has a wide spectrum of activity against fungi and bacteria and is essentially nontoxic and very gentle to the skin
* Miconazole (e.g., Dermazole—Allerderm/ Virbac)—Effective against *Malassezia* yeasts in addition to dermatophytes
* Lime sulfur (in a 2.5% solution)—Quite safe but has a disagreeable odor and can stain white haircoats
* Captan—Marketed to control garden fungi but has long been used by breeders, pet owners, and veterinarians in a 0.25% solution for the treatment of dermatophytosis; although it is relatively safe, it is a potent contact sensitizer in people and therefore should only be used by individuals that are properly protected and gloved
* Enilconazole (Imaverol—Janssen; available in Europe)—Used as a wash in a dilution of 1:50 on four occasions at 3 day intervals

Povidone-iodine and benzoyl peroxides also exert some antifungal activity.

It is important to treat all animals in the household simultaneously, once or twice weekly for at least 6 weeks, until the problem is controlled. It is also important that the individual doing the dips or baths wear rubber gloves to avoid contagion.

Griseofulvin is the most common systemic medication used for dermatophytosis, and treatment must be continued after an apparent clinical cure has been achieved (at least 6 weeks). If the microsize preparation (e.g., Fulvicin-U/F®—Scher-

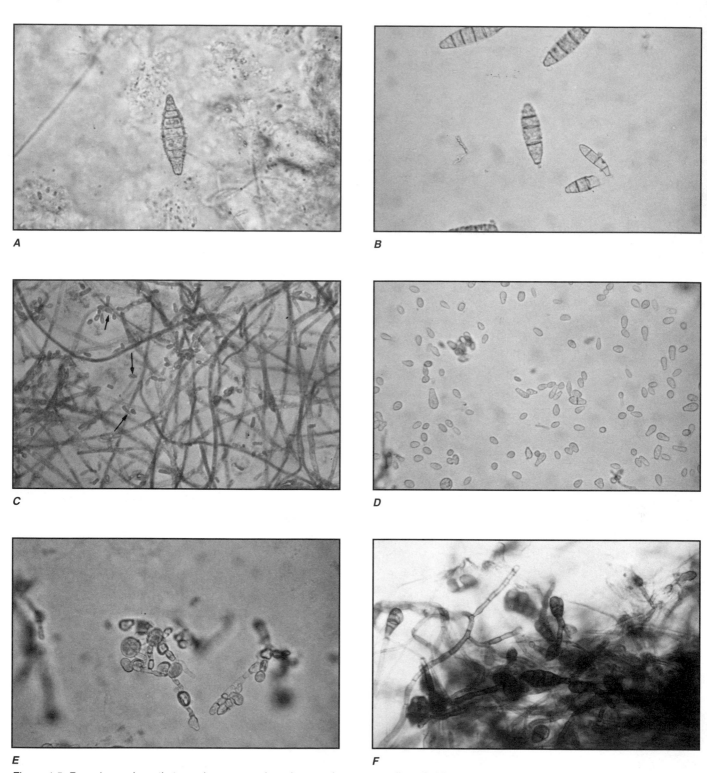

Figure 4-5. *Fungal organisms that may be recovered on dermatophyte test medium.* **A**, Microsporum canis: *macroconidia with a thick wall and more than six cells;* **B**, Microsporum gypseum: *macroconidia with a thin wall and six or less cells;* **C**, Trichophyton mentagrophytes: *tear drop–shaped microconidia* (arrows); **D**, Trichophyton terrestre; **E**, Epidermophyton floccosum; **F**, Alternaria; **G**, Aspergillus; **H**, Cladosporium; **I**, Trichothecium; **J**, Trichophyton verrucosum; **K**, Trichophyton georgia.

ing-Plough Animal Health) is used, it is important to give it with a fat meal, such as corn oil, to enhance its absorption. The dosage for this form of the drug is 50 mg/kg/day; the dosage can be split into a twice daily regimen to lessen the incidence of side effects. The ultramicrosize prepara-

tion (e.g., Gris-PEG®—Herbert Laboratories) does not require fat supplementation. The dosage for this form of the drug is 5 to 10 mg/kg once daily. Gastrointestinal distress, including vomiting and diarrhea, is not unusual in animals treated with griseofulvin. Griseofulvin can cause birth defects,

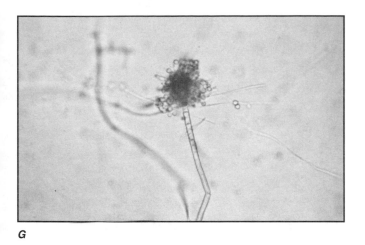

G

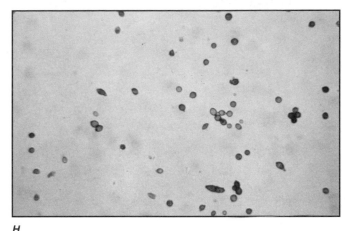

H

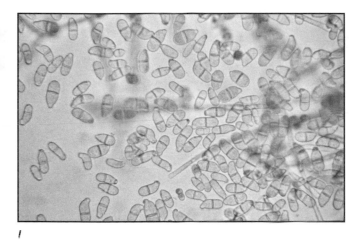

I

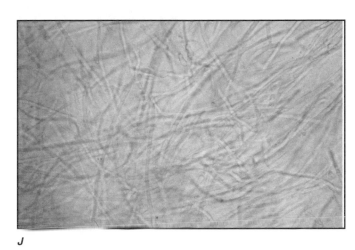

J

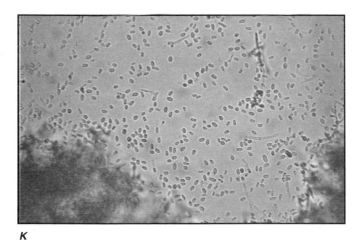

K

Figure 4-5. Cont'd.

and it should not be administered to pregnant animals. Cats appear to be particularly susceptible to toxicity, and purebred cats may be unusually sensitive to the side effects of griseofulvin; care should be exercised when administering it to Siamese, Abyssinian, and Himalayan breeds. Idiosyncratic reactions in cats include anemia,

leukopenia, thrombocytopenia, jaundice, pyrexia, depression, ataxia, and pruritus. To monitor cats for adverse reactions, a pretreatment feline immunodeficiency virus titer should be evaluated and red cell, white cell, and platelet counts as well as liver function tests should be evaluated every 2 weeks throughout treatment. Administration of the drug should be discontinued immediately if signs of toxicity develop.

Ketoconazole (Nizoral®—Janssen Pharmaceutica) is sometimes used in very chronic or resistant cases at doses of 10 mg/kg sid or bid. Side effects include anorexia, vomiting, diarrhea, weight loss, and liver abnormalities. Blood counts and liver function profiles should be performed every 2 weeks throughout treatment. Itraconazole (Sporanox—Janssen) has been useful in cats with dermatophytosis (50 mg every 1 or 2 days, with food) that were resistant to griseofulvin or experienced drug-related side effects with it. Itraconazole appears to be less toxic in cats than ketoconazole but shares all the same potential side effects. Treatment should therefore be monitored as for keto-

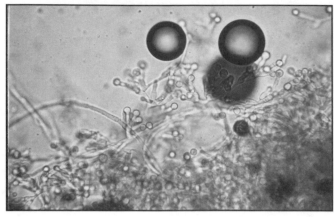

A

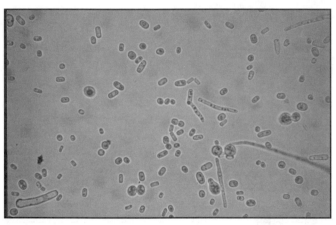

B

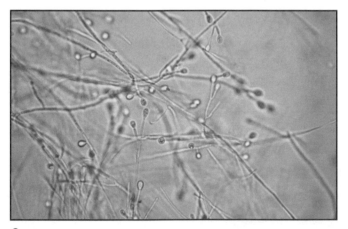

C

*Figure 4-6. Common contaminants on fungal cultures. **A**, Scopulariopsis; **B**, Geotrichum candidum; **C**, Scedosporium (Monosporium) apiospermum.*

SUITABLE ANTIFUNGAL CREAMS AND OINTMENTS	
Miconazole	Naftifine
Econazole	Ciclopirox olamine
Tioconazole	Ketoconazole
Clotrimazole	Sulconazole
Oxiconazole	Haloprogin

SUITABLE ANTIFUNGAL WASHES	
Chlorhexidine	Enilconazole
Lime sulfur	Captan
Povidone-iodine	Benzoyl peroxide

SUITABLE ENVIRONMENTAL DISINFECTANTS	
Chlorhexidine	Enilconazole
Chlorine	Iodine
Quaternary ammonium	Formaldehyde

any building or room that houses infected animals could potentially be a source of infection for humans or other animals. Brushes, bedding, transport cages, and other paraphernalia are all potential sources of infection or reinfection. Fungi have even been cultured from dust, heating vents, and furnace filters.

It is relatively easy to kill dermatophyte fungi on hard surfaces. A 1:10 dilution of household bleach kills these organisms on contact. This is suitable for kennels, runs, litterboxes, floors, and walls. Cages should be cleaned once daily with a 1:4 dilution of chlorhexidine solution, which is less likely to irritate the skin of animals. Disinfectants that contain chlorine, iodine, or quaternary ammonium compounds are also suitable for cleaning runs and cages if chlorhexidine is not available. Enilconazole (Clinafarm—Janssen; currently available in Europe) is also suitable for the environmental cleansing of dog kennels. Brushes, bedding, combs, and toys should be disinfected or destroyed. All grooming utensils should be disinfected with a dilute solution of household bleach or formaldehyde, all bedding should be laundered, and carpets and furniture should be thoroughly vacuumed. A list of suitable environmental disinfectants is presented in the third box above.

conazole. Even when using systemic treatments, antifungal dips are an important aspect of therapy, because they reduce environmental contamination.

Environmental decontamination remains the most difficult aspect of treating dermatophytosis because fungal spores can survive on shed hairs in the environment for up to 18 months. Therefore,

CONTROLLING DERMATOPHYTOSIS IN MULTIPLE PET HOUSEHOLDS

1. Separate known infected animals from uninfected animals and house them in an area that can be easily disinfected (e.g., crate, room with tiled floor).
2. Clip infected animals close to the skin, removing as much fur as possible. Fur should be burned or bagged in plastic for disposal. Disinfect all grooming utensils thoroughly, and bag them in plastic.
3. Try to identify any carrier animals with toothbrush cultures and house them with infected animals.
4. Bathe all animals (infected and noninfected) with an antiseptic.
5. Consider griseofulvin administration in infected animals, 50 mg/kg/day for 6 weeks; in uninfected animals, prophylactic dosage of 50 mg/kg/day for 2 weeks.
6. Clean premises as thoroughly as possible, using chlorine bleach (1:10) on hard surfaces and steam-cleaning carpets. Disinfect all cages and carriers with chlorhexidine solution diluted 1:4 in water. Where available, consider enilconazole (Clinafarm—Janssen) environmental treatments.
7. Repeat dermatophyte cultures on all household animals every 2 weeks. Continue treatment of infected animals for 1 full month past the time when all animals are culture-negative.

GUIDELINES FOR TREATING INFECTED CATTERIES

1. Cats from infected catteries should not be sold, shown, or sent on breeding loans. No new additions should be made either.
2. Clip the entire haircoat, including whiskers, and repeat monthly until the infection has cleared. Infected hairs should be burned, and all grooming utensils and clothing, as well as the room used for the procedure, should be thoroughly disinfected.
3. Commence topical treatment with an antifungal shampoo and continue with an appropriate antifungal dip. Chlorhexidine (e.g., Nolvasan®—Fort Dodge Laboratories; Chlorhexiderm—DVM) is the most appropriate product and should be used twice weekly. If warranted, spot treatment can be done with topical ointments or creams. The most appropriate products for this are miconazole (e.g., Conofite®—Pitman-Moore) and clotrimazole (e.g., Lotrimin®—Schering; Veltrim®—Miles), both prescription items.
4. Starting 6 weeks after therapy has been commenced and every 2 weeks thereafter, perform dermatophyte cultures on at least 25% of cats, using different animals each time. The culture material can come from lesional areas or ideally from combing the entire coat with a sterile toothbrush and gently touching the bristles to the agar surface.
5. If fungi are still cultured after 8 weeks, griseofulvin should be given to all nonpregnant queens and kittens over 12 weeks of age. Blood panels (i.e., blood counts, liver function tests) should ideally be monitored because of the possibility of toxicity. Continue treatment until 2 weeks after the point when *all* cats are culture-negative.

Dealing with contamination of carpets and furniture is a formidable challenge. Carpeted areas and furniture should be vacuumed at least once weekly, and the vacuum bag should be discarded after each use. Steam cleaning carpets does not eliminate fungi unless combined with an antifungal disinfectant such as chlorhexidine or chlorine bleach. It is important to check for color-fastness before treating large areas. All heating and cooling vents should be vacuumed and disinfected. Furnaces should be cleaned by a commercial company with high power suction equipment and filters should be changed often.

Guidelines for control of dermatophytosis in multiple pet households are presented in the box above. When dermatophytosis becomes enzootic in catteries, control can be particularly difficult. The guidelines in the box at right should be considered in those circumstances.

YEAST INFECTIONS

Yeast infections in dogs and cats are usually the result of *Malassezia pachydermatis* (formerly *Pityrosporon canis)*, which is found in the ear canals, anal sacs, vagina, and rectum. It is considered a normal resident of the skin and an opportunistic pathogen. It tends to cause complications in animals with other problems, especially allergies and

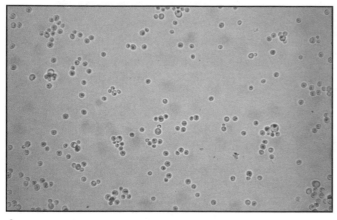

A

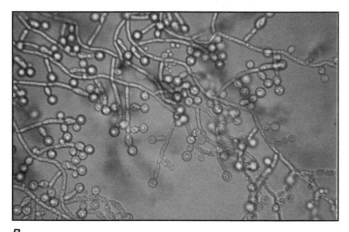

B

Figure 4-7. **A** and **B**, Candida albicans. *Note chlamydiospore production on bile agar in* **B**.

keratinization disorders, and in those who have received prior antibiotic administration. Breeds at increased risk include basset hounds, dachshunds, cocker spaniels, springer spaniels, and German shepherds. West Highland white terriers often have *Malassezia* dermatitis concurrently with epidermal dysplasia syndrome. There might be an allergic component to the problem or some defect in the immune process that allows the disorder to occur. Clinically, animals with these yeast infections are pruritic and musty smelling and most often the ears, face, feet, belly, thighs and neck are affected. *Candida albicans* (Figure 4-7), the common human yeast infection, is relatively rare in dogs and cats. When it does occur, it often involves the mucous membranes of the mouth, rectum, vagina, prepuce, and, occasionally, the nail beds.

Diagnosis

The diagnosis of yeast infections in dogs and cats requires histopathologic evidence of tissue

---

PROTOCOL FOR CULTURING YEASTS

1. Use sterile scalpel blades or swabs to collect surface debris for culture.
2. For deep lesions, consider biopsy and culturing tissue.
3. Inoculate sample onto Sabouraud dextrose agar.
4. Incubate at 30° C and 30% humidity.
5. Check daily for growth for at least 7 days.

---

invasion. The demonstration of these organisms in surface discharges, skin scrapings, or microbial cultures provides supportive evidence only. *Malassezia pachydermatis* can be recovered from the ears of about 50% of normal dogs so culture alone does not confirm a diagnosis.

Cytology is a quick and easy way to demonstrate yeasts. Material swabbed from the ear canals, skin surface, or interdigital area can be applied to a clean microscope slide and heat-fixed for a few seconds. Appropriate stains (e.g., Wright's stain, new methylene blue, Diff-Quik) can enhance the organisms to demonstrate the characteristic oval and sometimes budding yeast forms. Hyphae are noticeably absent with *Malassezia* infection. *Candida* often displays budding blastoconidia and pseudohyphae. Samples can also be collected by impression smear or skin scrapings. Yeasts are usually seen adequately with the high dry objective, but oil immersion may be necessary to clearly depict them. Finding one or more yeasts per oil immersion field is significant but does not necessarily imply that the yeasts are the primary cause of the skin disorder.

Histopathologic evaluation of biopsies is the best way to prove causation in yeast infections because the organisms can be observed directly and their relationship to the skin surface can be established. Most yeasts are observed in the stratum corneum but, occasionally, penetration into the epidermis can be observed. Routine stains are usually sufficient to demonstrate yeasts but highlighting with PAS or Gomori's methenamine silver (GMS) stains are sometimes used to demonstrate the organisms more clearly.

Culture for yeasts (see box above) is performed as for dermatophytes, but it is best to use Sabouraud dextrose agar because not all yeasts grow on dermatophyte test media. *Malassezia* yeasts typically grow in 3 to 4 days as yellow-orange colonies. *Candida* yeasts grow as cream-colored colonies in 2 to 7 days. Ideally, yeast cultures should be performed at 30° C and 30% humidity. Following successful culture, samples should be taken from the colonies for microscopic examination and yeast identification.

Treatment

Direct treatment targets the underlying cause, but specific treatment for the yeasts may be accomplished if necessary. *Malassezia* can be effectively treated with ketoconazole twice daily for 30 days and the use of selenium sulfide or chlorhexidine shampoos. Topical miconazole preparations (e.g., Dermazole—Allerderm/Virbac) and povidone-iodine rinses have also been advocated, if warranted. The treatment of choice for candidal infection is systemic and topical nystatin.

INTERMEDIATE FUNGAL INFECTIONS

Intermediate mycoses are deeper than the superficial infections but remain in the dermis and subcutaneous fat, rather than affecting the internal organs the way the systemic fungi can. The fungi that cause the intermediate mycoses are usually harmless, common soil-dwelling microbes that are "inoculated" into the skin by thorns, sticks, or anything that might cause a puncture wound. Even harmless fungi such as bread molds can cause problems if they are introduced into cuts or sores. This does not happen very often, probably because the immune system is very efficient at finding and removing these microbes before they do any real harm.

In general, the intermediate mycoses are not considered to be contagious because they are simply saprophytic organisms that are accidentally introduced. The notable exception is sporotrichosis in cats (see Plate IV-6), which can be spread by relatively casual contact; bite wounds and scratches are not required.

Because the intermediate mycoses consist of so many "normal" fungi, there is no easy way to categorize them but they are often described with respect to:

- Visual appearance (e.g., mycetoma)
- Histopathologic staining characteristics (e.g., phaeohyphomycosis, hyalohyphomycosis)
- Families to which they belong (e.g., zygomycosis, phycomycosis)

- Fungi names (e.g., aspergillosis, pythiosis, sporotrichosis)

Most fungal infections have similar features, including nodules, granulomatous reactions, and, often, fistulous tracts; nevertheless, most affected animals seem healthy.

Within this category some fungal look-alikes are included. Pythiosis is caused by *Pythium insidiosa*, a member of the Protista, and protothecosis is caused by *Prototheca wickerhamii* and *P. zopfi*, variants of green algae.

Diagnosis

Histopathologic, cytologic, and culture characteristics of the intermediate mycoses are presented in Table 4-1.

Biopsy is the most expedient way of making a diagnosis. Even with regular hematoxylin and eosin (H&E) staining, most of the intermediate mycoses have very characteristic changes. They elicit a granulomatous reaction in the dermis and subcutis, and many display characteristic hyphal and/or conidial forms. When necessary, special fungal stains (e.g., GMS, PAS, AOG) or immunologic preparations can be used to confirm the diagnosis.

Cytology is often used in the diagnosis of nodular skin diseases, but only occasionally is it helpful in confirming a diagnosis of intermediate mycosis. Many of the organisms exist in their hyphal forms in tissue and are difficult to aspirate. Sporotrichosis is most likely to have organisms that can be identified with cytology (Figure 4-8); these are more commonly recovered from cats than from other species.

Culture is often helpful at confirming the identity of the causative microbe but, when viewed on its own, its findings have the potential to be misleading. Organisms causing intermediate mycoses are common in the environment and also are common contaminants on fungal cultures. When attempting fungal cultures, the surface of the skin should first be disinfected and the sample for culture should be taken by biopsy. The biopsy should be added to a solution of sterile saline until it can be transferred to culture media. It must be remembered that the organisms are present in the dermis and subcutis, not in the surface scale. Another option for culturing exists if fistulous tracts are present. By squeezing the skin around a nodule to express discharge from the tract, a reliable sample can be collected

TABLE 4-1

HISTOPATHOLOGIC, CYTOLOGIC, AND CULTURE CHARACTERISTICS OF INTERMEDIATE MYCOSES

DISORDER	HISTOPATHOLOGIC CHARACTERISTICS	CYTOLOGIC CHARACTERISTICS	CULTURE CHARACTERISTICS
Eumycotic mycetoma	Septate, pigmented mycelia, chlamydospores, "grains"	Fungal hyphae and chlamydospores	Colonies with single conidia borne at the tips and sides of simple conidiospores *Curvularia:* Conidia are 25 × 10 μm
Hyalohyphomycosis	Septate, nonpigmented mycelia, branching at acute angles	Thick (4–6 μm) septate hyphae and conidiophores	*Aspergillus:* Green; conidia are 3–7 μm *Penicillium:* Blue-green; conidia are 3.0–3.3 μm × 2.8–3.5 μm
Phaeohyphomycosis	Septate, pigmented mycelia	Pigmented hyphae	*Cladosporium:* Green-brown; ellipsoidal conidia are 8–15 × 4–16 μm
Phycomycosis	Broad, sparsely septate hyphae	Broad, nonseptate hyphae	*Mucor:* White-gray; sporangiospores are 5–10 μm *Rhizopus:* Dark sporangia; spores are 9–11 μm; large columella
Prototecosis	Sporangia, 2–11 μm; larger organisms have thick walls and characteristic internal septations; not apparent without fungal stains (e.g., GMS, PAS)	Yeastlike	Cream-colored; yeastlike colonies within 72 hours
Pythiosis	Broad, nonseptate hyphae (4.5–5.5 μm); not apparent without fungal stains (e.g., GMS, PAS)	Fungal elements present only occasionally	Similar to phycomycosis; sporulation not evident with standard cultural techniques Tissue specimens preferred
Rhinosporidiosis	Large sporangia (up to 400 μm)	6–8 μm organisms; deeply basophilic spherules	Requires tissue culture
Sporotrichosis	Round to oval cells producing 3–6 μm buds; occasionally 4–8 × 1–2 μm "cigar bodies"; often not apparent without fungal stains (e.g., GMS, PAS)	Pleomorphic, 2–3 × 3–6 μm with 1–2 buds. Rarely found, except in cats	Dimorphic; can grow as yeast or mold At 25° C: brown-black mycelial colony producing conidia At 37° C: elongated, budding yeast

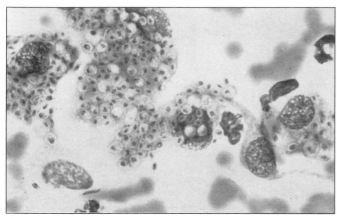

Figure 4-8. Sporothrix schenckii: *Direct smear of exudate from sporotrichosis lesion with numerous phagocytized yeast bodies (high power). (Courtesy of Nita Gulbas, Phoenix, Arizona.)*

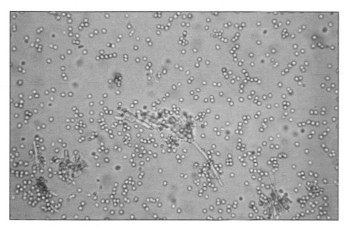

Figure 4-9. Penicillium.

TREATMENT OPTIONS FOR THE INTERMEDIATE MYCOSES, OTHER THAN SURGERY

Disorder	Medical Treatment Options
Eumycotic mycetoma	Miconazole Ketoconazole
Hyalohyphomycosis	Ketoconazole Enilconazole Itraconazole Nystatin Thiabendazole Flucytosine
Phaeohyphomycosis	Amphotericin B
Phycomycosis	Amphotericin B
Prototothecosis	Amphotericin B Nystatin Gentamicin
Pythiosis	Immunotherapy Amphotericin B Metalaxyl
Rhinosporidiosis	Dapsone
Sporotrichosis	Itraconazole Ketoconazole Amphotericin B Sodium iodide

with a sterile swab. It should then be immediately inoculated onto appropriate fungal culture media (e.g., Sabouraud dextrose agar) or transport media if it is to be sent to a laboratory. DTM is not suitable for the growth of these fungi as their growth is often inhibited by the cycloheximide in the medium. Samples should be incubated at 30° C and 30% humidity and examined daily for evidence of growth. All growth is to be examined microscopically for exact identification.

Ancillary tests may be performed, depending on the organism suspected and the clinical signs that are apparent. For instance, hyalohyphomycosis, especially that attributable to aspergillosis, may involve the nasal cavity; therefore skull radiographs may show decreased turbinate density and increased soft tissue density in affected nasal cavities and maxillary or frontal sinuses. An agar gel double diffusion test correlates well with infec-

tion, although it does cross-react with *Penicillium* (Figure 4-9). Counterimmunoelectrophoresis (CIEP) has also been used to demonstrate the presence of systemic antibody against *Aspergillus fumigatus*. For cases of gastrointestinal pythiosis, a barium series may reveal thickened bowel wall and strictures.

Treatment

The best treatment, if possible, is to surgically excise all infected tissue. Fungi create walls around themselves (granulomas) that prevent drugs from reaching the fungi and having any real effect on them. If surgery is not possible, the medical therapies shown in the box above can be attempted but are only infrequently effective.

TABLE 4-2

SYSTEMIC FUNGAL DISEASES

NAME	ORGANISM RESPONSIBLE	CYTOLOGIC CHARACTERISTICS OF ORGANISM
Blastomycosis	*Blastomyces dermatitidis*	Round, double-contoured wall; 8–10 μm; no capsule
Coccidioidomycosis	*Coccidioides immitis*	Large, double-walled spherules; 10–80 μm
Cryptococcosis	*Cryptococcus neoformans*	Large mucoid capsule; budding; 5–15 μm
Histoplasmosis	*Histoplasma capsulatum*	Intracellular; 2–4 μm

---

TABLE 4-3

SYSTEMIC ANTIFUNGAL AGENTS

AGENT	ACTION	DOSAGE/ROUTE	COMMENTS
Griseofulvin (microsize)	Fungistatic	50–150 mg/kg PO	Feed with fat meal; teratogenic; bone marrow suppression
Griseofulvin (ultramicrosize)	Fungistatic	35–65 mg/kg sid PO	No fat meal required
Potassium iodide (SSKI)	Sporicidal	Dogs: 40 mg/kg tid Cats: 20 mg/kg bid	Sporotrichosis; vomiting; depression
Flucytosine	Fungicidal	60 mg/kg tid PO	Candidiasis; cryptococcosis; rapid resistance and mutations; used in combination with other drugs
Amphotericin B	Fungistatic	Dogs: 0.25–0.5 mg/kg in dextrose 3× weekly IV Cats: 0.15 mg/kg in dextrose 3× weekly IV	Systemic mycoses; used in combination with amphoketaconazole or flucytosine; nephrotoxic; anemia; phlebitis, hypokalemia
Ketoconazole	Fungistatic	2.5–15 mg/kg bid PO	Systemic mycoses, candidiasis, dermatophytosis; inappetence; hepatotoxic
Itraconazole	Fungistatic	10 mg/kg sid	

SYSTEMIC FUNGAL INFECTIONS

The systemic mycoses (Table 4-2) were so named because infection with these fungi usually affects internal organs rather than being limited to the skin. The four fungi that are part of the systemic mycoses and the conditions they result in are:

- *Blastomyces dermatitidis*—Blastomycosis
- *Coccidioides immitis*—Coccidioidomycosis
- *Cryptococcus neoformans*—Cryptococcosis
- *Histoplasma capsulatum*—Histoplasmosis

Systemic fungal infections are very serious disorders that can occur when pets and humans inhale infectious spores from the environment. They are considered noncontagious, although blastomycosis has been transmitted, albeit very rarely, from dogs to humans via bite wounds.

All of the systemic mycoses except for cryptococcosis have quite regional distributions. In some areas exposure to these microbes is considered commonplace. Many animals are exposed to infectious spores, but the majority develop inapparent infections and recover completely. When animals are stressed or otherwise immunocompromised, however, full-blown and potentially fatal infections may result. Most dogs and cats develop respiratory infections after inhaling the spores, following which the infection spreads to other organs, including the skin.

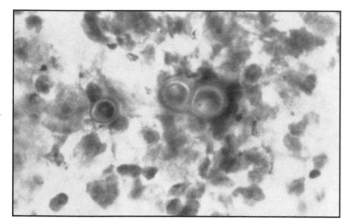

Figure 4-10. Blastomyces dermatitidis: *Large thick-walled budding yeasts with double-contoured walls seen on cytology. (Courtesy of Patrick McKeever, University of Minnesota, Minneapolis.)*

A list of systemic antifungal agents is presented in Table 4-3.

BLASTOMYCOSIS (see Plate IV-7)

Blastomycosis is caused by the soil organism *Blastomyces dermatitidis*, which normally resides in areas drained by rivers in the eastern United States and parts of southern Canada. The most endemic areas include the Great Lakes and the Ohio, Mississippi, and Missouri River valleys. Dogs, cats, and humans become infected by inhaling chlamydiospores from mold colonies present in contaminated soil. Most affected animals have respiratory signs (e.g., bronchopneumonia) but may also have problems related to the skin, eyes, and bones. If the saliva becomes contaminated, a potential concern arises regarding transferring the infection to humans via bite wounds.

Most affected dogs are less than 5 years of age and greater than 40 lb in weight. Sporting dogs and hounds, including coonhounds, pointers, and weimaraners, have an increased incidence (and exposure). The disease incidence in dogs is higher (perhaps by as much as 10 times) than in humans. In contrast, cats are only occasionally infected.

Diagnosis

The approach to diagnosis often involves thoracic radiography, histopathology/cytology, and blood tests. Radiography may be very suggestive, especially if there is evidence of alveolar and interstitial disease and hilar lymphadenomegaly. Cytologic preparations made from skin lesions or lymph nodes and stained routinely (e.g., Diff-Quik, new methylene blue, Wright's, Giemsa) may

reveal the round, 8 to 10 μm organisms with thick double-contoured cell walls but no capsule (Figure 4-10). Histopathologic evaluation may demonstrate the organisms within granulomatous reactions, and special stains (GMS, PAS) and fluorescent antibody "tagging" may facilitate localization of the fungi.

Serology offers important diagnostic potential; the agar gel immunodiffusion test is probably the best blood test currently available. This immunologic test has a sensitivity and specificity of over 90% in canine blastomycosis. Unfortunately, it has not proved to be useful in the diagnosis of feline blastomycosis. In dogs the complement fixation test is considered positive at levels of greater than 1:16, whereas titers of 1:16 are considered "suspicious." Complement fixation titers are less useful because canine serum is often anticomplementary and cross-reactions exist with histoplasmosis. An enzyme-linked immunosorbent assay and CIEP have been shown to be both sensitive and specific in the dog but are not yet widely available.

In-house fungal culture to diagnose blastomycosis is not recommended because of its potential to infect laboratory personnel. If cultures are needed, they should be performed with biopsy samples, aspirates, or discharge from fistulous tracts. Cultures may need to be incubated for 1 month before diagnostic yeast forms are evident.

Pets with blastomycosis may also have a variety of nonspecific clinicopathologic changes such as anemia, neutrophilia, and, rarely, hypocalcemia.

Treatment

Patients with systemic blastomycosis are often treated with either ketoconazole or amphotericin B. In most instances, regardless of the form of treatment selected, therapy must go on for a minimum of 3 months. Patients that survive the first week of therapy have a reasonably good prognosis. Animals with severe respiratory involvement may die within the first few days of treatment because of respiratory failure.

Ketoconazole (e.g., Nizoral®—Janssen Pharmaceutica) is an oral broad-spectrum antifungal agent that reaches therapeutic levels in all body tissues except the brain, testes, and eyes. The regular dose may need to be increased if there is neurologic involvement. Ketoconazole is excreted via the bile into the digestive tract and exits the body in the stool. There are few side effects associated with ketoconazole administration, although coat color changes are frequently reported. Monitoring should include a complete blood count and biochemical profile on a monthly basis.

Amphotericin B (e.g., Fungizone®—E. R. Squibb & Sons) is a polyene antibiotic that must be administered intravenously. It is reconstituted with either sterile saline or 5% dextrose/water. (Amphotericin B must not be added to solutions that contain electrolytes, as colloid aggregation occurs.) Once reconstituted, it is stable for about 1 week if refrigerated and protected from prolonged exposure to light. Preferably, a catheter is used to administer amphotericin B because perivascular injection is extremely irritating and can cause phlebitis. The reconstituted drug is usually added to 0.5 to 1 L of 5% dextrose/water and given over a period of 6 to 8 hours. If ketoconazole is added to the regimen, the total amount of amphotericin given can often be halved. This is significant because the side effects of amphotericin B include nephrotoxicity, anemia and hypokalemia. Patients should be monitored weekly or twice weekly to evaluate blood counts, liver and kidney function, urinalyses and electrolytes (especially potassium). Creatinine levels are particularly important, and treatments are not normally given if creatinine values are more than 3 mg/dl.

While patients are on therapy with either ketoconazole or amphotericin B, radiographic and cytologic evaluation should be done on a monthly basis to monitor progress. The agar gel immunodiffusion test is not a reliable indicator of the success of treatment. Animals deemed "cured" should still be reevaluated every 3 to 6 months to guard against relapse.

COCCIDIOIDOMYCOSIS (see Plate IV-8)

Coccidioidomycosis (valley fever, oidiomycosis) is caused by the organism *Coccidioides immitis*, which is typically found in the lower Sonoran life zone of the southwestern United States (California, Arizona, New Mexico, Texas, Nevada, Utah), Mexico, and parts of Central and South America.

Dogs and cats acquire the infection by inhaling arthrospores from contaminated soil. Within the body, the arthrospores develop into spherules, which are the pathogenic form of the fungus. Although the spherules are relatively fragile, infected animals that are buried after death can contaminate the soil for up to 6 years.

It is not unusual for animals in endemic areas to be exposed to the fungus, but most only develop inapparent infection, recover spontaneously,

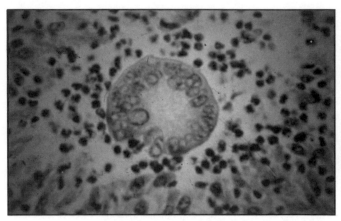

Figure 4-11. Coccidioides immitis: *Spherules with endospores in an aspiration biopsy of a lymph node (high power). (Courtesy of Robert Wilkins, Cenvet Laboratories, New York, New York.)*

and develop lifelong immunity. Others develop serious infections that often involve the bones, internal organs, skin, eyes, and heart. Clinical signs include cough, lameness, fever, and lymphadenomegaly. Dogs are affected more often than cats, and most are less than 5 years of age.

Diagnosis

Coccidioidomycosis is supportively diagnosed by radiography, cytology/histopathology, blood tests, and fungal cultures. Thoracic radiographs may show a diffuse interstitial pattern, and hilar lymphadenomegaly is a common finding.

Cytologic preparations of draining skin lesions, pleural fluid and lymph node aspirates may reveal the large 10 to 80 μm double-walled spherules that are diagnostic for the condition. On histopathologic analysis of biopsies these spherules are found to contain endospores amid pyogranulomatous tissue (Figure 4-11). Identification of the organisms may be enhanced with silver, PAS, or fluorescent antibody stains.

Fungal culture may be a helpful diagnostic test but should only be performed by commercial laboratories. The fungal growth that forms can infect laboratory personnel and must be handled appropriately. Although growth may be evident within 3 to 4 days, 2 weeks are often necessary for sporulation.

Serology is an important diagnostic tool for coccidioidomycosis. The agar gel immunodiffusion (precipitin) test is usually positive within 10 to 14 days of infection and begins to wane 4 to 6 weeks later. The complement fixation test may climb to 1:16 or above within 8 to 10 weeks of infection and remain elevated for many months. Therefore, early in the course of the disease, the precipitin test is usually positive and the complement fixation test is negative. With early active infection, both tests are positive. Later in the disease, the precipitin test is negative and the complement fixation test remains positive for many months. Once again, the limitations of complement fixation tests in the dog are that about 25% of canine serum is anticomplementary and there is some cross-reactivity with histoplasmosis and blastomycosis.

Treatment

The treatment of choice for coccidioidomycosis is ketoconazole. While on therapy, blood counts and liver function tests should be performed on a monthly basis. The minimum period for treatment is 3 months, but most animals require 4 to 12 months of therapy before the disease is arrested.

Lameness and osteomyelitis are frequent complications of coccidioidomycosis, and additional caution is frequently necessary. Although the organism is not directly transferable between infected and noninfected animals or humans, it can convert to its infectious form on suitable materials outside the body. For example, casts and bandages that are soaked with discharge can be a health risk for individuals handling the items. To guard against the risk of contagion, bandages should be changed at least every 24 hours to avoid sporulation of the organism.

Radiography and complement fixation titers are performed monthly during therapy, and treatment is discontinued when titers are 1:8 or less and there is evidence of disease resolution. Following discontinuation of therapy, monitoring should be continued every 3 to 6 months.

CRYPTOCOCCOSIS (see Plate IV-9)

Cryptococcosis is caused by *Cryptococcus neoformans,* a relatively ubiquitous organism. It is believed to be spread by pigeon droppings, in which the infective form can survive for up to 5 years. As for the other systemic mycoses, the fungi may attack the respiratory system and spread to the skin, central nervous system, bone, and other organs. This systemic mycosis affects cats more often than dogs.

Cryptococcosis is introduced into the body by inhalation; occasionally, it enters via the digestive tract. As with the other systemic mycoses, young animals are affected more often. The average age

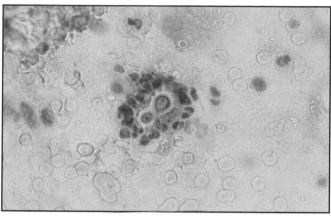

Figure 4-12. Cryptococcus neoformans: *Budding yeast in a direct smear of exudate (high power). (Courtesy of Robert Wilkins, Cenvet Laboratories, New York, New York.)*

for infection is 5 years in cats and 3 years in dogs. Many animals are exposed to the organism, but most are not systemically infected. Most infected animals presumably have some degree of dysfunction with respect to cell-mediated immunity.

The clinical picture of cryptococcosis differs somewhat between dogs and cats. Most dogs have signs of pulmonary disease similar to the other systemic mycoses. Cats often develop upper respiratory complications, including sneezing and nasal discharge. Internal involvement might include the skin, eyes, brain, and lymph nodes.

Diagnosis

Cytology is the most expedient way of diagnosing cryptococcosis. Impression smears from nasal discharges or aspirates from eyes, cerebrospinal fluid, or skin nodules may reveal the 5 to 15 μm organisms with their large mucoid capsule. Budding is often noted (Figure 4-12). With Gram stain, the capsule appears red; with India ink, the organism is unstained but is silhouetted against a dark background. Wright's stain or new methylene blue may also be used.

Histopathology may be necessary if the organism cannot be recovered on cytologic preparations. Histopathologic findings include granulomatous dermatitis, panniculitis, and, usually, the presence of many organisms. Methenamine silver, Mayer's mucicarmine, or PAS are often useful stains to highlight the organism within tissue.

Radiography may be supportive but is rarely confirmatory. Changes may be seen within the sinuses or the pulmonary parenchyma.

Culture of exudate, aspirates, transtracheal washes and urine may reveal organisms. Growth is normally evident in 2 to 14 days. As with other systemic mycoses, cultures should be performed in commercial laboratories so as not to place hospital personnel at risk.

Serology is available to detect the presence of cryptococcal capsular antigen in blood, cerebrospinal fluid, urine, and other body fluids. Titers of 1:16 or greater are considered positive. Cross-reactivity with toxoplasmosis is a consideration, especially in the evaluation of cats.

Treatment

The treatment of choice for cryptococcosis in the dog is a combination of amphotericin B and flucytosine. Flucytosine, an oral antifungal agent, is convenient because it reaches high levels in the central nervous system and lessens the amount of amphotericin B (a much more toxic compound) needed. Some side effects have been associated with flucytosine, however. It may have a mild impact on the liver, bone marrow, and gastrointestinal tract. Although it is not toxic to the kidneys, it is excreted by them and doses need to be adjusted in patients with kidney disease. Flucytosine cannot be used alone because resistant strains develop rapidly, often within 3 weeks. Ketoconazole is the treatment of choice in the cat and is also useful in the dog, especially considering the risks associated with amphotericin B use. Patients should be monitored routinely, as discussed in the sections on blastomycosis and coccidioidomycosis. The measurement of cryptococcal antigen on a monthly basis is sometimes helpful in deciding when to stop therapy. Sometimes high titers persist despite marked clinical improvement, however.

HISTOPLASMOSIS

Histoplasmosis is caused by *Histoplasma capsulatum*, which is most prevalent around the Great Lakes and the Mississippi, St. Lawrence, and Ohio River valleys. Fungal spores may be deposited in the soil by contaminated droppings of birds and bats. The organisms grow in the top 1 to 3 cm of soil. Infection occurs by breathing in microaleuriospores.

Exposure to the organism is not rare in endemic areas, and yet only a small percentage of dogs and cats develop severe infection. The two main manifestations of the disease in dogs are chronic diarrhea and pneumonia. In cats the most common signs are weight loss, lethargy, anemia, fever, and, in about half of affected cats, respiratory and gastrointestinal signs. Dermatologic signs are only seen in about 10% of affected animals.

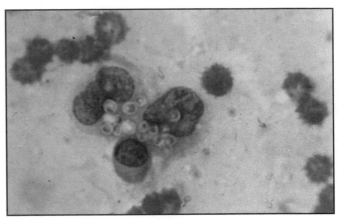

Figure 4-13. Histoplasma capsulatum: *Yeast phase phagocytized by macrophages in aspiration biopsy of a lymph node (high power). (Courtesy of Robert Wilkins, Cenvet Laboratories, New York, New York.)*

Diagnosis

Cytology is a valuable aid in diagnosing histoplasmosis. The 2 to 4 μm organisms are found intracellularly within members of the mononuclear-phagocyte series (e.g., monocytes, macrophages, histiocytes; Figure 4-13). Aspirates of the bone marrow or buffy coat examination may be helpful if there is concurrent anemia or leukocytosis. Occasionally, organisms can be found in peripheral blood cells. Lymph node aspiration and transtracheal washes are other important sources of organisms. Fecal smears can be revealing if there is evidence of large bowel disease. The organisms stain well with Giemsa or Wright's preparations.

Histopathology is sometimes helpful, especially if there is gastrointestinal involvement. Gastrointestinal, liver, spleen, or lymph node biopsy may reveal the organism. PAS stains are preferable to H&E in terms of highlighting *Histoplasma* organisms.

Serology is often less helpful in confirming histoplasmosis. Evaluations for precipitin and complement-fixing antibodies are often falsely negative in dogs and cats with histoplasmosis. Notwithstanding, the agar gel immunodiffusion (precipitin) test may be positive in infected dogs. Complement fixation titers of at least 1:32 are considered positive in the dog, and a titer of 1:16 is often considered suspicious. A fourfold rise in titers from paired serum samples helps to confirm the diagnosis. Roughly 25% of canine serum is anticomplementary and there is some cross-reactivity between histoplasmosis, blastomycosis, and coccidioidomycosis. Neither serum test is useful for diagnosing histoplasmosis in the cat.

Radiography is helpful in judging the extent of disease involvement in patients with histoplasmosis. Radiographs may reveal hepatosplenomegaly, thickened bowel walls, diffuse interstitial pneumonitis, and hilar lymphadenomegaly.

Ancillary tests on animals with histoplasmosis are often important because of the likely involvement of the bone marrow, liver, bowel, and other organs. Blood counts may reveal anemia and leukocytosis, and blood chemistries may show elevations in serum alkaline phosphatase, bilirubin, and sulfobromophthalein (BSP) retention and decreases in serum albumin. With progressive bowel disease, there also may be evidence of malabsorption.

Treatment

The treatment of choice for histoplasmosis is ketoconazole. Without treatment the condition is usually progressive and fatal. In cases that appear resistant or nonresponsive, amphotericin B may be used, although its potential for side effects is high.

RECOMMENDED READINGS

Ackerman L: Feline cryptococcosis. *Compend Contin Educ Pract Vet* 10:1049–1055, 1988.

Ackerman L: *Practical Canine Dermatology.* Goleta, CA, American Veterinary Publications, 1989.

Ackerman L: *Practical Feline Dermatology.* Goleta, CA, American Veterinary Publications, 1989.

Carakostas MC, Miller RI, Gossett KA: Clinical laboratory evaluation of deep mycotic diseases in dogs. *J Small Anim Pract* 25:687–693, 1984.

Jackson JA: Immunodiagnosis of systemic mycoses in animals: A review. *JAVMA* 188(7):702–705, 1986.

Macy DW: Systemic mycoses, in Morgan RV (ed): *Handbook of Small Animal Practice.* New York, Churchill Livingstone, 1988, pp 963–974.

Medleau L, Chalmers SA: Resolution of generalized dermatophytosis without treatment in dogs. *JAVMA* 201(12):1891–1892, 1992.

Medleau L, Kuhl KA: Dealing with chronic recurring dermatophytosis. *Vet Med,* pp 1101–1104, Nov 1992.

Medleau L, Ristic Z: Diagnosing dermatophytosis in dogs and cats. *Vet Med,* pp 1086–1091, Nov 1992.

Medleau L, White-Weithers ME: Treating and preventing the various forms of dermatophytosis. *Vet Med,* pp 1096–1100, Nov 1992.

Nesbitt GH, Ackerman LJ (eds): *Dermatology for the Small Animal Practitioner.* Trenton, NJ, Veterinary Learning Systems, 1991.

Pedersen NC: *Feline Infectious Diseases.* Goleta, CA, American Veterinary Publications, 1988.

Plant JD, Rosenkrantz WS, Griffin CE: Factors associated with and prevalence of high *Malassezia pachydermatis* numbers on dog skin. *JAVMA* 201(6):879–882, 1992.

Puccini S, Valdre A, Papini R, Mancianti F: In vitro susceptibility to antimycotics of *Microsporum canis* isolates from cats. *JAVMA* 201(9):1375–1377, 1992.

Rudmann DG, Coolman BR, Perez CM, Glickman LT: Evaluation of risk factors for blastomycosis in dogs: 857 cases (1980–1990). *JAVMA* 201(11):1754–1759, 1992.

Wolf AM, Troy GC: Deep mycotic diseases, in Ettinger S (ed): *Textbook of Veterinary Internal Medicine.* Philadelphia, WB Saunders, 1989, pp 341–372.

CHAPTER FIVE

Diagnosis and Management of Immunologic Skin Diseases

*I*mmunologic skin diseases consist of an array of conditions, ranging from allergies to autoimmune diseases, in which an aberrant immune response is involved. Many diseases that have an immunologic basis involve other factors as well and are discussed in other chapters (e.g., bacterial hypersensitivity, which has both bacterial and immunologic components, is dealt with in Chapter 3 and hormonal hypersensitivity is covered in Chapter 6).

INHALANT ALLERGIES

Allergic inhalant dermatitis (atopy) is the animal equivalent of hay fever; dogs, cats, and horses are commonly affected. Most affected animals react to a variety of inhaled substances, including:

- Tree, grass, and weed pollens
- Molds
- House dust
- House dust mites
- Feathers
- Dander

Most allergic pets develop pruritus as a result of their allergies; other clinical signs may also occur.

Though the mechanics of development of allergies are not well understood, it is clear that susceptibility to inhalant allergies is an inherited trait. Any animal, purebred or mutt, may be affected by inhalant allergies.

Inhalant allergies are "immediate" hypersensitivity reactions; that is, animals respond adversely within 15 minutes of exposure to an allergen. The reaction is believed to be related to mast cell degranulation, which in turn is associated with allergen-specific immunoglobulin E (IgE) or a subtype of immunoglobulin G (IgGd).

The fact that not all plants that pollinate cause clinical allergies must be considered in the selection of allergens for testing. The allergen must be buoyant to become airborne, be of a certain size and weight (5,000 to 60,000 daltons and 2 to 60 μm) to reach the proper level in the respiratory tract, and be present in significant quantities. Also, each allergen (such as a pollen) has several allergenic fractions (epitopes) that are quite specific. Only about 1% of the total weight of an allergen is actually the allergenic moiety.

Many pollens can travel at least 30 miles in the wind and can cause problems to pets even in the inner city. Of the 1 billion pollen grains capable of being produced by a single ragweed plant, only 1 μg of pollen (10 ng of allergen) per day needs to be inhaled to induce hay fever symptoms in a susceptible individual.

Clinical Signs

Unlike humans, allergic pets rarely show respiratory signs. Atopic dogs usually first begin to show signs between 6 months and 3 years of age (see Plate V-1). In time, such chronic and secondary changes (e.g., infections, thickening of the skin, increased pigmentation; see Plate V-2) may become prominent.

The clinical signs of an allergic pet can be demonstrated on a seasonal or year-round basis, depending on the allergen. The most common sign is chewing at the feet, and constant licking may stain the haircoat with a rust-like hue. Other pruritic areas include the flanks, groin, and axillae. Whereas humans with allergies characteristically sneeze, allergic pets develop pruritus. They lick, chew, scratch, and have decreased resistance to infection. Many animals rub their faces on carpeting, furniture, or other available surfaces. Inhalant allergies are also one of the most common causes for recurrent ear infections. Self-traumatized areas may develop recurrent bacterial infections ("hot spots"). Cats may have additional problems such as pinpoint scabbing (miliary dermatitis) or the development of hairless lumps (eosinophilic plaque).

A very common manifestation of allergy in dogs is otitis externa. Although this disorder may be complicated by bacterial and yeast infections, the underlying problem in most cases involves inflammatory changes associated with allergy. In cats miliary dermatitis, eosinophilic plaque, and symmetric alopecia may also reflect an underlying allergy (see Plate V-3).

Diagnosis

Inhalant allergies are diagnosed with either intradermal allergy tests or with the new in vitro tests. Currently, the intradermal allergy tests are considered to be superior. The intradermal allergy tests measure the ability of injected allergen to bind to allergen-specific immunoglobulin on the surface of mast cells and to cause actual mast cell degranulation. In vitro tests simply measure the relative levels of allergen-specific IgE in the bloodstream. The concordance between skin tests and blood tests is only about 50%.

Intradermal Allergy Tests

Before allergy testing is performed, it is important to ensure that substances that can influence the test are not in the system. These substances include:

- Corticosteroids
- Antihistamines
- Tranquilizers (including acepromazine, oxymorphone, ketamine/Valium®—Roche Laboratories)
- Hormones

Actual withdrawal times have not been established for dogs and cats, but some general guidelines do exist. Most antihistamines should be withdrawn at least 10 days before testing. Regarding corticosteroids, it has been shown that a 5 week course of oral prednisolone can influence the

hypothalamic-pituitary axis (HPA) for 2 weeks. Therefore, even when a short course of corticosteroid is given, a minimum withdrawal time of 2 weeks is suggested. With injectable forms of corticosteroid or with long-term administration, a minimum of 4 weeks' withdrawal time is recommended. These are only minimum withdrawal times; actual times may be many months, depending on how long the pet was treated and how potent and long-lasting the preparation used was.

The allergens used for intradermal allergy testing are selected based on regional prevalence and the allergenic potential of each item. (Figure 5-1 presents a sample allergy testing form listing 60 different allergens.) Some allergens are more problematic than others. For instance, flowering and blossoming plants are often insect pollinated rather than wind pollinated and pollen levels for these plants are less likely to become significant other than on a very local basis. On the other hand, most grass, tree, and weed pollens can travel up to 30 miles in the wind. If a regional allergy test kit is to be formulated, it is worthwhile to consult a veterinary dermatologist or a human allergist for recommendations.

All allergens used for testing should be individualized unless they are clearly cross-reactive. For instance, many of the grasses (e.g., June grass, orchard grass) share common allergens and can be combined into one test solution. Other grasses (e.g., Bermuda grass, Johnson grass) possess unique allergens and should be tested separately. Most of the trees, weeds, and molds are antigenically distinct (e.g., maple trees are not related to oak trees, ragweed is not related to English plantain or sheep sorrel, *Aspergillus* molds are not related to *Rhizopus* molds) and should be tested for separately. The same cautions are true for blood tests, which often inappropriately group allergens for convenience rather than accuracy. Grouping of unrelated allergens can result in false-positive or false-negative scores. For example, if 1000 protein nitrogen units (PNU) per ml is the desired testing strength, what happens when four allergens are grouped? If each allergen contributes 250 PNU per milliliter of testing solution (to total 1000 PNU/ml) and they do not cross-react, the likelihood is that 250 PNU of even a strong allergen is not sufficient to elicit a significantly positive score. On the other hand, if each of the allergens contributes 1000 PNU per milliliter, the total allergen load of 4000 PNU/ml is likely to cause positive reactions even in many nonallergic animals. An appropriate allergy test should

CLIENT: _____   PET: _____

ACCT: _____   DATE: _____

ALLERGENS	RESULTS							
1. SALINE								
2. HISTAMINE								
3. ASH (2-4)								
4. ELM (3-9)								
5. MULBERRY (3-5)								
6. OLIVE (4-5)								
7. PALM (4-6)								
8. PECAN (4-5) HICKORY								
9. JUNIPER (1-4)								
10. AZ CYPRESS (2.3)								
11. MESQUITE (4-6)								
12. WALNUT								
13. MT. CEDAR (12-1)								
14. OAK (4-5)								
15. BERMUDA (3-20)								
16. JOHNSON (5-9)								
17. KORT GRASS								
18. RYE								
19. BROME (3-6)								
20. SALTGRASS (4-9)								
21. GOLDENROD (8-9)								
22. KOCHIA (7-9)								
23. DANDELION								
24. DOCK/SORREL								
25. LAMBS QUARTER (4-10)								
26. ENGLISH PLANTAIN (2-4)								
27. PIGWEED (5-11)								
28. BAYBERRY								
29. MARSHELDER (7-10)								
30. COCKEL BUR (7-10)								
31. RUSSIAN THISTLE (7-10)								
32. SAGEBRUSH								
33. FRANSERIA (3-5) (DESERT RAGWEED)								
34. W. RAGWEED (8-10)								
35. S. RAGWEED (8-10)								
36. BURROBRUSH (3-4)								
37. SALT BRUSH (5-10)								
38. ALTERNARIA								
39. ASPERGILLUS								
40. PENICILLIUM								
41. HORMODENDRUM								
42. HELMINTHOSPORIUM								
43. PHOMA								
44. PHIZOPUS								
45. BERMUDA GRASS SMUT								
46. JOHNSON GRASS SMUT								
47. KAPOK								
48. FLEA								
49. CAT								
50. HOUSEMITE (D FARINAE)								
51. HOUSEDUST								
52. STAPH								
53. BEEF								
54. PORK								
55. FISH								
56. MILK								
57. EGG								
58. SOY								
59. CORN								
60. WHEAT								

Figure 5-1. Example of allergy testing form.

include at least 40 to 60 individual or appropriately grouped allergens. It is unlikely that testing with less than 25 individual allergens is of any real value.

There are many different protocols for allergy testing, and the concentration of allergen used and the amount injected can vary as well. Allergen concentration can be measured in one of two systems:

- The weight/volume (w/v) system measures the weight of defatted allergen in a given volume of diluent.
- The PNU system measures the amount of protein precipitated by phosphotungstic acid.

These two systems measure different parameters and are not interchangeable. For most pollen allergens an aqueous solution of 1:1000 w/v or 1000 PNU is used for intradermal injection. For some molds (e.g., *Rhizopus)*, house dust, and environmental allergens, 1:2000 w/v or 250 to 500 PNU is used. House dust mites, both *Dermatophagoides farinae* and *D. pteronyssinus*, are often tested at 250 PNU but recent evidence suggests that false-positive scores may occur at doses as low as 25 PNU.

The actual amount that is injected intradermally by allergists varies from 0.02 ml (a minimal bleb) to 0.1 ml. Allergen extract used for animals must not include glycerin because even small amounts have been shown to cause irritation in dogs. Allergens that have been diluted to testing concentrations should be replaced on a monthly basis. Also, testing allergens stored in plastic syringes in the refrigerator lose potency quickly; the proteins in the allergens adhere to the plastic barrel of the syringe, lowering the concentration of allergen in the liquid being injected. Whenever possible, testing allergens should be drawn up into syringes the day of testing rather than being stored in syringes for later use.

With the animal lying on its side, a rectangular patch is shaved on the side of the chest with a no. 40 clipper blade and various potentially allergenic substances are injected into—not beneath—the skin; that is, the injections are given intradermally rather than subcutaneously (Figure 5-2). The area used for testing should not be scrubbed, and soaps or disinfectants should not be applied.

If tranquilization or anesthesia is needed, only certain types are acceptable. Xylazine (e.g., Rompun®—Miles), although usually not a preferred tranquilizing agent, does not affect test results and is the tranquilizer of choice for allergy

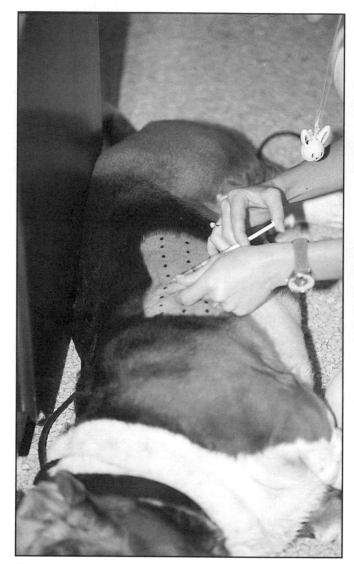

Figure 5-2. Intradermal injection of allergens.

testing. Side effects of this drug include bradycardia, heart block, and a potentially severe drop in blood pressure. Its effects can be reversed by yohimbine (e.g., Yobine®—Lloyd Laboratories) after the procedure has been completed. Recently, tiletamine/zolazepam (Telazol®—Fort Dodge Laboratories) has also been found to be a suitable tranquilizer with fewer side effects (hypersalivation, tachycardia) than xylazine. It is administered at doses of 4 mg/kg IV. If recovery is accompanied by dissociation or increased muscle activity, acepromazine or butorphanol can be given to make the recovery smoother. Injectable barbiturates or inhalation anesthetics are suitable, if needed. Most other tranquilizers (including acepromazine, chlorpromazine, and promethazine) and narcotics (including morphine and meperidine) affect test scores. Even atropine can result in mast cell degranulation and histamine release, which can cause false-positive reactions.

CAUSES OF FALSE-POSITIVE AND FALSE-NEGATIVE SKIN TESTS	
False-Positive Results	**False-Negative Results**
Extracts too strong	Drug or hormone interference
Contamination of extracts	Outdated or impotent extracts
Hypersensitive patient	Dilution or grouping of allergens
Presence of irritants (e.g., glycerin)	Air injected into skin
Effect of drug (e.g., atropine, narcotic)	Subcutaneous rather than intradermal injection

The entire allergy test should be completed in less than 15 minutes (preferably less than 10 minutes) because the reactions are time sensitive. The response is evaluated 15 minutes after completing the test. This insures that all reactions are at least 15 minutes old but not more than 30 minutes old. With positive reactions the area tested becomes swollen, red, and elevated (see Plate V-4), whereas with negative reactions any changes fade away. Reactions can be graded subjectively or measured for a more objective score. To aid in comparison, a positive control (histamine, a substance to which all animals should react) and a negative control (saline, a substance to which no animals should react) are used. Reactions involving an area whose diameter is at least 3 mm greater than the negative control area are considered positive.

Allergy testing should be done by someone who performs it regularly enough to reliably identify potential allergens and recognize false-positive and false-negative reactions (see box above). Many practitioners refer patients to clinics equipped to perform such procedures. Positive reactions on a skin test only indicate sensitivity to a particular allergen. It is up to the pet owner and the veterinarian to decipher this information so that it is relevant to the particular animal tested.

Blood Tests

Blood tests have been developed to measure the amount of circulating allergen-specific antibody (IgE) in serum. Unfortunately, most IgEs are bound to mast cells in the skin or basophils in the blood and do not float freely in the bloodstream for easy harvesting and measurement. Also, circulating levels of allergen-specific IgE do not necessarily correlate with levels in the skin. It also appears evident that conditions other than allergy (e.g., parasitism) can cause elevations of serum IgE.

Enzyme-linked immunosorbent assay (ELISA) and the radioallergosorbent test (RAST) are commercially available for evaluating the presence of allergy antibodies in blood in the dog. In the cat the demonstration of what may be IgE has been quite recent; currently, the value of this test is unknown. Studies have shown, however, that cats have an antibody with characteristics of IgE that cross-reacts with canine IgE. A recent study comparing intradermal and ELISA allergy tests concluded that the blood test should not be used to confirm a diagnosis of allergy or to identify allergens for hyposensitization because of a severe lack of test specificity. In-house serum tests are now available to help predict the likelihood of allergies and the need for more comprehensive testing. Research to date has failed to substantiate any value for this form of testing.

The potential value of these in vitro allergy tests should not be totally discounted, however. These tests have some worth in circumstances when a dermatologist is not available to do skin testing, when an animal cannot be shaved for the test, or when the skin is too inflamed for skin testing to be done. It should not be surprising that normal, nonallergic pets and pets with conditions other than allergy may have elevated levels of IgE to one or more allergens on blood testing; like any serum profile, this is a set of laboratory values and not a truly diagnostic test.

Recently, a basophil degranulation test has also been evaluated for the diagnosis of allergies in dogs. Basophils are white blood cells that are related to mast cells found in the skin. They can bind immunoglobulin in the same fashion as mast cells, providing a more definitive measure of allergic sensitivity than do blood tests measuring only allergen-specific IgE. When allergens bind to allergy antibodies on the surface of a basophil, they cause degranulation, the same way that mast cells release their contents in the skin. The test exposes a patient's blood sample (10 ml GTT [green top tube]) to different dilutions of allergens, and reactions are considered positive when the basophils lose their granules and become unstained. This is compared with an allergen-free control. The test can be quantitated by using an ELISA assay to detect the histamine released by basophils (e.g., Histamine Release Test—Hollister-Stier).

The test has some limitations:

- The test must be completed within 24 hours of blood collection.
- The test is adversely affected by corticosteroid administration.
- Because dogs do not have a high proportion of basophils in their blood, samples may need to be enriched in basophils by use of a density gradient.

When these technical difficulties are appropriately addressed, the basophil degranulation test may become an excellent in vitro diagnostic test for allergies in dogs and cats.

Treatment

The treatment of inhalant allergies can be specific or supportive. Having the dog or cat avoid inhalant allergens is the ideal solution but is rarely practical. Because allergens can originate many miles from the home environment, local control is seldom effective, although it may help ameliorate clinical signs.

Immunotherapy (allergy shots, hyposensitization, desensitization) involves serial subcutaneous injections of progressively larger amounts of allergen to make the pet less sensitive to, or more tolerant of, the effects of the allergen on its system. The majority of treated animals respond favorably, but the process can sometimes take up to a year before a benefit is seen in animals that do respond. Whereas testing allergens must be aqueous and are diluted to average concentrations of 1:1000 or 1000 PNU, treatment concentrations are much higher and may involve alum-precipitated antigens or aqueous allergens with or without propylene glycol. As a general rule, animals rarely receive more than 20,000 PNU (1:20) per injection. The best results usually occur when animals are treated with high potency extracts formulated on the basis of specific skin test scores. There is little doubt, however, that some pets improve with extracts formulated on the basis of grouped blood tests or even random selection of allergens.

Although the risks of anaphylactic reactions to immunotherapy injections are quite low,

adverse reactions should be treated as potential emergencies. Animals should remain at the hospital for 20 minutes after each injection of the series and be monitored by owners at home over the next 2 hours. Reactions should be treated as follows:

Reaction	Treatment
Mild	Fast-acting oral antihistamine
Moderate	Injectable antihistamine—e.g., diphenhydramine hydrochloride (1 to 2 mg/kg IV or IM) Moderate-dose corticosteroid—prednisolone (2 mg/kg PO), starting 12 to 24 hours after initiation Epinephrine (0.15 ml of 1:1000 solution SC at site)
Severe	Epinephrine (0.01 mg/kg of 1:1000 solution IM or SC repeated every 15 to 20 minutes while monitoring) Intravenous fluid—lactated Ringer's solution (50 to 150 ml/kg over several hours) Rapid-acting corticosteroid—e.g., prednisone sodium succinate (10 to 25 mg/kg IV) Oxygen therapy (in selected cases)

Symptomatic therapy with antihistamines, fatty acid supplements, and corticosteroids may be necessary initially to keep animals comfortable while awaiting the benefits of immunotherapy. Immunotherapy is based on the results of allergy testing, and the more specific form of testing (intradermal allergy testing) often gives the best results.

Antihistamines (Table 5-1) are commonly used as allergy treatment in pets as well as humans. These drugs are estimated to relieve the itchiness of allergies in perhaps 30% of cases. This may not seem like a large percentage, but most antihistamines have few side effects other than drowsiness. Some of the newer antihistamines are even nonsedating. In dogs and cats it appears that substances other than histamine, such as proteolytic enzymes, leukotrienes, serotonin, and kinins, may be responsible for pruritus; thus it is not surprising that antihistamines do not work in all cases.

Nonprescription antihistamines that can be purchased by pet owners include chlorpheniramine maleate (e.g., Chlor-Trimeton®—Schering-Plough HealthCare Products) and diphenhy-

TABLE 5-1

ANTIHISTAMINES

CLASS	GENERIC	TRADE NAME	ADMINISTRATION
Phenothiazine	Promethazine	Phenergan® (Wyeth-Ayerst)	0.2–1.0 mg/kg tid
	Trimeprazine	Temaril® (Herbert Laboratories)	1–2 mg/kg bid
Ethanolamine	Diphenhydramine	Benadryl® (Parke-Davis)	1–2 mg/kg bid–tid
	Clemastine	Tavist® (Sandoz Pharmaceuticals)	0.05–0.1 mg/kg bid
Alkylamine	Chlorpheniramine	Chlor-Trimeton® (Schering-Plough HealthCare Products)	0.5–2 mg/kg bid–tid
Ethylenediamine	Pyrilamine	Triaminic® (Sandoz Pharmaceuticals)	1–2 mg/kg bid–tid
Piperazine	Hydroxyzine	Atarax® (Roerig)	2.2 mg/kg tid
Piperidine	Terfenadine	Seldane® (Marion Merrell Dow)	2–5 mg/kg bid

dramine hydrochloride (e.g., Benadryl®—Parke-Davis). In some countries, clemastine (e.g., Tavist®—Sandoz Pharmaceuticals) and terfenadine (e.g., Seldane®—Marion Merrell Dow) are also nonprescription items. Hydroxyzine hydrochloride (e.g., Atarax®—Roerig) and trimeprazine tartrate (e.g., Temaril®—Herbert Laboratories) are prescription antihistamines that have been used in dogs and cats. Most antihistamines have not been approved for use in pets, and standardized dosages have not been calculated. The fact that one antihistamine does not work in an animal does not mean that all will fail. Often many different antihistamines must be tried before one is found that is helpful.

Recently, the piperidine compound 4-[3-[4-[bis(4-fluorophenyl) hydroxy-methyl]-1-piperidinyl]propoxy] benzoic acid (AHR-13268—A. H. Robins) was given to allergic dogs and found to be beneficial in about one-third of cases. Side effects were minimal, and the compound had an advantage over regular antihistamines in that it only needed to be given once a day.

Essential fatty acids (EFAs)—especially the omega-3 and omega-6 fatty acids—have been shown to be beneficial in perhaps 20% of allergic dogs. The omega-3 fatty acids (e.g., eicosapentaenoic acid [EPA]) are derived from alpha-linolenic acid and are found in a variety of marine lipids, especially fish oils. Omega-6 fatty acids (e.g., gamma-linolenic acid) are derived from linoleic acid and are found in a variety of plant lipids, especially evening primrose oil, borage oil, blackcurrant seed oil, or sunflower seed oil. These essential fatty acids are different from the regular essential fatty acids (linoleic acid, alpha linolenic acid, arachidonic acid) found in most retail products and are thought to work by bypassing a defective enzyme in animals and humans with inhalant allergies. Other mechanisms of action have also been postulated. For example, recent studies have suggested that atopic dogs may have a higher degree of fat malabsorption than normal dogs. Eicosapentaenoic acid competes with arachidonic acid for metabolism and results in the formation of noninflammatory prostaglandins and leukotrienes. Gamma-Linolenic acid may interfere with the production of inflammatory mediators, raising the allergic threshold for pruritus. The fatty acids used for supplementation are often more successful at relieving the inflammation associated with allergy, rather than pruritus. Products including both omega-3 and omega-6 fatty acids are important therapies for allergic dogs and cats because they may lessen inflammation and have minimal, if any, side effects. Products suitable for veterinary use and available from veterinarians that include both functional omega-3 and omega-6 fatty acids include DermCaps (DVM) and EFA-Z Plus® (Allerderm/Virbac).

Corticosteroids (glucocorticoids) markedly reduce pruritus but also are associated with many potential side effects. When large doses of corticosteroids are given orally or by injection, especially for long periods, the adrenal glands stop producing cortisol and may atrophy. Simultaneously, the other tissues of the body are subjected to the abnormally high levels of corticosteroids being administered. This commonly results initially in increased thirst, increased urination, increased hunger, and, occasionally, abnormal behavior. These problems are seen in most animals and are usually more inconvenient than dangerous. Long-term use may result in diabetes mellitus, decreased resistance to infection, decreased thyroid and growth hormone levels, decreased threshold for seizure activity, fluid retention, and deposition of fat in the liver. Corticosteroids should be used cautiously, especially in young or pregnant animals or those with diabetes mellitus, epilepsy, heart or kidney disease, infectious diseases, osteoporosis, or ulcers in the digestive tract.

If the allergy season is short, the product is suitable for alternate day administration, and the amount required to control clinical signs is small, corticosteroid therapy poses very little danger apart from transient side effects. When possible, alternate day therapy should be instituted so that the adrenal glands have an opportunity during the "off" day to produce cortisol, thus lessening the possibility of adrenal atrophy. Only certain corticosteroids (e.g., prednisone, triamcinolone) may be used on an alternate day basis; these should always be the first choice of therapy. Long-acting injectable forms of corticosteroids are a much less desirable alternative. Though corticosteroids can sometimes be used safely, alternatives should always be considered.

Environmental control is usually aimed at limiting exposure to offending allergens. Different approaches are used for pollen allergies, mold allergies, and house dust allergies. For pollen allergies, keeping the animal indoors most of the day is partially effective. Though air conditioners do little to remove air-borne allergens, they limit pollen exposure because doors and windows are kept closed when they are in use. In temperate climates pollen allergies are often seasonal, reflecting the pollination periods of the different plants. In warmer climates pollination periods are usually longer.

There is circumstantial evidence that pets can absorb some allergens directly through the skin. If this is true, dogs and cats roaming in environments containing allergens to which they have sensitivities would be doubly exposed. Not only would they breathe in the pollens and molds, but they would also absorb the substances directly through the skin. In light of this, allergic animals should be bathed in cool water with colloidal oatmeal shampoo after they have played outdoors on lawns or in fields. Not only does the bathing soothe the skin directly, but it washes away any pollens or molds on the skin or haircoat.

Pets with mold allergies may benefit from efforts to limit their exposure to molds in the home environment. Humidifiers, vaporizers, dehumidifiers, and air conditioners may develop growths of mold and should be periodically cleaned. Depending on the type of mold, spores may be dispersed by rainfall, humidity, or winds. Usually, there are as many molds inside a home as outside. Indoor mold growth and spore levels are directly related to relative humidity in the range of 30% to 70%. Below 30% humidity little interior mold growth can occur. A crude method of detecting problem mold areas is to put saucers containing potato slices just covered by water in various places around the home. Comparing the rate and amount of mold growth roughly indicates problem areas.

Adequate ventilation is essential to prevent mold growth in attics or roof crawl spaces. Basements should be well lit and well ventilated. Basement floors and walls should be treated with mold-resistant paint. Fungicides can be sprayed in problem areas to limit mold growth, if necessary. Pillows and mattresses are also a source of molds. Pillows ideally should be made of synthetic fibers or chipped foam, and mattresses should be encased in zippered protectors that can be removed and laundered. Bedding should be cleaned frequently. House plants should be removed because they harbor large numbers of molds. If they cannot be removed, their mold content can be reduced by covering the soil surface with aquarium tank filter charcoal bits. An aquarium can also be a source of mold. An algicide should be added to tank water and any immersed items periodically cleaned with chlorine bleach and detergent. Obviously, all objects need to be thoroughly rinsed before being replaced in the tank.

It is impossible to completely eradicate house dust and house dust mites from a home, but these can be controlled. Control measures should be most stringent in areas where the allergic pet spends most of its time. The stuffing of any pet bedding should be of a synthetic material. Kapok, feathers, wool, and horsehair should be avoided. Cotton is good but not as hypoallergenic as synthetics. Bedding should be frequently washed. In rooms with carpeting, kapok-stuffed furniture, or house plants severe reactions in dust-allergic pets can occur. Animal hair and dander attract dust, so rooms frequented by pets are often dusty. Therefore keeping pets well groomed is important. Dust-allergic animals that share a home with other animals are also likely to be more affected.

Because a home heating and cooling system can trap significant amounts of dust, ducts and filters should be periodically cleaned. Electrostatic filters help reduce the amount of dust in the air by about 80% but cannot produce a dust-free environment. High efficiency particulate air (HEPA) filters can clear over 95% of pollens, molds, yeasts, bacteria, and viruses in the air, and, when coupled with a charcoal filter, remove most of the dust. This is the best choice for treating the household environment. A household relative humidity between 30% and 50% is best because house dust mites cannot reproduce at humidities below 60%. A hygrometer, available from most hardware stores, allows easy monitoring. Household vacuuming should be done with a canister or cylindric type of vacuum cleaner, as the upright bag types return much of the dust passing through the bag to room air. Water trap vacuum cleaners collect dust in water instead of an air bag so dust is not being continually recirculated into the air. Central vacuum systems with proper ventilation to the outside are also beneficial.

ADVERSE REACTIONS TO FOODS

Adverse reactions to foods are often labeled as "food allergies," but there is a distinction between actual hypersensitivity and intolerance:

- Food hypersensitivity refers to an immune-mediated reaction to a dietary component.
- Food intolerance refers to any abnormal physiologic response to a food that is not immunologic in nature.

Because it is rarely determined whether a pet has intolerance or allergy, the term "adverse reaction to a food" is preferred as it does not presuppose an etiology.

Unlike inhalant allergies, "food allergy" may result from several different mechanisms, including type I, type III, or type IV hypersensitivity reactions. Hypersensitivity responses to ingested antigens are precise. Any influence that alters the antigenicity of dietary components, such as cooking, processing or digestion, can significantly alter the reaction of an animal to a food.

Food intolerance can result from metabolic problems (e.g., gluten or wheat sensitivity), pharmacologic reactions (e.g., to serotonin, histamine, saurine, lectins in foods), idiosyncracies (e.g., to egg whites, tomatoes), or even toxicities (e.g., caused by preservatives, dyes, flavorings). These mechanisms are rarely considered in veterinary practice, and their ultimate significance is only hypothesized. For example, gluten enteropathy in Irish setters (which has many features in common with celiac disease in humans) results in diarrhea but can be resolved completely with a gluten-free diet. Lactose intolerance is anticipated in dogs and cats. After puppies are weaned, their levels of lactase (needed to break down the milk sugar lactose) are only about 10% of those found in younger animals. It is therefore not surprising that they cannot tolerate large quantities of milk.

Many foods contain or cause the release of histamine. Animals that ingest these foods can have clinical signs that might be easily confused with food allergy. Some foods, especially fish-based diets, contain large amounts of histamine. Lack of refrigeration can lead to even higher levels of histamine as the amino acid histidine in the diet is converted to histamine. Common histamine-releasing foods include egg whites, fish, shellfish, strawberries, and tomatoes.

Food toxicity or food poisoning has also been reported in pets. Some cases are straightforward, but others require diagnostic acumen. For instance, onion poisoning has been reported in cats. Food additives such as benzoic acid or propylene glycol may also have toxic consequences.

Clinical Signs (see Plates V-5 and V-6)

The clinical signs of adverse food reactions vary considerably and can affect not only the skin but the digestive system, respiratory system, and the nervous system as well. The cutaneous clinical signs can be impossible to distinguish from inhalant allergies or a variety of parasite infestations. Noncutaneous manifestations are less common but might include vomiting, diarrhea, pruritus ani, flatulence, sneezing, asthma-like conditions, behavioral changes, and seizures. Adverse food reactions are often overlooked by owners because the problems do not necessarily coincide with feeding times or because the pet had been fed the diet for years without problems. Adverse reactions develop over time, and, depending on the mechanism, they may occur minutes, hours, or days after a meal is ingested.

Diagnosis

Adverse food reactions are best diagnosed by performing an exclusion diet trial, sometimes referred to as a hypoallergenic diet trial. There is usually little benefit in distinguishing hypersensitivity from intolerance, unless an underlying problem needs to be addressed.

Hypoallergenic Diet Trial

Many misconceptions exist about exclusion (hypoallergenic) diet trials and how they should be performed. Pets cannot be allergic to ingredients to which they have never been exposed; thus what is hypoallergenic for one animal is not necessarily so for another. Depending on the ingredients in commercial foods in the pet's diet and additional foodstuffs that may have been provided by owners, the purpose of the test diet is to "exclude" all dietary ingredients to which the pet has ever been exposed. Improvement of the condition during the trial suggests a diet-related component involving one or more ingredients in the pet's previous diet.

There is nothing intrinsically "hypoallergenic" about lamb. Lamb is only hypoallergenic if it has never been fed to a pet. Since there are now over 20 lamb-based diets on the market, lamb is becoming less and less suitable as a test diet. Similarly, a commercial lamb-based diet that provides other ingredients (e.g., corn, wheat, chicken, etc.) is unlikely to be hypoallergenic because most animals have been fed the other ingredients at some point in their lives.

The search for a hypoallergenic protein source becomes more and more difficult as owners begin to routinely feed lamb-based diets to their pets. Nevertheless, if lamb has never been part of the animal's diet, using ground lamb (or lamb baby food for small dogs and cats) is sufficient. Otherwise, rabbit, venison, or other wild game may be needed for the trial. Chicken, beef, and tofu (soy) are not suitable for a hypoallergenic diet trial. Rice is used as the carbohydrate component unless it has been part of the previous dietary regimen, in which case potatoes are used instead.

For dogs the meal is prepared by mixing one part protein with two parts carbohydrate and allowing free access to fresh (preferably distilled) water. Treats, snacks, vitamins, chew toys, and even flavored heartworm-preventive tablets must not be given during the trial. Cats should be given protein and carbohydrate sources in equal ratios. This makes taurine deficiency a less likely possibility. Most homemade hypoallergenic diets are not nutritionally sound, and long-term feeding can result in deficiencies. Particularly troubling is the poor calcium-to-phosphorus ratio, which can cause skeletal disease in young dogs if fed for more than 4 weeks. Homemade hypoallergenic diets intended to be fed for more than 4 weeks should be appropriately supplemented with additive-free nutrients.

The diet must be fed for a minimum of 4 weeks (8 weeks is suggested by some investigators). Pretrial fasting (48 hours) and enemas are often recommended if an abbreviated trial (e.g., 2 weeks) is desired by the owner. To prevent accidental exposure to allergens, pets must not be allowed to eat the feces of other household pets.

Commercial "hypoallergenic diets" are more convenient and nutritionally balanced but much less sensitive than homemade diets at identifying food allergies. It is estimated that 10% to 20% of food-allergic animals fed a commercial preparation continue to have problems. Therefore commercial diets are better used for management—rather than diagnosis—of food allergies.

At the conclusion of the hypoallergenic diet trial, two scenarios are possible:

- If there has been no improvement, it is exceedingly unlikely that the pet's problems are diet related. The regular diet may be resumed.
- If there has been substantial improvement, the regular diet should be fed for a meal or two. If the problem is indeed diet related, the clinical signs previously reported should reappear. If the animal's condition does not worsen, the improvement seen on the diet trial was coincidental.

Skin and Blood Testing

Allergy testing with either skin tests or blood tests is not recommended for animals with suspected adverse food reactions. Results of these tests are accurate less than 20% of the time. This is not surprising because not all adverse food reactions are immunologic in nature and those that are may not necessarily be mediated by IgE. Moreover, positive test scores, especially on the blood tests, are often misleading rather than helpful.

Gastroscopic Testing

Gastroscopic food sensitivity testing (GFST) is a new procedure being studied to identify adverse responses to foods. Similar to intradermal allergy testing, this procedure introduces food allergens to the surface of the stomach lining and monitors for responses of edema, erythema, mucus secretion, and hyperperistalsis.

Patients are anesthetized and an endoscope is inserted into the stomach. A piece of disposable tubing is passed through the endoscope and then 0.5 ml of each food extract (1:1000 or 1000 PNU/ml) is dripped onto the dependent gastric surface. Reactions are recorded after 5 minutes.

There appears to be reasonably good correlation between GFST, diet history, and clinical response, but the ultimate usefulness of this test has yet to be determined. To its advantage the procedure is a rapid means of identifying food sensitivity in some cases. To its disadvantage it requires anesthesia, expensive instrumentation, and an experienced endoscopist and it cannot detect all cases of adverse food reaction.

Treatment

Animals with documented adverse reactions to foods do not need to be kept on homemade diets indefinitely. In fact, long-term use of homemade diets should be discouraged because they are difficult to balance nutritionally. Most animals can be maintained on commercial hypoallergenic diets, if necessary. Optimally, pets should be challenge fed with individual food ingredients to determine which ones are causing problems. One ingredient is added to the diet trial in small amounts for 5 to 7 days, and the animal is observed for any reactions. If the ingredient causes problems immediately, it does not need to be tested further; a minimum of 5 days is needed, however, to determine that an ingredient is not causing the problem. The individual ingredients to be tested include beef, chicken, pork, soy (tofu), corn, milk, fish (halibut or mackerel), veal, rice, liver, and wheat (bread). Based on the results of this study, an acceptable ingredient list can be formulated and a suitable commercial diet selected that is hypoallergenic for that specific animal.

CONTACT DERMATITIS

Contact eruptions are rare in pets, no doubt because the skin surface is generally covered with fur.

There are two types of contact eruptions:

ETIOLOGIC AGENTS OF IRRITANT CONTACT DERMATITIS IN DOGS AND CATS	
Chemicals and Ions	**Materials and Products**
Chrome	Wool
Nickel	Synthetic fibers
Iodine	Rubber
Formaldehyde	Plastic
Dyes	Cleaning materials
Finishes (floor, fibers)	Polishes
Oleoresins	Leather
Sterols	Vehicles for drugs
Antioxidants	Flea collars
	Fertilizer

- Allergic contact dermatitis
- Irritant contact dermatitis

The substances responsible for allergic contact dermatitis are small haptens that bind to carrier proteins in the epidermal cells, forming an allergenic complex. Substances that can cause contact sensitivity in dogs include plants, medications (e.g., topical antibiotics, local anesthetics, shampoos, flea products), fibers (wool, synthetics), leather, disinfectants, carpet deodorizers, and plastics (see box above).

Irritant contact dermatitis results from contact with irritating substances that would affect any pet, not just allergic ones. Animals with sensitive skin may be affected especially by many products that do not cause allergic reactions but rather inflammation as a result of irritation. Shampoos, detergents, disinfectants, and salt on roadways are examples of substances that can irritate the skin.

Clinical Signs

The clinical signs associated with contact eruptions involve inflammatory reactions in the sparsely haired areas of the body (Figure 5-3). The muzzle, lips, ventral area, and perineum are most prone to eruptions. Densely haired areas of the body appear clinically normal. In fact, a sharp line of demarcation is often evident at the hairline, where the inflammation abruptly stops.

Diagnosis

Skin scrapings, fungal culture, bacterial culture, biopsy, intradermal allergy testing, and

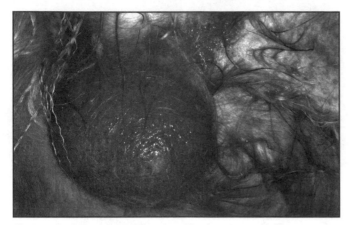

Figure 5-3. Scrotal dermatitis caused by a contact eruption.

hypoallergenic diet testing do not confirm a diagnosis of contact eruption, but they do help eliminate other possibilities. Even biopsies are not specific for contact eruptions, although some microscopic changes are consistent with the condition.

Patch testing is the preferred method for diagnosing contact eruptions, but it is seldom used in practice. The closed patch test commonly used in humans is rarely used in dogs or cats. The fur is shaved in a rectangular patch on the side of the chest. A series of contact allergens are applied to the skin and covered with an occlusive dressing. The test is read in 48 hours. Commercial contact allergens that may be important in dogs and cats include carba rubber mix, thiuram mix, epoxy resin, mercapto rubber mix, nickel sulfate, and colophony. A commercial patch test kit used with Finn chambers is available from Hermal Pharmaceutical Laboratories. An open patch test can be performed by applying chemical extracts or vehicles directly to the skin surface. The major problem is obtaining the extracts or vehicles of suspected contact allergens in a concentration that can produce an allergic reaction and be nonirritating.

Therapy

The treatment of choice for contact eruptions is to avoid the contact allergen responsible for the reaction. If complete avoidance is not possible, every effort should be made to minimize exposure; in many cases the life-style of the dog or cat must be changed to minimize the contact time with the primary allergen. When it is not possible to avoid the offending material or chemical, a low dose, alternate day maintenance regimen of corticosteroid may be required. Frequent cleansing baths can remove the contact allergens, and topical corticosteroids may also be helpful.

DRUG ERUPTIONS

Drug eruptions are adverse reactions to medications and can result from administering a drug orally, parenterally, topically, or as an inhalant. Although drugs can cause immune-mediated adverse reactions, problems can arise from nonimmunologic mechanisms as well. For instance, cancer chemotherapy can cause hair loss in some animals as it does in humans. Using antibacterial agents indiscriminately can result in the overgrowth of other microbes. In most cases, however, the adverse response to a drug involves an immunologic reaction and all four types of hypersensitivity can be involved. This complicates determining an accurate diagnosis. Antibiotics (especially trimethoprim-sulfonamides and penicillins) are a primary cause of drug eruptions. Doberman pinschers are particularly prone to hypersensitivity reactions to trimethoprim-sulfonamides. Neomycin, one of the most common components of topical medicaments, is another common cause of contact drug eruptions. There appears to be a spectrum of drug eruptions:

- Drug eruption is used to refer to relatively benign presentations.
- Erythema multiforme is used to refer to more major conditions.
- Toxic epidermal necrolysis is used to refer to extremely severe cases.

Clinical Signs

The clinical appearance of a drug eruption is highly variable depending on the mechanism of damage involved. If a drug evokes a type I (immediate) hypersensitivity reaction, the clinical signs might mimic those of inhalant allergies, food allergies, or flea bite hypersensitivities. Reactions to topical preparations (e.g., a medicated shampoo) are usually localized to the areas where the shampoo actually came into contact with the skin, and the dermatologic signs do not usually appear until days after the bathing. For example, a necrolytic dermatitis has recently been reported in miniature schnauzers that were bathed with natural or tarsulfur shampoos. A topically applied drug eruption is suspected to be responsible, and a genetic predisposition also appears likely.

Because the clinical appearance of a dog or cat with a drug eruption is so variable, history becomes increasingly important. Clinical signs in dogs include maculopapular eruptions, erosions and ulcers (see Plate V-7), pustules, or scaling.

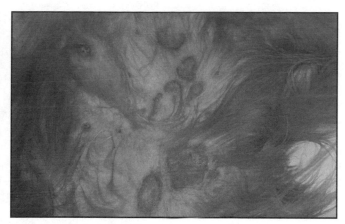

Figure 5-4. Erythema multiforme.

Other clinical signs reported in cats include miliary dermatitis, urticaria/angioedema, ulceration, and symmetric alopecia. Fixed drug eruptions are rare in dogs and initially involve edema, followed by uniformly well-circumscribed, erythematous lesions. The most common cause of fixed drug eruptions is reaction to diethylcarbamazine, the daily heartworm preventive.

Most cases of erythema multiforme and toxic epidermal necrolysis are serious manifestations of drug eruptions, although they can also be caused by infections or internal diseases. Animals with erythema multiforme (Figure 5-4) are usually presented with papules, urticarial plaques, raised erythematous lesions (including serpentine patterns and "doughnuts"), and blisters. Erythema multiforme major (Stevens-Johnson syndrome) is a more dangerous form, and oral ulcers are a typical part of the presentation. Toxic epidermal necrolysis is an even more severe condition involving painful, ulcerative lesions, resembling burns (see Plate V-8).

Diagnosis

Taking a complete history is the most important diagnostic test for drug eruption because there are no confirmatory tests. Any drug, even those commonly used (e.g., heartworm preventive), can cause eruptions. Affected animals may not have a history of recent drug administration. Drug eruptions can also occur following long-term administration of a drug that has not previously caused problems.

Histopathologic evaluation of biopsies is the best means of establishing a diagnosis in suspected cases because telltale changes often suggest drug eruption. Biopsies are critical for cases of erythema multiforme and toxic epidermal necro-

lysis, where the histopathologic changes are even more profound; in these cases full hematologic and biochemical studies are warranted because of possible internal involvement.

Treatment

The only suitable treatment for long-term remission is drug withdrawal and avoidance of further use of the suspected offender or any related drugs. The use of topical corticosteroids and antihistamines may ameliorate some of the clinical signs, but there is little evidence that they improve or shorten the course of the disorder. Even though the role of systemic corticosteroids is controversial, they frequently are used in management protocols. Pets with toxic epidermal necrolysis require intravenous fluid therapy in addition to corticosteroids and antibiotics.

AUTOIMMUNE SKIN DISEASES

The autoimmune skin diseases are a group of immunologic diseases in which the body attacks and destroys some of its own tissues. Sometimes the process is an intentional mistake, but in other cases the tissue is simply an innocent bystander in an immunologic war zone.

Usually, the body can distinguish its own tissues as "self" because of unique surface markers on each cell of the body; everything else is considered "nonself" and is targeted for destruction by the body's immune system. Occasionally, however, the body creates autoantibodies and directs its defenses against one or many of its own tissues. If the target tissue is not very critical, the process may go unnoticed. If the target organ becomes compromised in its function, however, the clinical picture recognizable as autoimmune disease results. With diseases such as systemic lupus erythematosus, the target tissues may include joints (rheumatoid arthritis), blood cells (autoimmune hemolytic anemia), or skin. For most of the other autoimmune diseases discussed in this chapter, the target tissues are usually limited to parts of the skin.

LUPUS ERYTHEMATOSUS

Lupus erythematosus is a multisystemic disease in which autoantibodies circulate in the bloodstream and target different tissues for injury.

CRITERIA FOR DIAGNOSING SYSTEMIC LUPUS ERYTHEMATOSUS[a]

- Characteristic skin lesions
- Erosive-ulcerative mucocutaneous lesions
- Nonerosive polyarthritis
- Hemolytic anemia, leukopenia, and/or thrombocytopenia
- Proteinuria and characteristic kidney disease
- Generalized lymphadenomegaly
- Fever of unknown origin that is unresponsive to antibiotics
- Pleuritis, pneumonitis, pericarditis, or myocarditis
- Polymyositis or polymyalgia
- Petechiae, purpura, or vasculitis
- Positive ANA test, LE cell test, or Coombs' test
- Characteristic histopathologic findings
- Characteristic immunopathologic findings (lupus band)

[a]Requires four or more of these features.

CONDITIONS THAT MIGHT PRODUCE A POSITIVE ANA TEST

Aural hematoma	Inhalant allergies
Autoimmune hemolytic anemia	Keratoconjunctivitis
	Myeloma
Cancer	Pemphigus
Cholangiohepatitis	Rheumatoid arthritis
Demodicosis	Systemic lupus
Endocarditis	erythematosus
Glomerulonephritis	Thyroiditis
Heartworm disease	Thrombocytopenia

There are two variants of the disorder in animals:

- Systemic lupus erythematosus (SLE), in which autoantibodies target internal as well as surface tissues
- Cutaneous lupus erythematosus (also known as discoid lupus erythematosus), in which damage is localized to the skin

The cause of lupus erythematosus is currently unknown but it appears to result from hyperactivity of the immune system. The autoantibodies produced are directed against nuclear or cytoplasmic constituents, red blood cells, white blood cells, clotting cells and factors, and ribonucleic acids. Some evidence suggests that the disorder may be associated with interaction of a virus with a disturbed immune system in a genetically predisposed host. Collies, Shetland sheepdogs, and Doberman pinschers are some of the breeds commonly affected.

Clinical Signs

The most common clinical findings in dogs with SLE are arthritis, fever that is unresponsive to antibiotics, kidney disease (glomerulonephritis) with protein loss in the urine, anemia, and skin disease. Many other syndromes have also been reported in association with this disorder; SLE can thus masquerade in a number of different forms

of disease. The skin disorders seen with SLE are diverse and may include scaling (dandruff), red rashes, scarring, hair loss, loss of pigment, and ulceration of the mucous membranes (mouth, nose, anus, vulva, penis, nail beds; see Plate V-9).

Cutaneous (discoid) lupus erythematosus appears to be a benign variant of SLE, in which there is no internal damage. The most common presentation is a red, scaling facial rash. Often there is also a loss of pigment inside the nostrils, which helps to distinguish cutaneous lupus erythematosus from other causes of facial dermatitis (see Plate V-10). In the past many cases of this benign disorder have likely been misdiagnosed as "collie nose."

Diagnosis (see box at left)

No single diagnostic test can confirm all cases of lupus erythematosus. The most common test used is the antinuclear antibody (ANA) test, which detects antibodies directed against cell nuclei. The ANA test is significantly positive in over 75% of dogs with active SLE. (The titer at which the ANA test is considered significant differs with each laboratory performing the test.) By itself the test cannot be used to confirm a diagnosis because many other diseases also produce positive ANA tests (see box above). The ANA test is negative in cases of cutaneous lupus erythematosus.

The lupus erythematosus (LE) cell test (see box on p. 127) is more specific than the ANA test but is only positive about 60% of the time in cases of SLE. It is negative in cases of cutaneous lupus erythematosus. The test is subjective as the determination is made entirely by the technician as to what constitutes an LE cell. Conditions that can cause a positive LE cell test include autoimmune hemolytic anemia, rheumatoid arthritis, lymphosarcoma, lymphoblastic leukemia, pulmonary granulomatosis, and warfarin poisoning.

LE CELL PREPARATION

1. Collect blood in heparinized blood tube (GTT).

2. Shake tube slightly to damage the white blood cells, exposing them to any autoantibody present.

3. Place one to two drops of blood on a microscope slide and apply coverslip.

4. LE cells are white blood cells that engulf exposed nuclei.

Biopsies for histopathology and immunopathology are often critical to making a diagnosis of either systemic or cutaneous lupus erythematosus. Both disorders usually show characteristic changes at the junction between the dermis and the epidermis. This is often referred to as an interface dermatitis, which consists of either lichenoid infiltrates of mononuclear cells or hydropic degeneration of epidermal basal cells. When biopsies are submitted for direct immunofluorescence testing or immunoperoxidase testing, antibody deposits are usually found in this junctional zone, and are referred to as a "lupus band." This finding is common to both the systemic and cutaneous variants.

Treatment

The treatment of lupus erythematosus requires suppressing the immune response to a level that is not harmful. This is an involved process, because it is also not desirable to oversuppress the immune system; if this happens, the body cannot effectively defend itself from viruses, bacteria, parasites, and other problems and becomes more susceptible to infections. Also, the drugs used to suppress the immune system cause side effects.

The treatment of cutaneous (discoid) lupus erythematosus need not be as aggressive as that for systemic lupus because the disorder does not put the pet's health status at risk. Treatment options usually include mild to moderate doses of corticosteroids (0.25 to 1.0 mg/kg/day), vitamin E (100 to 400 IU bid), and protection from sun exposure. Although ultraviolet light does not cause lupus, it can lead to scarring and ulcerative changes on skin already affected by cutaneous lupus erythematosus. Affected pets should avoid peak sunlight hours or wear protective coverings or sunblocks. A new therapy that appears to have much merit is the combination of tetracycline and niacinamide. Both medications are given at 500 mg tid. When clinical signs are in complete remission, administration can often be decreased to once or twice daily.

Because SLE is a potentially fatal disease, treatment must be more aggressive. Immunosuppressive doses of prednisone (2.2 to 6.6 mg/kg/day) combined with chemotherapies such as azathioprine (Imuran®—Burroughs Wellcome) and cyclophosphamide (Cytoxan®—Bristol-Myers Oncology) are often necessary. Blood counts, organ profiles, and urinalysis are monitored frequently for evidence of side effects or disease progression.

PEMPHIGUS

Pemphigus is used to described those conditions that result in "blisters" within the epidermis. The blisters are rarely evident clinically because of the thinness of the epidermis of dogs and cats. Scaling, pustules, erosions, and ulcers are more commonly seen than blisters.

There are four variants of pemphigus in dogs and cats:

- Pemphigus foliaceus
- Pemphigus erythematosus
- Pemphigus vulgaris
- Pemphigus vegetans

Clinical Signs

The presentation of each variant of pemphigus differs slightly:

- Pemphigus foliaceus, the most common form in dogs and cats, causes generalized scaling that often starts on the face and head (see Plate V-11). Clusters of pustules are often noted that in most cases evolve from vesicles (blisters). In many cases the footpads also become hyperkeratotic.

- Pemphigus erythematosus is a benign variant of pemphigus foliaceus, in which the changes usually remain localized to the face and head.

- Pemphigus vulgaris is more aggressive and causes damage deeper in the epidermis. Clinical signs include erosions and ulcers, often involving the mouth and other mucous membranes (see Plate V-12).

- Pemphigus vegetans, a benign variant of pemphigus vulgaris, is primarily a facial dermatitis characterized by crusts, scales, erosions, and hair loss.

None of the variants of pemphigus affect internal organs. Pemphigus vulgaris often affects the mucous membranes of the mouth, rectum, prepuce, and conjunctivae.

Diagnosis

Routine blood tests are not helpful in diagnosing pemphigus. ANA and LE cell tests should be negative. The diagnosis is based on characteristic cytologic, histopathologic, and immunopathologic findings. Fine needle aspirates of intact pustules may reveal pink, round epidermal cells admixed with neutrophils. These acantholytic keratinocytes are highly suggestive of pemphigus. They may also be found in impression smears made from erosive or ulcerative lesions, once the crust cover has been removed.

Multiple, carefully chosen biopsies should be entrusted to a competent pathologist with a special interest in dermatology. The pathologist will likely uncover diagnostic changes in about 80% of cases. Biopsies of early lesions, especially pustules, may reveal intact blisters within the epidermis, in which are found granulocytes and acantholytic keratinocytes. The location of the blister within the epidermis helps determine which variant of pemphigus is present. Pemphigus foliaceus and pemphigus erythematosus cause superficial (subcorneal) blisters, whereas pemphigus vulgaris and pemphigus vegetans cause deep (suprabasilar) blisters.

Biopsies collected for immunopathology should be taken from areas adjacent to lesions because inflammation destroys the antibodies in tissue. The samples are placed in Michel's solution for transport to specialized facilities for immunofluorescence testing. Immunoperoxidase testing can be done on regular paraffin-embedded tissue but is not commonly available from most laboratories. Immunopathology may be exciting and "high tech," but it rarely provides more information than do routine biopsies alone. Of biopsy-confirmed cases of pemphigus, only about 60% have positive immunopathologic results.

Treatment

The treatment of pemphigus depends on the variant involved and the extent of disease. Pemphigus erythematosus and pemphigus vegetans are usually localized and relatively benign; on the other hand, pemphigus vulgaris and pemphigus foliaceus can be extensive and aggressive. Pemphigus vulgaris is usually the most harmful variant because it can also cause ulcers on mucous membranes.

Prednisone is the initial treatment of choice because of its rapid onset of action, low cost, and ready availability. The doses used (2.2 mg/kg/day) are immunosuppressive but often less than those used for cases of systemic lupus erythematosus. Nevertheless, corticosteroids alone are effective in only 50% of cases because of their side effects or failure to induce remission. They usually need to be combined with chemotherapies (e.g., azathioprine, cyclophosphamide) or gold (chrysotherapy). Small dogs and cats may be effectively managed with prednisone combined with chlorambucil.

PEMPHIGOID

Pemphigoid means pemphigus-like. Bullous pemphigoid (the principal variant) shares many similarities with pemphigus vulgaris. The main difference between pemphigoid and pemphigus is that the blisters of pemphigoid form beneath the epidermis rather than within the epidermis.

Two variants of pemphigoid that have been recognized in dogs and cats are:

- Bullous pemphigoid (aggressive variant)
- Cicatricial pemphigoid (benign variant)

Clinical Signs

Bullous pemphigoid is clinically similar to pemphigus vulgaris. Animals with this disorder are presented with transient blisters, crusts, and ulcerations (see Plate V-13). The blisters and pustules may be more apparent in this disorder than in pemphigus because they occur deeper in the skin.

Cicatricial (mucous membrane) pemphigoid is a chronic blistering disease that preferentially affects the mucous membranes of the mouth and eyes. This disorder is not commonly associated with skin disease.

Diagnosis

The diagnostic tests useful for pemphigus are also useful for pemphigoid. The distinction between bullous pemphigoid and cicatricial pemphigoid is made on the basis of clinical findings. The cytology, histopathology, and immunopathology are identical for the two variants.

Cytologic preparations may reveal neutrophils within blisters but not acantholytic keratinocytes, the hallmarks of pemphigus. Carefully chosen biopsies should show clefts in the area immediately beneath the dermal-epidermal junction. This is a deeper location than the intraepidermal blisters seen with pemphigus. Immunopathology may reveal antibody and/or complement deposits in the area between the dermis and epidermis.

Treatment

The treatment of pemphigoid is identical to that of pemphigus and includes corticosteroids and adjuvant chemotherapy with azathioprine, chlorambucil, cyclophosphamide, and chrysotherapy. Cicatricial pemphigoid usually does not require such drastic therapy and may respond to topical corticosteroids or 1% to 2% cyclosporine preparations.

VASCULITIS

Vasculitis is an inflammatory disorder of blood vessels that can result from several very different mechanisms. As such, it is a convenient descriptive term but does not imply a diagnosis. The most common causes of vasculitis are infections, immunologic reactions, systemic or chronic diseases, and injection site reactions (especially to rabies vaccines). Most vasculitis syndromes are associated with immune complex deposition in the blood vessel walls. They have also been associated with parvovirus infection in puppies, Rocky Mountain spotted fever, drug reactions (e.g., sulfa hypersensitivity in Doberman pinschers), bacterial hypersensitivity, lupus erythematosus, and polyarteritis.

Clinical Signs

Because vasculitis can affect small or large blood vessels, the clinical presentation is not always the same. The process frequently affects the most dependent parts of the body (i.e., the parts that hang lowest), and the feet and ears. The classic feature is an elevated bruise, referred to as a "palpable purpura." Erosions and ulcers are usually present at some stage of the process, and the areas heal with a depressed scar. Systemic involvement can also occur and affect the heart, kidneys, gastrointestinal tract, and brain.

Injection site vasculitis and panniculitis are not uncommon. The principal culprit is usually a killed rabies vaccine (e.g., Imrab—Merieux). A roughly circular patch of smooth hair loss appears at the site of injection 6 to 8 weeks after vaccination. The condition is not associated with pain or medical consequences.

Polyarteritis is a rare form of vasculitis that has been principally described in young beagles. Affected animals usually have fever, cervical pain, anorexia, and a host of other signs. There are many similarities to Kawasaki syndrome in humans.

Diagnosis

The diagnosis of vasculitis relies on histopathologic and sometimes immunopathologic evaluation of biopsies. This can provide important clues toward identifying the ultimate cause and can also provide evidence to link the condition with other immune-mediated disorders. If the biopsy suggests an infectious cause, microbial cultures and appropriate serology can be conducted. If the biopsy suggests an immune-mediated etiology, ANA, rheumatoid factor, and circulating immune complex (CIC) tests may be warranted.

Dogs with polyarteritis (systemic necrotizing vasculitis) have a syndrome clinically distinct from types of vasculitis that cause only dermatologic problems. Blood should be collected for a complete blood count and electrolyte and biochemical profiles. Typical findings are nonregenerative anemia, hypoalbuminemia, and leukocytosis with mature neutrophilia. Cerebrospinal fluid evaluation often reveals neutrophilic pleocytosis and elevations of protein concentration. If pups succumb to the disorder, the diagnosis can be confirmed by postmortem examination.

Treatment

The treatment of vasculitis is individualized, depending on the cause:

- Bacterial hypersensitivity vasculitis can be managed by appropriate antibiotic therapy.
- Vaccination site vasculitis often requires no treatment at all, but owners may request surgical excision of the affected area for cosmetic reasons.
- Immune-mediated vasculitis responds best to azathioprine (Imuran®—Burroughs Wellcome), dapsone (Avlosulfon—Ayerst), or corticosteroids.

• Treatment for polyarteritis requires immuno-suppressive doses of prednisone because of the systemic effects of the disease.

UVEODERMATOLOGIC (VOGT-KOYANAGI-HARADA) SYNDROME

The cause of uveodermatologic syndrome is currently unknown, but it may represent an autoimmune attack against pigment-producing cells (melanocytes) or an abnormal response to a viral infection. The term Vogt-Koyanagi-Harada syndrome is derived from the three individuals who described the ophthalmic, dermatologic, and neurologic manifestations in humans.

Clinical Signs

The condition is characterized by a serious eye disorder (granulomatous panuveitis) and concurrent loss of pigment from the nose, lips, eyelids, and, occasionally, the entire body. Unlike humans, dogs rarely have any neurologic involvement. Most affected animals are young adults.

Diagnosis

The diagnosis of Vogt-Koyanagi-Harada syndrome relies on histopathologic evaluation of biopsies of affected tissues. There is a pronounced inflammatory reaction at the dermal-epidermal junction, in which histiocytes (modified macrophages) are the predominating cell type (a very definitive feature of the disease). It has also been proposed that titers of antiretinal antibodies may be helpful in diagnosis. Normal dogs usually have serum titers of 1:25 to 1:50, whereas those with this syndrome have much higher titers (e.g., over 1:100).

Treatment

Treatment must be commenced immediately, or irreversible blindness could result. The mainstays of therapy are systemic corticosteroids and perhaps topical cyclosporine. The goal of therapy is to stop disease progression. Pigmentation may return in some cases.

ALOPECIA AREATA

Alopecia areata is a rare disorder characterized by a localized area of hair loss because of lim-ited autoantibody production against hair follicles in the anagen (growing) phase.

Clinical Signs

The main sign of alopecia areata is a discrete, well-circumscribed area of baldness, which is probably frequently mistaken for dermatophytosis (ringworm). The hairless patch may remain as is or expand, or hair may regrow spontaneously. There is no medical significance associated with this condition.

Diagnosis

Alopecia areata may be suspected clinically, but histopathologic examination of biopsies is needed for confirmation. Early in the clinical course, there may be a conspicuous lymphocytic "swarm of bees" around growing hair bulbs. Once the inflammation has subsided, diagnosis is more difficult.

Treatment

Treatment for alopecia areata is not necessary because it is a cosmetic concern rather than a medical problem. Sometimes the hairs regrow spontaneously. Intralesional corticosteroids or topical minoxidil (Rogaine®—Upjohn) can be contemplated if owners desire intervention.

SJÖGREN'S SYNDROME

Sjögren's syndrome is a sicca complex characterized by dry eyes (keratoconjunctivitis sicca) and dry mouth (xerostomia), coupled with an autoimmune connective tissue disease. The dermatologic manifestations of this syndrome are similar to those of erythematosus, warranting speculation that they might be related in some way.

Clinical Signs

The most common presentation involves keratoconjunctivitis sicca, and so more cases are initially presented to ophthalmologists than to dermatologists. The cutaneous manifestations resemble those of lupus erythematosus (e.g., hair loss, keratinization disorders, erythema, induration).

Diagnosis

The diagnosis of keratoconjunctivitis sicca can be made by measuring tear production. Confirming Sjögren's syndrome as the cause of keratoconjunctivitis sicca requires appropriate biopsies. Biopsy of the lacrimal glands shows periductal or diffuse mononuclear cell invasion, fibrocytic replacement of acinar elements, and lymphoid nodules. In studies of dogs with keratoconjunctivitis sicca, 42% had a positive ANA test and 34% were positive for rheumatoid factor.

Treatment

Corticosteroids have long been the mainstay of conventional therapy for Sjögren's syndrome, but recently topical cyclosporine has been found to be very effective and is associated with fewer side effects. Parotid duct transposition (a surgical procedure that reroutes a salivary duct under the skin to the corner of the eye so saliva can replace tear film and lubricate the eye surface) has been effectively utilized for cases of keratoconjunctivitis sicca. Unfortunately, with Sjögren's syndrome there is also salivary gland involvement; the procedure is unlikely to improve the situation and is not appropriate for dogs with this syndrome.

JUVENILE CELLULITIS

Juvenile cellulitis (puppy strangles) previously was thought to be bacterial in nature, but recent studies suggest an immune-mediated etiology. Dachshunds, golden retrievers, Labrador retrievers, and pointers are most commonly affected.

Clinical Signs

The condition affects young puppies; the face and head are commonly swollen and inflamed (see Plate V-14). Knotted lymphatics, enlarged submandibular lymph nodes, facial cellulitis, and draining tracts are commonly observed. Scarring is a usual sequela.

Diagnosis

Biopsies are consistent with cellulitis, but in most cases bacterial infection is secondary rather than primary. Bacteria recovered on cultures are likely contaminants or opportunistic invaders.

Treatment

The treatment of choice is prednisone (2.2 mg/kg/day) for approximately 2 weeks. The condition usually responds completely with little

chance of recurrence. Prophylactically, a bactericidal antibiotic (e.g., cephalexin, oxacillin) is prescribed to manage any bacterial component that may be present.

STERILE PYOGRANULOMA

Sterile pyogranuloma was once thought to be a bacterial infection but is now presumed to have an immune-mediated etiology based on histopathologic findings and response to corticosteroids. Great Danes, St. Bernards, Newfoundlands, dachshunds, Chinese Shar peis, pit bull terriers, and English bulldogs appear to be predisposed.

Clinical Signs

The condition presents as firm, red, nodular lesions between the toes or on the face (see Plate V-15). The nodules may enlarge, ulcerate, or form draining tracts.

Diagnosis

Although animals with the condition are frequently said to have "interdigital cysts," the histopathologic presentation is granulomatous and not cystic. Bacterial cultures are sterile or yield secondary contaminants.

Treatment

The treatment of choice is anti-inflammatory therapy with prednisone and/or azathioprine (Imuran®—Burroughs Wellcome).

TREATING IMMUNE-MEDIATED DISORDERS

The standard of treatment for immune-mediated disorders is prednisone. It is inexpensive, readily available, effective, and has been in use for a long time. In the past human patients with immune-mediated diseases usually died from complications of the conditions. Since the advent of corticosteroids, however, most of these patients now succumb to side effects of their treatment.

Dogs and cats produce cortisol, a natural corticosteroid from the adrenal glands at the top of their kidneys. Although it was once thought that dogs and cats have different circadian rhythms for cortisol secretion, it is now known that cortisol production is episodic for both species and does not fluctuate based on time of day. Cortisol is

TABLE 5-2

LENGTH OF ACTION OF SYSTEMIC CORTICOSTEROIDS

TYPE	LENGTH OF ADRENAL SUPPRESSION	DRUG	RELATIVE ANTI-INFLAMMATORY EFFECTS[a]
Short acting	<36 hours	Hydrocortisone	1
		Prednisone	4
		Prednisolone	4
		Methylprednisolone	5
		Triamcinolone	5
Long acting	>60 hours	Dexamethasone	10–20
		Betamethasone	10–20
		Flumethasone	≥20
Residual	2–4 weeks	Triamcinolone acetonide	NK[b]
		Methylprednisolone acetate	NK
		Betamethasone dipropionate	NK

[a]When compared with hydrocortisone on a milligram-to-milligram basis.
[b]Not known.

equivalent in strength to hydrocortisone, and prednisone is five times as potent. Physiologic doses of prednisone for dogs are 0.2 mg (1 mg of hydrocortisone or cortisol) per kilogram of body weight per day. Therefore, a 10 kg (22 lb) dog produces the equivalent of 2 mg of prednisone each day. When prednisone is administered in doses 10 times higher than physiologic levels (2.2 mg/kg), the immune system is suppressed. Lesser doses (usually 0.25 to 1.0 mg/kg) are used to manage inflammatory conditions such as allergies or arthritis.

When greater than physiologic doses of corticosteroids are given over a long period, the adrenal glands may atrophy and become incapable of responding to the body's need for cortisol production. At the same time, the glucocorticoids that are being administered as medication affect virtually every other tissue of the body. Commonly, corticosteroid administration causes increased thirst, increased urination, and increased hunger, but the effects that are not seen are much more dangerous. Long-term corticosteroid use can result in diabetes mellitus, recurrent infections, osteoporosis, liver disease, and a host of other ills. Because of these potential side effects, corticosteroids should be used cautiously, especially in young animals, pregnant females, and animals with diabetes mellitus, kidney or heart disease, infectious

diseases, or gastrointestinal ulceration. Ideally, long-term administration of corticosteroids should be given on an alternate day basis to provide the adrenals with the opportunity to produce cortisol and to give the body a day of rest from the high levels of steroid administered.

The choice of corticosteroid used is as important as the dosage; some formulations can cause much more damage at lower doses than others. For most skin problems only prednisone and triamcinolone are suitable for long-term oral use. Repository forms of corticosteroids (e.g., methylprednisolone acetate) are inappropriate for long-term use in dogs but are important anti-inflammatory agents in cats. Products containing dexamethasone, betamethasone, or flumethasone are rarely, if ever, needed to manage dermatologic conditions. Hydrocortisone is the steroid of choice for topical use.

The choice of corticosteroid is complicated by the fact that most preparations are combined with another agent to affect absorption and excretion. Sodium phosphate and succinate esters are very water soluble, quickly attain high blood levels, and are quickly excreted. These preparations (e.g., prednisolone sodium succinate [Solu-Delta Cortef®—Upjohn]) are often administered to animals in shock because of their quick effect. On the other hand, acetate, diacetate, and acetonide esters

TABLE 5-3

CHEMOTHERAPEUTIC AGENTS

AGENT	ACTION	ADMINISTRATION	COMMENTS
Prednisolone	Immunosuppressive	Taper if possible	Polydipsia, polyuria, polyphagia; increased susceptibility to infection; delayed wound healing
Cyclophosphamide	Alkylating agent; immunosuppressive	50 mg/m^2; 1.5 mg/kg 3–4 days per week	Leukopenia, hemorrhagic cystitis
Chlorambucil	Alkylating agent; immunosuppressive	0.2 mg/kg sid	Usually no adverse effects
Azathioprine	Antimetabolite	2.2 mg/kg sid or every 2 days PO	Leukopenia; thrombocytopenia; vomiting; use with caution in cats
Vincristine	Vinca alkaloid	0.5 mg/m^2 weekly or alternate weeks	Anemia; leukopenia; stomatitis
Methotrexate	Antimetabolite	$2.5–15 \text{ mg/m}^2$ sid IV, IM, PO	Anemia; gastrointestinal disturbances
Aurothioglucose (chrysotherapy)	Immunosuppressive	Test dose: 1–5 mg IM Maintenance dose: 1 mg/kg weekly IM	Thrombocytopenia; stomatitis; dermatitis; nephritis
Gold sodium thiomalate (chrysotherapy)	Immunosuppressive	Same as above	Same as above
Dapsone (Avlosulfon— Ayerst)	Enzyme interference	1.1–1.5 mg/kg bid–qid; taper to every 2 days	Thrombocytopenia; anemia
Cyclosporine	Cyclic polypeptide	10–30 mg/kg sid	Vomiting; dermatitis
Vitamin E	Antioxidant	200–400 IU bid PO	

are poorly water soluble, slowly absorbed, and slowly excreted. For example, methylprednisolone is roughly equivalent to prednisone in potency, but methylprednisolone acetate (e.g., Depo-Medrol®—Upjohn) has prolonged effects and side effects. Length of action of commonly used corticosteroids is presented in Table 5-2.

Several chemotherapeutic agents are used in the management of immune-mediated diseases (Table 5-3). Azathioprine (Imuran®—Burroughs Wellcome) is a chemotherapeutic agent that has become commonplace in the management of immune-mediated diseases. It is converted to 6-mercaptopurine in the liver and must be used cautiously in animals with liver disease. Cats appear to be particularly prone to its toxic effects. Other side effects include bone marrow suppression, gastrointestinal disturbances, and hepatic dys-

function. It is typically given at 1.1 to 2.2 mg/kg on alternating days with prednisone. There is a lag of 3 to 5 weeks before its effects are clinically evident.

Monitoring is an important aspect of therapy with azathioprine. Initially, liver function tests and blood counts should be performed twice weekly for the first 2 weeks and then weekly for the next 2 weeks. If no problems occur during the first month, blood tests can be repeated every 1 to 3 months as needed. Elevations of serum alkaline phosphatase are to be anticipated and need to be interpreted in light of other liver function enzymes, such as alanine transaminase.

Chlorambucil (Leukeran®—Burroughs Wellcome) is a synthetic alkylating agent used in cancer therapy. Recently, it has also proved to be useful in the management of several autoimmune diseases, especially in small dogs and cats. In many ways, chlorambucil has replaced cyclophosphamide (Cytoxan®—Bristol-Myers Oncology) as the alkylating agent of choice for immune-mediated skin diseases. Cyclophosphamide has a number of debilitating side effects, including hemorrhagic cystitis, leukopenia, thrombocytopenia, gastrointestinal disturbances, nephrotoxicity, hepatotoxicity, carcinogenicity, and hair loss. In comparison, the main concerns with chlorambucil are thrombocytopenia and lymphopenia. Anorexia, vomiting, and diarrhea usually resolve quickly when the drug dosage is decreased or when the drug is discontinued.

Chlorambucil (0.1 to 0.2 mg/kg) is given on alternating days with prednisone (2.2 mg/kg/day). Once disease is in remission, the doses of both drugs can be gradually decreased. Monitoring consists of weekly blood counts for the first month and then hematologic and biochemical profiles and urinalyses every 3 to 6 months as long as therapy continues. If the white blood cell count drops below 4,000/μl or the platelet count drops below 100,000/μl, the dosage should be reduced by 25% and monitoring should be more frequent.

Chrysotherapy uses gold as a therapeutic agent. In most cases it is given intramuscularly, but an oral form, triethylphosphine gold (auranofin [Ridaura®—SmithKline Beecham Pharmaceuticals) has also been evaluated. It is administered at 0.1 to 0.2 mg/kg every 12 hours. In the United States aurothioglucose (Solganal®—Schering) is the most common injectable product used, whereas in Canada and Europe gold sodium thiomalate (Myochrysine—Rhône Poulenc) is more popular. Therapy is initiated by giving two test doses a week apart by intramuscular injection. Cats and small dogs (less than 10 kg) are given 1 mg and then 2 mg injections; larger dogs receive 5 mg and then 10 mg a week later. If no adverse reactions are encountered, gold therapy is continued at 1 mg/kg weekly until a response is noted, following which therapy is tapered to alternate weeks and then monthly. Corticosteroids are given concurrently because the side effects are not additive with those of gold and because it takes many weeks of gold injections before any benefits are realized.

Monitoring of patients on gold therapy is critical. A complete blood count and urinalysis should be performed before each injection. Eosinophilia or proteinuria may signal impending toxicosis. Gold therapy can result in heavy metal poisoning, so the results of testing should be evaluated prior to injecting more drug.

Newer therapies for immune-mediated skin diseases include danazol and cyclosporine A. Danazol is an attenuated androgen that, in addition to other effects, reduces the number of immunoglobulin receptors on phagocytic cells. Danazol may allow more rapid tapering of glucocorticoid and azathioprine doses. Dosage is 3 mg/kg PO tid. Potential side effects include skin rash, elevated liver enzymes, and potential hepatotoxicity.

Cyclosporin A received worldwide acclaim as a breakthrough for transplant patients. Its main use in veterinary medicine has been as a topical therapy for immune-mediated keratoconjunctivitis sicca. It has been used systemically in the treatment of some autoimmune skin diseases but is inferior to the standard chemotherapies already in use. Cyclosporin A is given at 20 mg/kg/day PO. Side effects include nephrotoxicity, vomiting, diarrhea, lymphoplasmacytoid dermatitis, hepatotoxicity, gingival hyperplasia, infections, and intestinal intussusception.

RECOMMENDED READINGS

Ackerman LJ: Pemphigus and pemphigoid in the dog and cat. Part I. Pemphigus. *Compend Contin Educ Pract Vet* 7:89–97, 1985.

Ackerman LJ: Pemphigus and pemphigoid in the dog and cat. Part II. Pemphigoid. *Compend Contin Educ Pract Vet* 7:281–286, 1985.

Ackerman L: Pemphigus and pemphigoid in dogs and cats. Part I: Clinical signs, diagnosis and treatment. *Mod Vet Pract* 67:260–265, 1986.

Ackerman L: Pemphigus and pemphigoid in dogs and cats. Part II: A clinical survey. *Mod Vet Pract* 67:358–360, 1986.

Ackerman L: Diagnosing inhalant allergies: Intradermal or in vitro testing? *Vet Med* 83:779–788, 1988.

Ackerman L: Medical and immunotherapeutic options for treating atopic dogs. *Vet Med* 83:790–797, 1988.

Ackerman L: Autoimmune disorders, in Morgan R (ed): *Handbook of Small Animal Practice*, ed 2. New York, Churchill Livingstone, 1992, pp 991–996.

Ackerman L: Hypersensitivity disorders, in Morgan R (ed): *Handbook of Small Animal Practice*, ed 2. New York, Churchill Livingstone, 1992, pp 996–999.

Ackerman L: Adverse reactions to foods. *J Vet Allerg Clin Immunol* 1(1):18–22, 1993.

Allbritton AR: Clinical significance of ANA. *J Vet Allerg Clin Immunol* 1(1):12–14, 1993.

Beale KM, Kunkle GA, Chalker L, Cannon R: Effects of sedation on intradermal skin testing in flea-allergic dogs. *JAVMA* 197(7):861–864, 1990.

Bettenay S: Diagnosing and treating feline atopic dermatitis. *Vet Med*, pp 488–496, May 1991.

Boothe DM: Drug therapy in cats: Mechanisms and avoidance of adverse drug reactions. *JAVMA* 196(8):1297–1305, 1990.

Anderson RK: The diagnosis of atopic disease—Intradermal or in vitro testing. *J Vet Allerg Clin Immunol* 1(1):23–28, 1993.

Codner EC, Lessard P, McGrath CJ: Effect of tiletamine/zolazepam sedation on intradermal allergy testing in atopic dogs. *JAVMA* 201(12):1857–1860, 1992.

DeBoer DJ, Moriello KA, Pollet RA: Efficacy of AHR-13268, an antiallergenic compound, in the management of pruritus caused by atopic disease in dogs. *JAVMA* 53(4):532–536, 1992.

Grindem CB, Johnson KH: Systemic lupus erythematosus: Literature review and report of 42 new canine cases. *JAAHA* 19:489–503, 1983.

Halliwell REW: Comparative aspects of food intolerance. *Vet Med*, pp 893–899, Sept 1992.

Kaswan RL, Salisbury M-A: Canine keratoconjunctivitis sicca: Etiology, clinical signs, diagnosis, and treatment. Part I. Etiology and clinical signs. *J Vet Allerg Clin Immunol* 1(1):9–11, 1993.

Kern TJ, Walton DK, Riis RC, et al: Uveitis associated with poliosis and vitiligo in six dogs. *JAVMA* 187:408–414, 1985.

Kunkle GA: Contact dermatitis. *Vet Clin North Am* 18:1061–1068, 1988.

Kunkle G, Horner S: Validity of skin testing for diagnosis of food allergy in dogs. *JAVMA* 200(5):677–680, 1992.

McMurdy MA: A case resembling erythema multiforme major (Stevens-Johnson Syndrome) in a dog. *JAAHA* 26(3):297–300, 1990.

Medleau L, Shanley KJ, Rakich PM, Goldschmidt MH: Trimethoprim-sulfonamide-associated drug eruptions in dogs. *JAAHA* 26(3):307–311, 1990.

Miller WH Jr, Scott DW, Scarlett JM: Evaluation of an allergy screening test for use in atopic dogs. *JAVMA* 200(7):931–935, 1992.

Monier JC, Fournel C, Lapras M, et al: Systemic lupus erythematosus in a colony of dogs. *Am J Vet Res* 49:46–51, 1988.

Morgan RV, Abrams KL: Topical administration of cyclosporine for treatment of keratoconjunctivitis sicca in dogs. *JAVMA* 199(8):1043–1046, 1991.

Murphy CJ, Bellhorn RW, Thirkill C: Anti-retinal antibodies associated with Vogt-Koyanagi-Harada-like syndrome in a dog. *JAAHA* 27(4):399–402, 1991.

Panich R, Scott DW, Miller WH Jr: Canine cutaneous sterile pyogranuloma/granuloma syndrome: A retrospective analysis of 29 cases (1976–1988). *JAAHA* 27(5):519–528, 1991.

Rosser EJ Jr: Antipruritic drugs. *Vet Clin North Am* 18:1093–1099, 1988.

Roudebush P, Cowell CS: Results of a hypoallergenic diet survey of veterinarians in North America with a nutritional evaluation of homemade diet prescriptions. *Vet Dermatol* 3(1):23–28, 1992.

Scott DW: Localized scleroderma (morphea) in two dogs. *JAAHA* 22:207–211, 1986.

Scott DW, Walton DK, Manning TO, et al: Canine lupus erythematosus. I. Systemic lupus erythematosus. *JAAHA* 19:461–479, 1983.

Scott DW, Walton DK, Manning TO, et al: Canine lupus erythematosus. II. Discoid lupus erythematosus. *JAAHA* 19:481–488, 1983.

White SD, Rosychuk RA, Reinke SI, Paradis M: Use of tetracycline and niacinamide for treatment of autoimmune skin disease in 31 dogs. *JAVMA* 200(10):1497–1500, 1992.

White SD, Rosychuk RAW, Stewart LJ, et al: Juvenile cellulitis in dogs: 15 cases (1979–1988). *JAVMA* 195(11):1609–1611, 1989.

Wills JM: Diagnosing and managing food sensitivity in cats. *Vet Med* pp 884–892, Sept 1992.

Color Plates

PLATE I

I-1. Zinc-responsive dermatosis: Footpad hyperkeratosis and erythema.

I-2. Sebaceous adenitis (periappendageal dermatitis): Marked erythroderma and hair loss.

I-3. Epidermal dysplasia: Extensive hair loss, exfoliation, and erythema in a young dog.

I-4. Follicular dysplasia: Hair loss on the head and ears of a young Doberman pinscher.

I-5. Ichthyosis: Marked exfoliative dermatitis in a young dog with suspected ichthyosis. (From Ackerman LJ: A new approach to dermatologic diagnosis in the dog. *Vet Focus* 1:6–11, 1989.)

I-6. Canine acne: Alopecia and comedones on the ventral chin accompanied by focal erythematous ulceration and furunculosis.

I-7. Feline acne: Comedo formation on the anterior ventral chin. Note crust secondary to trauma at the posterior aspect of the lesion.

I-8. Footpad hyperkeratosis: Increased thickness of stratum corneum of the footpads.

I-9. Lichenoid-psoriasiform dermatitis: Papulonodular dermatitis with plaques in a springer spaniel. (From Ackerman LJ: A new approach to dermatologic diagnosis in the dog. *Vet Focus* 1:6–11, 1989.)

I-10. Cutaneous asthenia: Boxer with marked hyperextensibility of the skin. (Courtesy of Anthony Stannard, School of Veterinary Medicine, University of California, Davis.)

I-11. Cutaneous asthenia: A 1-year-old Siamese cat with marked hyperextensibility of the skin.

I-12. Dermatomyositis: Facial scaling, hair loss, and scarring in a young affected dog.

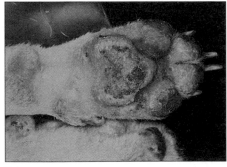

I-1

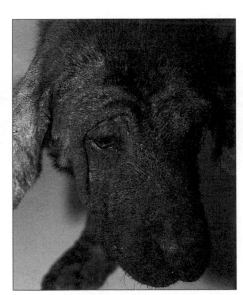

I-2

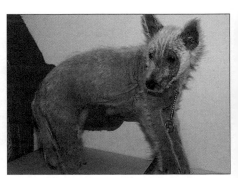

I-3

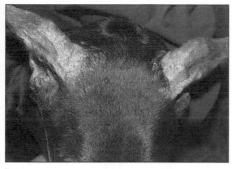

I-4

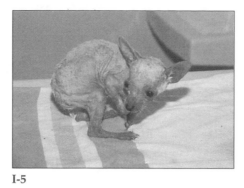

I-5

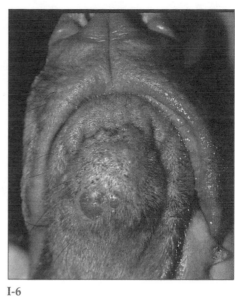

I-6

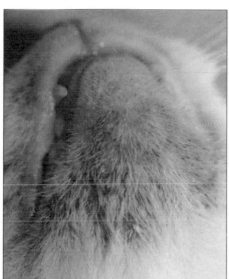

I-7

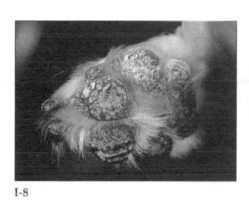

I-8

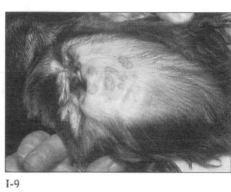

I-9

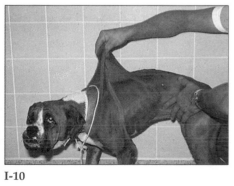

I-10

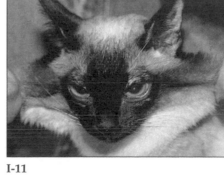

I-11

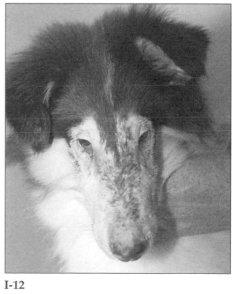

I-12

PLATE II

II-1. Flea dermatitis: Adult flea on an alopecic patch of dorsal caudal back.

II-2. Flea dermatitis: Multifocal, erythematous papules on the ventral abdomen.

II-3. Adult *Rhipicephalus* ticks feeding in the ear of a dog. (Reprinted from Lewis T: Ticks and associated diseases. *Pet Focus* 1:21–23, 1989, with permission.)

II-4. Generalized demodicosis: Patchy alopecia, hyperpigmentation, and focal excoriation with crusts on the face and neck of a 4-year-old dog.

II-5. Generalized demodicosis: Diffuse alopecia and erythema of the foot of a 6-month-old dog.

II-6. Sarcoptic mange: Severe diffuse crusting of the face of a 3-month-old dog.

II-7. Notoedric mange: Diffuse alopecia with scales and crusts on the head and dorsal neck of a cat. (Courtesy of Tom Willemse, State University of Utrecht, Utrecht, The Netherlands.)

II-8. Cheyletiellosis: Mild dandruff on the dorsum of a cat.

II-9. Myiasis: Multifocal ulcers after the removal of larvae from the lesions on the dorsal caudal back of a dog.

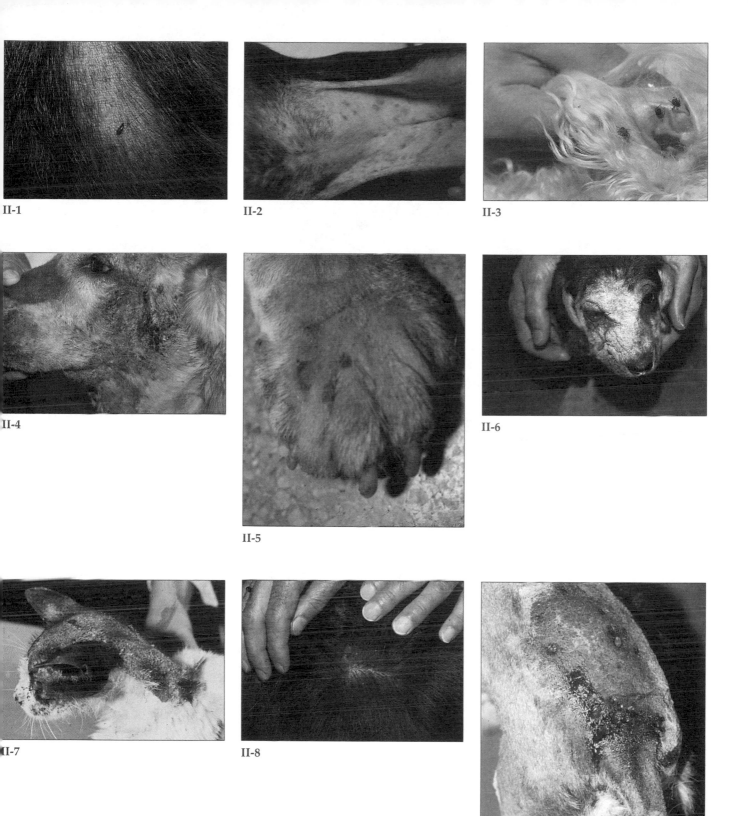

II-1

II-2

II-3

II-4

II-5

II-6

II-7

II-8

II-9

PLATE III

III-1. Pyotraumatic dermatitis: Erosion, erythema, and hair loss.

III-2. Lip fold pyoderma: Focal erythema and erosion on the lower lip.

III-3. Superficial folliculitis: Erythematous papules and pustules on the ventral area of a dog.

III-4. Deep pyoderma: Generalized multifocal ulceration on the trunk associated with furunculosis.

III-5. Cellulitis: Ulceration and swelling associated with a deep infection.

III-6. Actinomycotic mycetoma: Chronic induration, ulceration, and fistulation resulting from nocardiosis in a cat.

III-7. Bacterial granuloma: Chronic nodular dermatitis associated with impaired resistance to staphylococcal infection.

III-8. Atypical mycobacteriosis: Nodular facial dermatitis in a cat.

III-9. Perianal pyoderma: Multiple fistulous tracts dorsolateral to the anus.

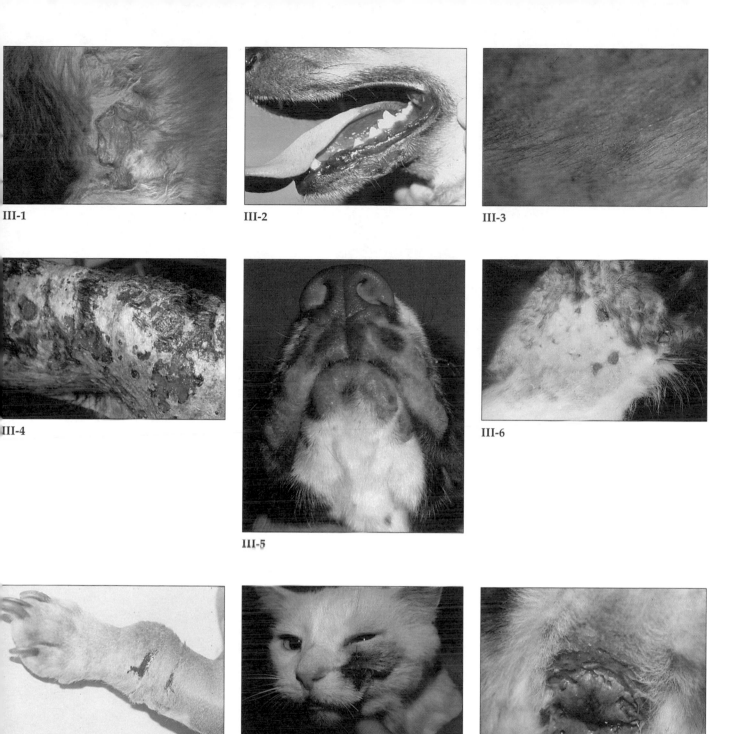

III-1

III-2

III-3

III-4

III-5

III-6

III-7

III-8

III-9

PLATE IV

IV-1. Dermatophytosis: *Microsporum gypseum* infection with alopecia and mild erythema of the dorsal head, neck, and shoulders of an adult dog.

IV-2. Dermatophytosis: *Microsporum canis* infection causing hair loss and scaling on the dorsum of the head of a kitten.

IV-3. Dermatophytosis: Scaling and hair loss as the only clinical signs in a cat.

IV-4. Contaminant growth on dermatophyte test medium in which the medium is red but the colony is not fluffy and white.

IV-5. Positive culture of a dermatophyte showing a white fluffy colony that turns the dermatophyte test medium red.

IV-6. Sporotrichosis: Multiple subcutaneous ulcerated nodules and crusting on the distal extremities of a cat. (Courtesy of Nita Gulbas, Phoenix, Arizona.)

IV-7. Blastomycosis: Granulomatous nodule on the lateral surface of the foot of a dog. (Courtesy of Al Legendre, University of Tennessee, Knoxville.)

IV-8. Coccidioidomycosis: Ulceration and fistulation on the head of a cat.

IV-9. Cryptococcosis: Multiple ulcerated granulomatous nodules on the face of a cat. (Courtesy of Nita Gulbas, Phoenix, Arizona.)

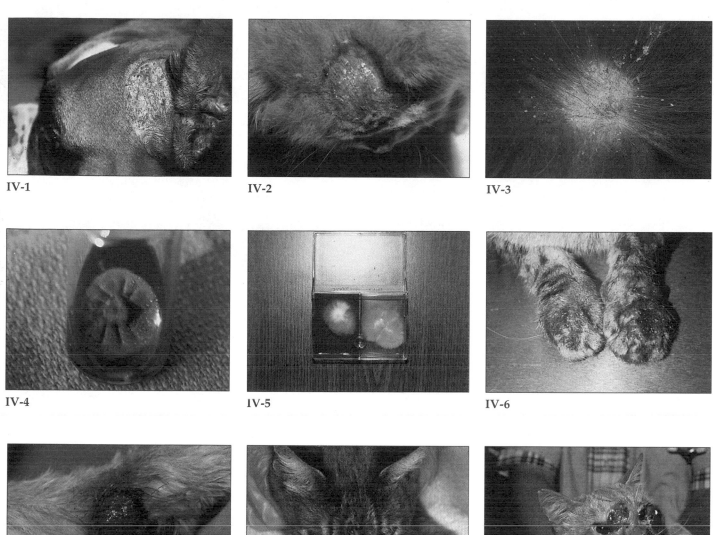

IV-1

IV-2

IV-3

IV-4

IV-5

IV-6

IV-7

IV-8

IV-9

PLATE V

V-1. Acute atopic dermatitis: Alopecia, diffuse erythema, and excoriation of axillae and ventral thorax.

V-2. Lichenification and hyperpigmentation associated with chronic allergic disease.

V-3. Feline allergic dermatitis associated with airborne allergens: Facial alopecia and excoriations.

V-4. Reactions seen 15 to 30 minutes after intradermal allergy testing in an allergic dog. (From Ackerman LJ: Inhalant allergies. *Pet Focus* 1:4–9, 1989.)

V-5. Facial swelling and erythema associated with an adverse food reaction in a Chinese Shar pei. (From Ackerman LJ: Inhalant allergies. *Pet Focus* 1:4–9, 1989.)

V-6. Erosions, ulcerations, and excoriations associated with beef hypersensitivity in a cat. (From Ackerman LJ: Food hypersensitivity: A rare, but manageable disorder. *Vet Med* 83:1142–1148, 1988.)

V-7. Drug eruption: Adverse reaction to tetracycline resulting in ulceration of the footpad.

V-8. Toxic epidermal necrolysis: Dorsal crusting associated with total epidermal necrosis in a linear pattern.

V-9. Systemic lupus erythematosus: Pronounced facial ulceration.

V-10. Cutaneous (discoid) lupus erythematosus: Hypopigmentation and ulceration of the planum nasale and anterior muzzle of a dog.

V-11. Pemphigus foliaceus: Diffuse alopecia, excoriation, and crusting of the dorsal muzzle, anterior face, and medial pinnae of a dog.

V-12. Pemphigus vulgaris: Crusting at the mucocutaneous junction.

V-13. Bullous pemphigoid: Ulceration on the ventral area of a dog.

V-14. Juvenile cellulitis: Erythema, induration, and erosions in a young dog.

V-15. Sterile pyogranuloma: Interdigital dermatitis of an immune-mediated nature.

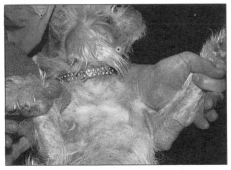

V-1

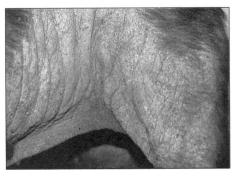

V-2

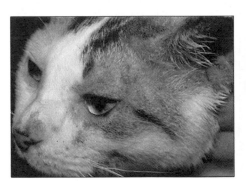

V-3

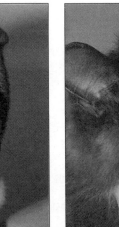

V-4

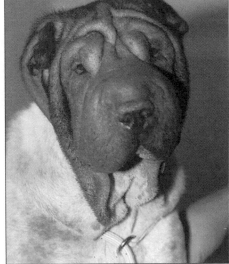

V-5

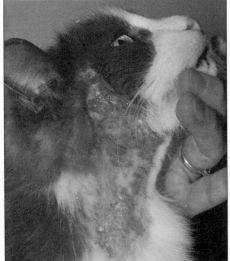

V-6

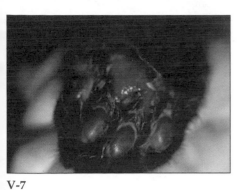

V-7

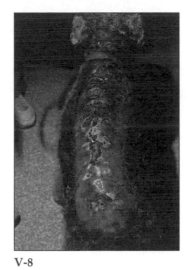

V-8

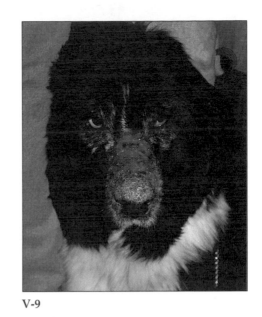

V-9

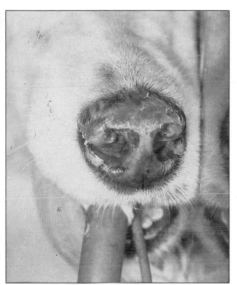

V-10

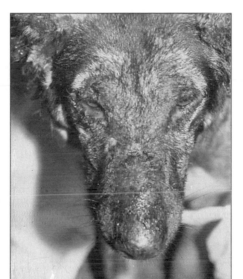

V-11

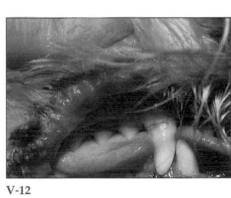

V-12

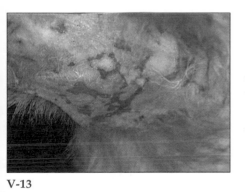

V-13

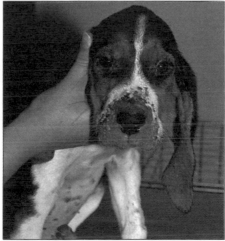

V-14

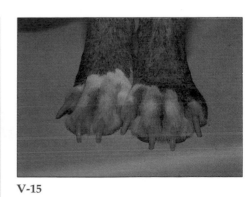

V-15

PLATE VI

VI-1. Hypothyroidism: Multifocal patches of hair loss and folliculitis.

VI-2. Hypothyroidism: Diffuse alopecia of perineum and posterior thighs of a dog.

VI-3. Hyperadrenocorticism: Total trunchal alopecia and hyperpigmentation.

VI-4. Hyperadrenocorticism: Calcinosis presenting as erythematous plaques in a dog.

VI-5. Adrenal sex hormone–related dermatosis (growth hormone–responsive dermatosis): Bilaterally symmetrical hair loss and intense hyperpigmentation.

VI-6. Hyperestrogenism: Partial alopecia and moderate hyperpigmentation of the perineum and posterior thigh of an intact female dog.

VI-7. Hypoestrogenism: Diffuse alopecia of ventral area and abnormal soft, smooth skin of a spayed weimaraner.

VI-8. Male feminizing syndrome: Bilaterally symmetrical alopecia, hyperpigmentation, and pendulous prepuce in a dog with a testicular Sertoli cell tumor.

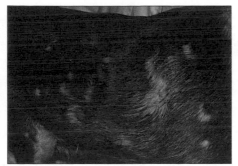

VI-1

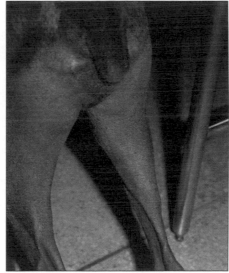

VI-2

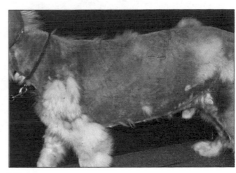

VI-3

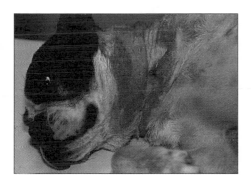

VI-4

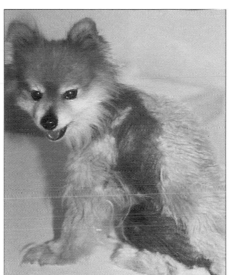

VI 5

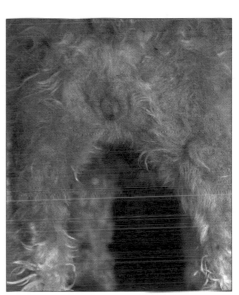

VI-6

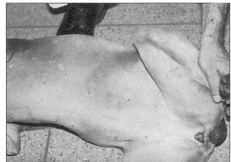

VI-7

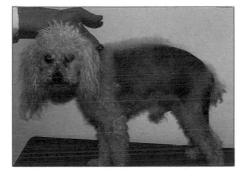

VI-8

PLATE VII

VII-1. Pyogranulomatous inflammation.

VII-2. *Blastomyces* organisms. (Sample courtesy of Judy Taylor, DVM, DVSc, University of Guelph.)

VII-3. Sarcoma from the lateral hock. (Sample courtesy of Judy Taylor, DVM, DVSc, University of Guelph.)

VII-4. Melanoma from the skin of a dog. (Sample courtesy of Judy Taylor, DVM, DVSc, University of Guelph.)

VII-5. Histiocytoma from the ear of a dog. (Sample courtesy of Judy Taylor, DVM, DVSc, University of Guelph.)

VII-6. Apocrine gland adenocarcinoma.

VII-7. Basal cell tumor with sebaceous differentiation. (Sample courtesy of Judy Taylor, DVM, DVSc, University of Guelph.)

VII-8. Deep granulomatous inflammation associated with a fungal infection.

VII-9. Most hormonal (endocrine) disorders cause the hair follicles to enter a resting (telogen) stage.

VII-10. Special stains may be used (e.g., PAS) to highlight certain cell types or microorganisms.

VII-11. Cancers may be identified histologically by the cell types involved.

VII-12. A biopsy allows the pathologist to evaluate all layers of the skin (epidermis, dermis, subcutaneous tissue, hair follicles, adnexa).

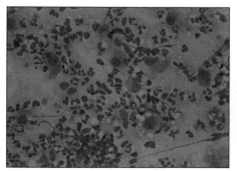

VII-1

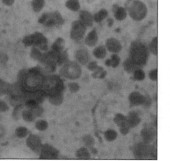

VII-2

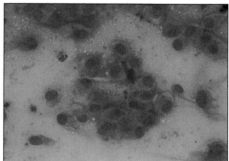

VII-3

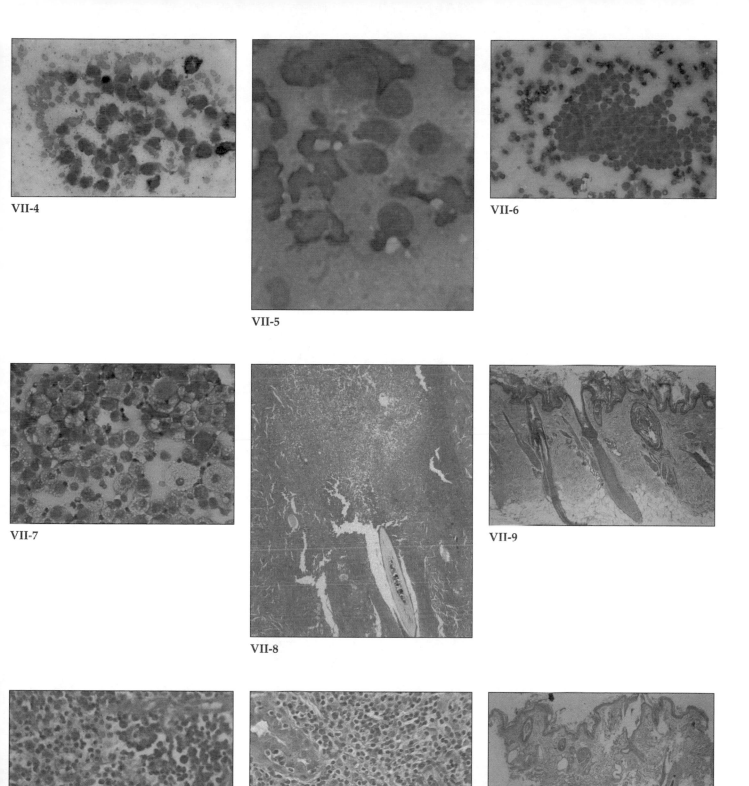

VII-4

VII-5

VII-6

VII-7

VII-8

VII-9

VII-10

VII-11

VII-12

PLATE VIII

VIII-1. Acanthosis nigricans: Axillary hyperpigmentation in a dachshund.

VIII-2. Acral lick dermatitis: Ulceration and induration on a limb.

VIII-3. Anal sac abscess: Taut abscess in the perineal region of a dog.

VIII-4. Indolent ulcer: Ulceration on the margins of the lips in a cat.

VIII-5. Indolent ulcer: Ulceration and thickening of the upper anterior lip of a cat. Note the eosinophilic granuloma on the hard palate *(arrow)*.

VIII-6. Eosinophilic plaque: Focal plaque with a moist, erythematous, ulcerative surface on the abdomen of a cat.

VIII-7. Linear granuloma: Linear pattern of multiple raised, dry, granulomatous lesions on the posterior thigh of a cat. (Courtesy of Paul Caciolo, St. Louis, Missouri.)

VIII-8. Canine lymphosarcoma: A dog with multiple discrete dermal nodules over the trunk and extremities.

VIII-9. Canine mast cell tumor: Solitary circumscribed tumor with a smooth surface on the stifle.

VIII-10. Feline mast cell tumor: Rapidly growing, ulcerated tumor on the face.

VIII-11. Nodular panniculitis: Multiple ulcerative draining subcutaneous nodules and associated crusting in the lateral flank and thigh regions of a dog.

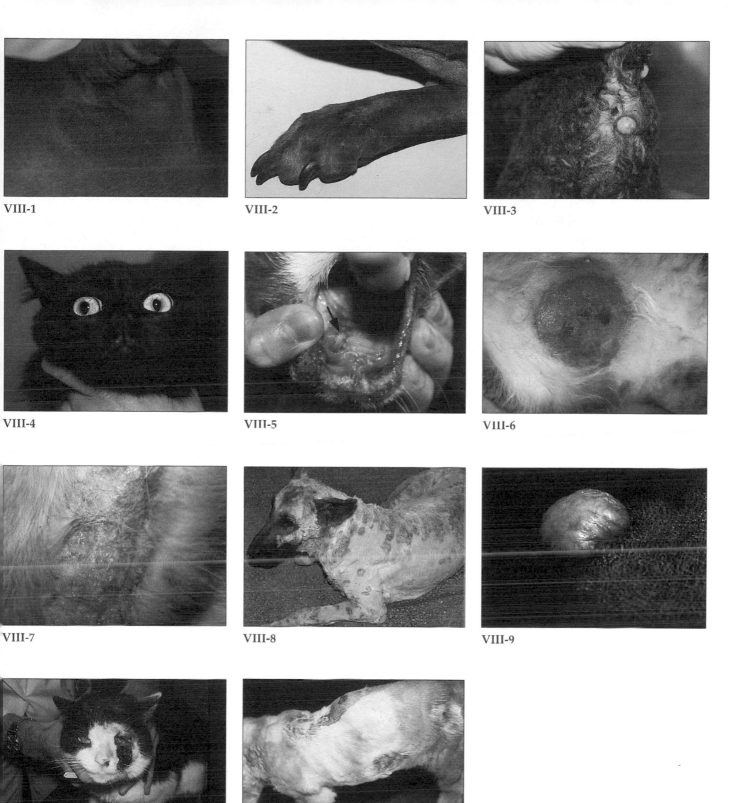

VIII-1

VIII-2

VIII-3

VIII-4

VIII-5

VIII-6

VIII-7

VIII-8

VIII-9

VIII-10

VIII-11

CHAPTER SIX

Diagnosis and Management of Endocrine Skin Disorders

*T*he endocrine system is a complex collection of glands that produce hormones and secrete them directly into the bloodstream. Some diseases (e.g., hypothyroidism) are caused when hormone levels are too low, some (e.g., Cushing's disease) are caused when levels are too high, and others (e.g., growth hormone–responsive dermatosis) may be an indirect reflection of disease.

Endocrine skin disorders discussed in this chapter include:

- Hypothyroidism
- Hyperadrenocorticism (Cushing's syndrome)
- Growth hormone–responsive dermatosis
- Sex hormone disorders

Most hormone systems have a negative feedback mechanism. When hormone levels in the blood are too high, the system stops producing hormones; when levels are too low, the system resumes production. For example, the hypothalamus produces a hormone (thyrotropin-releasing hormone [TRH]), which triggers release of another hormone (thyroid-stimulating hormone [TSH]) in the pituitary gland. TSH then triggers the release of actual thyroid hormones (thyroxine [T_4] and 3,5,3-triiodothyronine [T_3]). When thyroid hormone levels become too high, the process "turns off" until the levels become too low and the cycle starts over. This active process occurs every minute of every day for all hormones, complicating evaluation of hormone levels.

Because hormone levels in the blood fluctuate so widely throughout the day, one blood sample cannot be used as the basis for a diagnosis. Very often it is necessary to stimulate or suppress the system to see how high or low the levels can become or to perform more exacting tests.

HYPOTHYROIDISM

Hypothyroidism, a condition in which there are low levels of thyroid hormones in the blood, is the most commonly diagnosed endocrine disorder in dogs but is rare in cats.

TRH, which is produced in the hypothalamus of the brain, stimulates the pituitary gland, located at the base of the brain, to secrete another hormone, TSH. TSH stimulates the thyroid gland to produce two hormones, T_4 and T_3. Both of these hormones circulate in the blood tightly bound to proteins (principally albumin); only after being released are these now "free" hormones able to exert any effect. Approximately 99% of the hormone is tightly bound to protein and therefore is not active; only about 1% of the hormone is in its free active form. The bound portion serves as a reservoir of hormone, whereas the free portion actually does the work. At least one-third of all T$_4$ is later converted to T$_3$ or reverse T$_3$ (rT$_3$), mostly in the liver and kidneys. Although hypothyroidism may be attributable to low levels of either T$_4$ or T$_3$, T$_4$ is the more important hormone and the one most likely to cause hypothyroidism problems. This is true in spite of the fact that T$_3$ is three to four times more potent than T$_4$.

Common causes of hypothyroidism in dogs include:

- Lymphocytic thyroiditis—most common
- Idiopathic follicular atrophy (a degeneration of the thyroid tissue for no apparent reason)—second most common

Evidence now indicates that many cases of hypothyroidism have a genetic basis and many breeds are prone to developing hypothyroidism (see box at right). Thyroiditis usually starts between 1 and 3 years of age, progresses throughout middle age, and may only be clinically detectable later in life.

As animals lose thyroid reserve from continuing destruction of thyroid tissue, an important dynamic takes place. When the available or free levels of T$_4$ start to drop, the body compensates by having the pituitary gland secrete more TSH. This in turn results in production of more T$_4$. Because the levels of T$_4$ in the blood are normal, these animals often appear free of clinical signs and do not receive appropriate veterinary attention.

Many dogs evaluated for thyroid function have values that are not obviously hypothyroid or that are inconclusive. These dogs are referred to as having "borderline hypothyroidism," "nonthyroidal illness," or "euthyroid sick syndrome." Usually, the problem is not related to thyroid function. Many drugs (especially corticosteroids, sulfonamides, phenylbutazone, diphenylhydantoin, phenobarbital, diazepam, salicylates) profoundly influence the levels of thyroid hormones in circulation. In addition, any problem that causes animals not to eat properly for more than 2 days can dramatically affect thyroid hormone levels. Several diseases are also known to affect thyroid hormones levels (e.g., diabetes mellitus, Cushing's disease, kidney disease, liver disease, congestive heart failure). Animals with skin diseases are not more likely to have diminished thyroid function than those without skin problems, however. Because sex hormones can also profoundly affect testing, thyroid profiles are difficult to interpret in intact females up to 2 months following estrus (heat).

DOG BREEDS PRONE TO HYPOTHYROIDISM	
Afghan hound	Akita
Alaskan malamute	Boxer
Brittany spaniel	Chinese Shar pei
Chow chow	Cocker spaniel
Dachshund	Doberman pinscher
English bulldog	Golden retriever
Great Dane	Irish setter
Irish wolfhound	Newfoundland
Pomeranian	Poodle
Schnauzer	Vizsla

Clinical Signs

There are many misconceptions about the clinical signs associated with hypothyroidism in dogs and how it is best diagnosed. Roughly one-third of hypothyroid dogs do not have any skin problems. Despite the attention it receives, obesity is only rarely associated with hypothyroidism. Dogs often appear entirely normal until they have completely used up their reserve of thyroid hormone, which may take several years. The most common clinical signs of hypothyroidism in dogs are lethargy and recurrent infections.

When dogs have skin problems associated with hypothyroidism, hair loss and cutaneous infections are commonly seen (see Plate VI-1 and VI-2). The hair loss is noninflammatory and often bilaterally symmetrical. In large-breed dogs hair loss can involve the limbs, whereas in most other dogs it is confined to the trunk. Bacterial infections such as staphylococcal folliculitis may be associated with hypothyroidism because of an immune deficit.

Hypothyroidism is very rare in cats. Although congenital thyroid defects occur, most cases are the result of surgical removal of the thyroid glands as treatment for hyperthyroidism, a much more common feline disorder.

Diagnosis
Ancillary Tests

Over 50% of hypothyroid dogs have high blood cholesterol and often increased triglycerides and lipoproteins. A small percentage of affected dogs are anemic.

Measurement of total T_4 and T_3 is easy to perform and inexpensive but unreliable, because thyroid hormone levels fluctuate greatly throughout the day. At any one time thyroid levels may be normal in 30% to 60% of hypothyroid dogs and abnormal in 20% of normal dogs. This measurement also cannot detect dogs in early stages of disease in which the T_4 and T_3 levels are still in the normal range. T_3 should not be used alone to diagnose hypothyroidism because it is a poor measure of glandular function. Most T_3 is created by peripheral conversion from T_4. It is also the hormone most affected by nonthyroidal illnesses.

There is also some variation in normal thyroid levels related to age, breed, and sex. Puppies have total thyroxine concentrations two to five times the normal adult concentrations until about 4 months of age. After that time, levels continuously decrease with age. There is also some breed variability, and the greyhound has been shown to have lower T_4 levels and higher T_3 levels than mixed-breed dogs. As a general rule, small-breed dogs have higher concentrations of T_4 than do larger breeds. Finally, concentrations of T_4 and T_3 are consistently higher in bitches that are pregnant or in diestrus.

Radioimmunoassays

Radioimmunoassays (RIAs) are used at commercial laboratories for evaluating thyroid hormone levels. An enzyme-linked immunosorbent assay (ELISA) has been designed for in-clinic semiquantitative T_4 evaluation (CITE Semi-Quant T_4 Test—IDEXX). Although the assay has less sensitivity and greater variability than RIA, the convenience makes it an option worth considering for routine screening.

Free T_4 and T_3 Screening

Free T_4 and free T_3 tests measuring the active levels of T_4 and T_3 available to the tissues are done by specialized laboratories. Since only 1% of total serum levels are actually free hormone, the assay requires a relatively large quantity of serum (3 ml, RTT [red top tube]). Free levels are a much more sensitive indicator of hypothyroidism than are total levels, which fluctuate greatly throughout the day. Recent studies question, however, whether free levels of thyroid hormones provide more information about thyroid gland function than do total levels.

TSH STIMULATION TESTING
1. Collect blood for baseline serum levels of T_4 and T_3 (1 ml serum, RTT).
2. Reconstitute TSH with diluent provided.
3. Inject 0.1 IU TSH/kg IV.
4. Collect poststimulation samples (1 ml serum, RTT) 6 hours later if TSH was given IV, 8 to 12 hours later if TSH was given IM.
5. Carefully mark serum samples "pre" and "post" and forward to laboratory.
6. Levels in animals with hypothyroidism do not rise adequately in response to TSH. Normal animals meet or exceed normal limits set by testing laboratory.

TSH Stimulation Testing (see box above)

TSH stimulation is regarded as the classic diagnostic test for hypothyroidism because it measures the maximum output of thyroid hormones after stimulation of the thyroid gland. Baseline serum T_4 and T_3 levels are determined, TSH is injected intravenously, and a second blood sample is obtained in 4 to 6 hours. If the TSH was administered intramuscularly, the second sample should be collected in 8 to 12 hours. This test is useful as it measures the ability of the thyroid gland to respond to maximal stimulation, although TSH is expensive and difficult to obtain. It is less helpful in diagnosing secondary (pituitary) or tertiary (hypothalamic) causes of hypothyroidism, but these are quite rare compared with primary hypothyroidism. Once the TSH has been reconstituted, it can be refrigerated for up to 3 weeks to maintain its potency. Freezing can probably extend the potency of the product for up to 3 months, but this has not been rigorously studied.

TRH Stimulation Testing (see box on p. 140, left)

TRH stimulation is occasionally used when a stimulation test is required and TSH is not available (periodically, TSH has been in short supply and difficult to acquire). The TRH stimulates the pituitary gland to release TSH, which in turn stimulates the thyroid gland to release T_4 and T_3. TRH administration is not without risk; salivation, vomiting, tachycardia, tachypnea, pupillary dilatation, urination and defecation have all been reported. Apparently, short-term freezing (up to 3 months) does not adversely affect the potency of TRH.

TRH STIMULATION TESTING

1. Collect blood for baseline serum levels of T_4 and T_3 (1 ml, RTT).
2. Reconstitute TRH with diluent provided.
3. Inject 0.1 mg/kg TRH IV for dogs and 0.02 mg/kg for cats.
4. For dogs collect poststimulation sample (1 ml, RTT) 4 to 8 hours later. For cats collect second sample in 6 hours.
5. Carefully mark serum samples "pre" and "post" and forward to laboratory.
6. Levels in animals with hypothyroidism do not rise adequately in response to TRH. Normal animals meet or exceed normal limits. Postinjection levels may not be as high as those seen with TSH.

K VALUES PAIRING T_4 AND TSH STIMULATION

1. Collect blood for baseline serum levels of T_4 (1 ml, RTT).
2. Reconstitute TSH (e.g., Dermathycin—Burroughs Wellcome, Thytropar—Rorer) with diluent provided.
3. Inject 2.5 IU TSH intravenously in small dogs (less than 20 kg), 5.0 IU in large dogs (more than 20 kg).
4. Collect poststimulation sample 4 to 8 hours later (1 ml, RTT).
5. Carefully mark serum samples "pre" and "post" and forward to laboratory for assessment of T_4 levels.
6. Calculate $K = 0.5 \times$ baseline T_4 (nmol/L) + (T_4 poststimulation [nmol/L] – T_4 prestimulation [nmol/L]).
7. K less than 15 suggests hypothyroidism. Dogs with K above 30 are considered normal or unlikely to respond to treatment.

Predictive Formulas

Predictive formulas (K values; see box at right) have been proposed to increase the likelihood of correctly diagnosing hypothyroidism in dogs, but their ultimate usefulness is not definitively known. These formulas combine the results of two or more tests to provide a more balanced assessment. It is unlikely that they provide any greater insight into thyroid function than do other appropriate individual tests. It is important to calculate all values based on the units specified.

A second predictive formula proposes an association between free levels of T_4 and cholesterol as it is known that over 50% of hypothyroid dogs have elevated cholesterol levels. In this version of the formula:

$$K = 0.7 \times \text{Free } T_4 \text{ (pmol/L)} - \text{Cholesterol (mmol/L)}$$

Hypothyroid dogs often have K values of less than –4, whereas those with values greater than +1 are considered normal or unlikely to respond to treatment. The real value of these predictive formulas is still a matter of debate.

Measurement of Thyroid Autoantibodies

Thyroid autoantibodies refer to serum antibody levels directed against thyroid antigens, the thyroid hormones, and thyroglobulin. These can be measured on serum samples (1.5 ml, RTT) taken from hypothyroid "suspects" or from breeds at risk of developing autoantibody-associated hypothyroidism. Great Danes, Irish setters, and Old English sheepdogs having an increased occurrence of autoantibodies. High levels of autoantibody only indicate risk; they do not confirm a diagnosis. Roughly 50% to 60% of hypothyroid dogs have antithyroglobulin antibodies. The presence of antithyroglobulin antibodies (ATAs) alone is not an indicator of hypothyroidism; it merely suggests the presence of lymphocytic thyroiditis.

Autoantibody levels alone do not confirm a diagnosis but can be useful as part of a genetic screening program. Together with other thyroid profiles, the presence of anti–thyroid hormone antibodies might suggest a breeding prospect be reconsidered. It can also be used to screen animals at risk of developing the disease. Animals with normal thyroid function tests but antithyroid antibodies should be further screened every 6 months for onset of disease.

Dogs can also have circulating autoantibody that targets the thyroid hormones, especially T_3. Anti–thyroid hormone antibodies alone do not cause hypothyroidism. There is usually a compensatory increase in TRH and TSH. In dogs with T_3 autoantibodies but normal T_4 levels a compensatory mechanism appears to maintain normal levels of T_3 not bound to T_3 autoantibodies. In dogs with low total T_4, this mechanism is not operative and the presence of T_3 autoantibodies may actually aggravate the hypothyroid state. It is important to note that high circulating levels of these autoantibodies can interfere with RIA of regular thyroid hormones. They can bind a fraction of the radiolabeled hormone used in the procedure. Therefore, if routine RIA measurement reveals high levels of T_3 or T_4 in a patient, the presence of anti–thyroid hormone antibodies should be suspected.

TSH Assay

TSH assay is regularly used as a reliable test in humans, but a suitable canine and/or feline version is not available at present. Unfortunately, human test kits cannot reliably measure canine TSH and therefore are not useful.

Reverse T₃ Testing

Reverse T_3 is not a commonly run test of thyroid function but circulating levels are often increased when thyroid levels are decreased by processes other than thyroid disease. It is periodically used when thyroid levels are less than normal but hypothyroidism is not considered to be the primary disease state.

Treatment (see box at right)

Fortunately, treatment of hypothyroidism is simple, inexpensive, and very successful. It involves supplementing the hormone (T_4) that is lacking. Doses can be calculated based on body weight (20 µg/kg bid) or by body surface area (0.5 mg/m²). Supplementation with T_3 alone may provide sufficient hormone for most organs, but the brain and pituitary gland derive most of their T_3 from T_4 and may still manifest a deficiency. Therefore neither T_3 nor any combination product (including both thyroxine and triiodothyronine) is regularly used in the treatment of hypothyroidism.

Typically, patients are reevaluated after 6 weeks of therapy, with thyroid levels measured 4 to 8 hours after the morning dose is given (the time thyroid hormones are at their highest). Hair growth may be evident at 6 weeks, but several months are required for complete hair regrowth. For animals with recurrent skin infections, antibiotic therapy and hormone replacement should resolve the problem by 6 weeks. If levels are well into normal range, once daily dosing may be considered but most dogs are maintained on twice daily treatment for life. Levels should be measured annually to insure maintenance of the normal range and that the dosage does not require alteration.

TREATMENT REGIMEN FOR HYPOTHYROIDISM IN DOGS

1. Commence treatment with thyroxine on a twice daily schedule.
2. Measure thyroxine levels in 6 weeks. Blood should be collected between 4 to 8 hours after the morning dose was given.
3. Dosage and frequency of medication are adjusted as necessary.
4. Repeat thyroid profile annually. Alter medication as required.

Dogs sometimes benefit from thyroid replacement therapy even if they are not clinically hypothyroid because of the effects of thyroid hormones on other circulating hormones. Also, thyroid hormones may be involved in the regulation of fatty acid activity in serum as well as in the skin. In these dogs the improvement seen with replacement therapy is usually temporary.

HYPERADRENOCORTICISM (CUSHING'S DISEASE)

Hyperadrenocorticism, commonly called Cushing's disease or Cushing's syndrome, describes a condition in which the body produces too much cortisol, its own form of cortisone. Cortisol is produced in the adrenal glands, which are located at the top poles of the kidneys. Other hormones (including small amounts of sex hormones) are also produced by these glands.

The adrenals work on a negative feedback mechanism. When blood levels of cortisol are below normal, the hypothalamus releases corticotropin-releasing factor (CRF). The pituitary then releases adrenocorticotropic hormone (ACTH), which in turn causes the adrenals to release cortisol into the blood.

Hyperadrenocorticism can result from hyperactive diseases of the pituitary, hypothalamus, or adrenals. In addition, animals stressed by such chronic conditions as diabetes mellitus, liver disease, and kidney disease may have higher than "normal" cortisol levels. This is attributed to an adaptive change in the regulation of cortisol. Of the cases of natural Cushing's disease in dogs roughly 85% are caused by pituitary tumors and 15% are caused by tumors of the adrenal glands. These tumors are not necessarily malignant. In fact, most pituitary tumors are benign but result in

---

**DOG BREEDS PRONE TO
HYPERADRENOCORTICISM**

Boxer
Boston terrier
Poodle
Dachshund

---

the hypersecretion of ACTH, which in turn results in high levels of cortisol. About half of the adrenal tumors are malignant and half are benign. A list of dog breeds prone to hyperadrenocorticism is presented in the box above. In cats most cases are attributable to benign pituitary adenomas, though pituitary carcinomas have been reported.

Not all cases of Cushing's syndrome are attributable to natural causes. Hyperadrenocorticism that results from the administration of corticosteroid drugs is called iatrogenic Cushing's syndrome. Iatrogenic Cushing's syndrome can follow the use of injectable corticosteroids, tablets, liquids, eye drops, or topical preparations. The constant administration of corticosteroid-containing medications causes decreased ACTH stimulation because of negative feedback. This in turn results in adrenal atrophy and the inability of the adrenals to produce sufficient amounts of cortisol. Iatrogenic Cushing's syndrome is rare in the cat. Even injectable corticosteroids such as methylprednisolone acetate are unlikely to alter the hypothalamic-pituitary-adrenal (HPA) axis if used conservatively. Megestrol acetate (e.g., Ovaban®—Schering-Plough Animal Health) is capable of causing iatrogenic hyperadrenocorticism. As it is not licensed for use in the cat and is less frequently prescribed than in the past, fewer cases are being reported.

Clinical Signs

Hyperadrenocorticism can have many different effects on animals, with some more tolerant of changes in blood cortisols than others. Some animals are affected immediately, whereas others may have the condition for years before changes are evident. About two-thirds of cushingoid dogs have increased thirst (polydipsia), increased urination (polyuria), and increased hunger (polyphagia) associated with their disease. Perhaps as many as half of the cases have bilaterally symmetric alopecia that is not associated with any inflammation (see Plate VI-3). High blood pressure is

seen in approximately 60% of cases. Because corticosteroids interfere with the body's immune responses, affected dogs are often more susceptible to infection. Other clinical signs that might be seen include thinning of the skin, plugged hair follicles (comedones) on the underside, muscle atrophy, calcinosis cutis (see Plate VI-4), hepatomegaly resulting from fatty deposits, muscle weakness, exercise intolerance, and abnormal behavior. More bizarre symptoms may be evident if animals have large tumors associated with the disease that press on surrounding organs, especially within the brain.

In cats the clinical signs are often significantly different from those of dogs. One of the most common dermatologic manifestations of hyperadrenocorticism in cats is fragile skin. This can result in tearing of the skin or easy bruising. There may be partial or complete alopecia of the ventral area and/or flanks. Recurrent abscessation may also be a manifestation of Cushing's syndrome. Other possible changes include prominent superficial blood vessels, comedones, and hyperpigmentation.

Diagnosis

Hyperadrenocorticism can be suspected from the history, clinical signs, blood and urine test results, and skin biopsy, but confirmation requires measuring specific levels of the different hormones involved in this condition. A diagnosis is rarely possible with only one cortisol value. Often it is necessary to take a baseline measurement and then either stimulate or suppress the system to see how high or low the levels become.

Once the diagnosis of hyperadrenocorticism has been confirmed, the disease process must be localized to either the pituitary gland (hypophysis) or the adrenal gland.

Screening Tests for Cushing's Disease

Ancillary tests are often very helpful when Cushing's syndrome is suspected because so many different organ systems are affected by corticosteroid excess. Some findings that are suggestive of canine Cushing's disease include:

- Recurrent urinary tract infections
- Hyperglycemia
- Hypercholesterolemia
- Increased liver enzymes (serum alkaline phosphatase, serum alanine transaminase)

ACTH STIMULATION TESTING

In Dogs

1. Collect a blood sample (1 ml serum or plasma, RTT or GTT) for baseline cortisol.
2. Warm ACTH gel in vial by rolling gently in your hands or by immersing in warm (not hot) water. If synthetic ACTH is used, reconstitute it with diluent.
3. Aspirate liquified ACTH into syringe and administer 2.2 IU/kg to a maximum of 40 IU IM. If synthetic ACTH is used, inject 0.25 mg IM.
4. Collect second sample (1 ml serum or plasma, RTT or GTT) 2 hours later if ACTH gel was used and 1 hour later if synthetic ACTH was used and forward to laboratory.
5. Cortisol levels elevated significantly above the normal range for the laboratory suggest Cushing's syndrome but do not localize the disease process to pituitary gland or adrenal gland.

In Cats

1. Collect a blood sample (1 ml serum or plasma, RTT or GTT) for baseline cortisol.
2. Warm ACTH gel in vial by rolling gently in your hands or by immersing in warm (not hot) water. If synthetic ACTH is used, reconstitute it with diluent.
3. Aspirate liquified ACTH into syringe and administer 2.2 IU/kg to a maximum of 20 IU IM. If synthetic ACTH is used, inject 0.125 mg IM or IV.
4. Collect second sample (1 ml serum plasma, RTT or GTT) 2 hours later if ACTH gel was used and 45 to 60 minutes later if synthetic product was injected and forward to laboratory.
5. Cortisol levels elevated significantly above the normal range for the laboratory suggest Cushing's syndrome but do not localize the disease process to pituitary gland or adrenal gland.

Serum alkaline phosphatase and cholesterol levels are elevated in about 80% of canine cases. Although glucose levels may be elevated in about 50% of dogs with Cushing's syndrome, overt diabetes mellitus is only seen in about 15% of cases. Insulin resistance and glucose intolerance associated with hyperadrenocorticism sometimes resolve with proper treatment of the Cushing's syndrome. In dogs with limited pancreatic reserve, however, diabetes mellitus becomes a more likely sequela. A stress leukogram may also be evident in affected dogs. Finally, 85% of dogs with hyperadrenocorticism have dilute urine (specific gravity less than 1.007).

Cats with hyperadrenocorticism appear to be predisposed to hyperglycemia, hypercholesterolemia, and diabetes mellitus. Also, cats are not as likely as dogs to have significant elevations of serum alkaline phosphatase (evident in only 30% of feline cases) or serum alanine transaminase.

Radiographs might reveal hepatomegaly, osteoporosis, abnormal calcium deposits in tissues, or even calcified adrenal tumors. It is important to realize that mineral deposits occur often in the adrenal glands of cats and are not necessarily associated with Cushing's syndrome. Hypertension is present in about 60% of cushingoid dogs. Evaluations of this parameter will become more routine as instruments for measuring blood pressure become more commonplace in veterinary clinics. Elevated blood pressure can lead to thromboembolism, hypertension within the kidney, and congestive heart failure. Although hypertension sometimes resolves if the hyperadrenocorticism is successfully managed, antihypertensive medication is required in most cases. Although rarely available to veterinary practitioners, computerized tomography (CT) has been used to differentiate bilateral adrenal hyperplasia from unilateral adrenal neoplasia. Contrast-enhanced CT has even demonstrated pituitary masses.

Baseline cortisol levels are rarely diagnostic because levels fluctuate on a minute-to-minute basis and do not remain consistently elevated. A diagnosis can only be determined if the baseline cortisol is elevated significantly. Most laboratories process either serum or plasma to yield cortisol values.

ACTH stimulation (see box above) is a useful test because, although cortisol values fluctuate greatly throughout the day, an injection of ACTH stimulates the adrenals maximally to release their content of cortisol. This provides the likely "high point" that cortisols would achieve. Only increased adrenal mass can explain hypercortisolemia following ACTH injection. Increased adrenal mass could result from an ACTH-secreting pituitary tumor or from a neoplastic adrenal

LOW DOSE DEXAMETHASONE SUPPRESSION TESTING

In Dogs

1. Collect a blood sample (1 ml serum or plasma, RTT or GTT) for baseline cortisol.
2. Inject dexamethasone IV at 0.01 mg/kg.
3. Collect a blood sample (1 ml serum or plasma, RTT or GTT) for cortisol 3 to 4 hours after injection.
4. Collect a blood sample (1 ml serum or plasma, RTT or GTT) for cortisol 6 to 8 hours after injection.
5. The 6 to 8 hour cortisol value is most likely to be diagnostic. The sample taken at 3 to 4 hours demonstrates those animals whose levels are suppressed initially but eventually rebound by the end of the test.

In Cats

1. Collect a blood sample (1 ml serum or plasma, RTT or GTT) for baseline cortisol.
2. Inject dexamethasone IV at 0.01 mg/kg.
3. Collect a blood sample (1 ml serum or plasma, RTT or GTT) for cortisol 6 to 8 hours after injection.
4. Cats with non–adrenal-related illnesses (e.g., diabetes mellitus, chronic renal disease, congestive heart failure) may have inadequate suppression of cortisol with the low dose test.

gland. Some dogs with chronic diseases such as diabetes mellitus may have moderately enlarged adrenal glands as an adaptive process. ACTH stimulation is diagnostic about 85% of the time in dogs but less so in cats. Some drawbacks are that the adrenals of patients with iatrogenic Cushing's syndrome cannot be stimulated (because of negative feedback) and many animals with adrenal tumors fail to hyperrespond. The test also fails to differentiate between disease of the pituitary and disease of the adrenal gland. The main advantages are that ACTH stimulation testing is quick (less than 2 hours), inexpensive, and is the test of choice when monitoring therapy. It therefore provides a handy baseline.

Low dose dexamethasone suppression testing (see box above) measures how much the cortisol levels can be suppressed by a single, moderate burst of corticosteroid. Suppression in normal animals should result in quite low levels and should be maintained for at least 8 hours. Animals with increased adrenal mass attributable to tumors of either the adrenal gland or pituitary should recover from suppression more quickly or their levels may not be suppressed at all. The levels in roughly one-third of dogs with pituitary-dependent Cushing's disease initially are suppressed but rebound by 8 hours. The test is considered about 90% diagnostic, and normal dogs show significant suppression of cortisol levels for at least 8 hours. In dogs with Cushing's disease levels have recovered by that time, even if they were suppressed initially.

Dexamethasone suppression–ACTH stimulation testing was proposed as a combination test that could aid in the diagnosis of hyperadrenocorticism and the localization of the disease process. Unfortunately, the results of this test are often confusing and ambiguous and it is no longer recommended.

Urine cortisol:creatinine ratios provide a simple and quick screening test for Cushing's syndrome. The sensitivity of the test is excellent but the specificity of the test is quite low (about 25%). Therefore, although an increased urine corticosteroid-to-creatinine ratio does not diagnose Cushing's disease always, a normal value makes a diagnosis of Cushing's disease most unlikely. The test is performed by collecting a single voided urine sample, which is submitted to a diagnostic laboratory for determinations of urine cortisol and urine creatinine. These are performed with the same test kits used with serum samples. When both values are compared (in μmol/L), cortisol to creatinine ratios greater than 13.5 are considered diagnostic for Cushing's disease.

Alkaline phosphatase isoenzyme refers to a specific corticosteroid-induced isoenzyme of serum alkaline phosphatase in dogs. It is produced in the bile canalicular membranes of liver cells and tends to be associated with diseases causing hepatic lipidosis. This may be a convenient screening test but is not specific for Cushing's syndrome. Normal levels, however, suggest that a diagnosis of Cushing's disease is unlikely.

HIGH DOSE DEXAMETHASONE SUPPRESSION TEST

1. Collect a blood sample (1 ml serum or plasma, RTT or GTT) for baseline cortisol.
2. Inject dexamethasone IV at 0.1 to 1.0 mg/kg.
3. Collect a blood sample (1 ml serum or plasma, RTT or GTT) for cortisol 6 to 8 hours after injection.
4. Submit samples to laboratory for cortisol determinations. Appropriately label as "pre" and "post."
5. Animals whose levels are suppressed completely likely have pituitary disease. Those with adrenal cancers are least likely to show suppression. This test may be the best screening test for Cushing's disease in the cat.

METYRAPONE SUPPRESSION TESTING

1. Collect a blood sample (1 ml serum or plasma, RTT or GTT) for baseline cortisol and 11-DOC.
2. Give oral metyrapone at 25 mg/kg every 6 hours for four doses.
3. Collect a blood sample for cortisol and 11-DOC (1 ml serum or plasma, RTT or GTT) 6 hours after giving the last dose of metyrapone.
4. In cases of pituitary-dependent hyperadrenocorticism 11-DOC levels increase and serum cortisol levels decrease. In cases of adrenocortical tumor plasma cortisol decreases with no change in 11-DOC levels.

ENDOGENOUS ACTH ASSAY

1. Chill plastic blood tubes on ice.
2. Collect blood (12 ml) in chilled plastic tubes. If collected with glass tubes, quickly transfer to chilled plastic tubes.
3. Centrifuge at room temperature for 5 minutes.
4. Remove plasma from tubes and freeze it.
5. Ship by overnight service to laboratory, using freezer packs to keep samples cold.

Differentiating Pituitary from Adrenal Disease

The most common test used to distinguish between pituitary and adrenal disease is the high dose dexamethasone suppression test (see box above). The test is similar to the low dose dexamethasone suppression test but a much higher dose of corticosteroid is given. The premise is that tumors in the adrenals are more resistant to suppression by corticosteroid than are tumors in the pituitary. This test should only be used in animals in which the diagnosis of Cushing's disease has already been made. It must be used cautiously in diabetic animals because ketoacidosis, a serious complication of diabetes, can result from the higher dosage of corticosteroid administered.

Metyrapone suppression testing (see first box at right) is based on the premise that metyrapone suppresses an enzyme (11-beta-hydroxylase) that converts 11-deoxycortisol (11-DOC) to cortisol. Oral metyrapone (Metopirone®—CIBA Pharmaceuticals) is administered to animals and 11-DOC levels are then measured. Elevated levels of 11-DOC suggest pituitary disease; little or no change suggests an adrenal tumor.

Endogenous ACTH assay (see second box at right) is technically difficult to perform, but it does help differentiate pituitary from adrenal disease in confirmed Cushing's cases. It is important that the preliminary tests confirm the diagnosis because there is marked crossover between normal animals and those with pituitary-dependent Cushing's disease. In cushingoid dogs ACTH levels are elevated in pituitary-dependent disease and markedly decreased in adrenal-dependent disease. One of the major difficulties with this test is the careful sample handling that is required.

Treatment

Even though Cushing's disease is caused by a tumor in either the brain or the adrenal, there are many successful treatment options available. In humans both causes are treated surgically, but very few facilities are capable of performing pituitary microsurgery on dogs.

Mitotane (o,p′-DDD; Lysodren®—Bristol-Myers Oncology) is the most commonly used drug to treat pituitary-dependent hyperadrenocorticism. It is a selective toxin for the adrenal cortex and destroys the capability of the adrenal gland to produce too much cortisol. It does not address the problems in the pituitary gland.

**KETOCONAZOLE THERAPY
FOR CUSHING'S DISEASE**

1. Administer ketoconazole (Nizoral®—Janssen Pharmaceutica) orally at 10 mg/kg bid for 7 to 10 days.
2. Perform ACTH stimulation test and adjust dosage as necessary.
3. If more than 30 mg/kg is required to control cortisol levels, ketoconazole is not sufficient or there is inadequate absorption. Confirm malabsorption by collecting blood sample for ketoconazole levels 3 to 4 hours after administration.
4. If malabsorption of ketoconazole is confirmed, dissolve 400 mg ketoconazole in 10 ml of 0.1 M hydrochloric acid. Administer proper dosage in 30 ml of distilled, deionized water.

**MAINTAINING CORTISOL HOMEOSTASIS
DURING ADRENAL SURGERY**

1. Patient must be on intravenous fluids throughout surgery.
2. Administer intraoperative corticosteroids (3 to 5 mg dexamethasone or 25 to 50 mg prednisolone sodium succinate).
3. On first postoperative day, give prednisone 0.5 mg/kg bid.
4. Taper dosage to 0.2 mg/kg by end of first week.
5. Gradually wean off all medication by end of month.

Treatment is divided into (1) an induction stage and (2) a maintenance stage. Initially, the drug is given daily for a week; then an ACTH stimulation test is done to determine the status of cortisol production. Usually, 1 week of daily treatment is sufficient, and the maintenance stage consists of once a week therapy thereafter. Too much medication is potentially dangerous, and monitoring of cortisol levels is important. An ACTH stimulation test is done 3 months into treatment and then every 6 to 12 months after that. Most of the clinical problems associated with the disease should be resolved 3 months into therapy; if not, reevaluation is critical. If any side effects (e.g., vomiting, diarrhea, weakness, ataxia) are caused by oversuppression of cortisol levels, small amounts of prednisolone can be given or the treatment dose of mitotane can be altered. Some dogs become more resistant to mitotane with long-term use. As dogs are maintained for months and years, the dosage often needs to be increased and the interval may need to be shortened to twice weekly or even daily. Changes are made if cortisol values continue to climb during therapy. Mitotane is a chlorinated hydrocarbon and must be used cautiously in cats.

Ketoconazole, a drug more commonly used to treat deep fungal infections, is another potential treatment for pituitary-dependent Cushing's disease in dogs (see box above). In addition to its antifungal activity, it inhibits gonadal and adrenal steroid synthesis. It can also be used to stabilize dogs with adrenal tumors presurgically and as an alternative in animals that are resistant to or intolerant of mitotane. The disadvantage is that its effect on cortisol levels is transient, and so this somewhat expensive drug must be given twice daily rather than once weekly for maintenance. Ketoconazole is not effective for treatment of cats with Cushing's syndrome. Metyrapone has been used experimentally in cats and is another treatment option.

Adrenal tumors account for less than 15% of cases, and about half of those are malignant. Adrenal tumors should be surgically removed, if possible, but the surgery is not without risk. When the cancerous gland is removed, animals can go into shock and their blood levels of cortisol can drop precipitously. This is prevented by keeping patients on fluids containing corticosteroids before, during, and following surgery (see box above). Oral corticosteroids are used for about a month until the other, usually atrophied, adrenal gland has had time to recover and is producing sufficient amounts of cortisol. Unfortunately, about half of all dogs surviving surgery eventually succumb to complications including kidney failure, pneumonia, and thromboembolism. These animals probably have been released too soon from the hospital, more often a financial decision than a medical one.

GROWTH HORMONE–RESPONSIVE/ADRENAL SEX HORMONE–RELATED DERMATOSIS

Growth hormone–responsive dermatosis is a controversial endocrine disorder because the evidence that the primary problem is related to growth hormone is not very convincing. In fact, there is mounting evidence that the cause of the problem is actually aberrant adrenal sex steroids. Growth hormone is not regulated by the same thermostat-like negative feedback as are the thyroid and adrenal hormones but rather by intermediate insulin-like growth factors called somatomedins.

Growth hormone–responsive dermatosis was so named because it responded to treatment with growth hormone. In at least some dogs, however, it appears that a partial adrenal enzyme defect may be the actual culprit. Negative feedback would result in the excessive production of androgens by the adrenals. Much research remains to be done before any real conclusions can be made. In the interim, many now refer to the condition as "adrenal sex hormone–related dermatosis."

Clinical Signs

Males are much more commonly affected than females, and most affected animals are quite young, often 1 to 3 years of age. Various breeds are affected, but those predisposed include the chow chow, pomeranian, poodle, Airedale, Samoyed, American water spaniel, and keeshond. Affected animals start to lose hair on their trunks but the legs and head remain relatively spared. In time, the skin often becomes quite dark in the areas of hair loss (see Plate VI-5).

Diagnosis

Growth hormone stimulation testing (see box at right) is the most common diagnostic test used for this condition. (Because the ultimate cause has not been proven, this test is not helpful in all cases.) Drugs are given that stimulate maximal secretion of growth hormone, and the diagnosis is confirmed in those animals whose hormone levels are not stimulated adequately.

Sex hormone levels (especially those of sex hormones produced by the adrenal glands) have recently been implicated in so-called growth hormone–responsive dermatosis. Dehydroepiandrosterone sulfate (DHEA-S) and androstenedione are increased in many cases. In pomeranians the defect appears to be similar to late-onset 21-hydroxylase deficiency in humans.

Somatomedin C is a growth hormone intermediary, which may be reduced in cases of growth hormone–responsive dermatosis. At present, testing for this is not available from most diagnostic laboratories.

GROWTH HORMONE STIMULATION TESTING

1. Collect blood samples for baseline growth hormone levels.

2. Administer growth hormone stimulant, either xylazine (100 to 300 µg/kg IV), human growth hormone–releasing factor (1 to 5 µg/kg), or clonidine hydrochloride (10 mg/kg).

3. Collect postadministration blood samples at 15, 30, 45, and 60 minutes.

4. Send samples to specialized laboratories that perform this test. Affected animals have very low levels of growth hormone.

Treatment

Therapy of growth hormone–responsive dermatosis can be directed at correcting either growth hormone or sex hormone levels. Because the condition does not affect the health of the animal, treatment is only indicated for cosmetic reasons. Neutering is always an excellent recommendation; chow chows and Samoyeds respond especially well to this form of therapy.

Growth hormone can be used in therapy, but it is scarce and quite expensive. Although many regimens exist, growth hormone is usually administered twice weekly for 6 weeks or every other day for 3 weeks. Hair growth is expected within about 3 months. Treatment with growth hormone is not without risk, and diabetes mellitus may result because of the effect on insulin levels. Therefore blood glucose levels should be monitored throughout treatment.

Ketoconazole has been shown to affect sex hormone levels and has successfully managed cases of growth hormone–responsive dermatosis. Undoubtedly, its effect on adrenal hormones is the reason for its success.

Mitotane (Lysodren®—Bristol-Myers Oncology) is receiving attention for its success in treating cases of growth hormone–responsive dermatosis. It is likely effective because it modifies the interaction of hormones at hair follicle receptors, stimulating hair follicle growth. Mitotane has been particularly helpful in pomeranians, in which an adrenal enzyme deficiency has been documented. Treatment is usually initiated with an induction dose of 15 to 25 mg/kg/day for 5 to 7 days, following which maintenance therapy is instituted with 15 to 25 mg/kg every 7 to 14 days. ACTH stimulation tests should be performed after the first week of therapy and then every 3 to 6 months to insure that hypoadrenocorticism (Addison's disease) does not result.

SEX HORMONE DISORDERS

Types of sex hormone disorders seen in pets include:

- Hyperestrogenism
- Estrogen-reponsive dermatosis
- Testicular tumors
- Hormonal hypersensitivity

Hyperestrogenism results when blood levels of the female sex hormone estrogen become too high as a result of functional cysts on the ovaries, ovarian cancers, or administration of estrogen-containing drugs (e.g., diethylstilbestrol [DES]) to treat other conditions. Hair loss around the genitals, on the ventral area, and extending down the hind legs is seen (see Plate VI-6). Often the vulva and nipples are swollen because of the high circulating levels of female sex hormones. Itchiness, waxy ears, and a greasy, scaly haircoat are frequent secondary features of the disorder; heat cycles are irregular, prolonged, or suppressed. There may also be a history of previous endometritis or pyometra.

Diagnosis is made tentatively because it is very difficult to identify the cyst or tumor without surgery. Blood samples for estradiol and estrone levels are sometimes helpful. Plasma or serum levels of estrogens are not always elevated because there are many different estrogenic compounds that might be implicated. Also, the changes seen may not be the result of increased estrogens alone but rather involve an altered skin sensitivity to estrogens. Blood counts are evaluated as chronically high circulating estrogen levels cause bone marrow suppression. The preferred diagnostic test as well as treatment of choice is ovariohysterectomy.

Estrogen-responsive dermatosis (hypoestro-genism; see Plate VI-7) occurs when blood levels of estrogen are too low. It has never been documented, however, that animals with this condition are deficient in estrogen. Dribbling of urine (urinary incontinence) is common. There may be bilaterally symmetrical hair loss around the perineum and down the backs of the hind legs. Diagnosis is based on the history, clinical examination, and response to estrogen supplementation. Blood levels of estradiol and estrone are not helpful in evaluating ovariohysterectomized animals with this condition. Estrogens should be used cautiously because of possible suppression of bone marrow.

Testicular tumors sometimes secrete female sex hormones and result in hyperestrogenism in male dogs. The incidence is much higher in cryptorchid dogs. Clinical signs include perineal alopecia, gynecomastia, drooping of the prepuce, and other signs of feminization (see Plate VI-8). Diseases of the prostate gland and estrogen-induced bone marrow suppression are possible consequences of the disorder. Diagnosis is based on the history, physical examination, and response to castration. Because about 10% of these tumors are malignant and can metastasize, thoracic radiography and blood panels should be considered before surgery.

Hormonal hypersensitivity is a rare hormonal problem in which dogs develop hypersensitivity reactions to the hormones they produce, resulting in intense pruritus. Most of the itchiness is around the perineum and hind end, but it can be generalized. Ceruminous otitis and keratinization disorders may be other manifestations of the disorder. It is most commonly seen in females, especially those with a history of pseudopregnancy, cystic ovaries, or irregular heat cycles. The diagnosis can occasionally be confirmed by performing a modified allergy test in which estrogen (0.0125 mg), progesterone (0.025 mg), and testosterone (0.05 mg) are injected intradermally. Histamine and saline are used as controls. The sites are evaluated after 15 minutes and again in 48 hours. The itchiness is usually dramatically reduced within 10 days of neutering.

APPENDIX:
VETERINARY ENDOCRINE DIAGNOSTIC LABORATORIES

Animal Health Diagnostic Laboratory
P.O. Box 30076
Lansing, MI 48909-7576
(517) 353-6021

Animal Reference Pathology
P.O. Box 30095
Salt Lake City, UT 84130
(800) 242-2787

Auburn University Endocrine Diagnostic Laboratory
Department of Physiology and Pharmacology
College of Veterinary Medicine
Auburn University, AL 36849-5520
(205) 844-5403

California Veterinary Diagnostics
3911 West Capitol Avenue
West Sacramento, CA 95691
(916) 372-4200

Clinical Endocrinology Laboratory
College of Veterinary Medicine
University of Tennessee
Room A-105, Noyland Drive
Knoxville, TN 37916
(615) 546-6092

Colorado Veterinary Diagnostic Laboratory
Colorado State University
Fort Collins, CO 80523
(303) 491-1281

New York State College of Veterinary Medicine
Cornell University
P.O. Box 786
Ithaca, NY 14851
(607) 253-3900

Radionuclide and Hormone Radioimmunoassay
 Laboratory
University of Wisconsin
School of Veterinary Medicine
2015 Linden Drive West
Madison, WI 53706
(608) 263-5863

University of Minnesota Veterinary Diagnostic Laboratory
1943 Carter Avenue
St. Paul, MN 55108
(612) 625-9290

Veterinary Research Laboratories
333 West Merrick Road
Valley Stream, NY 11580
(800) 872-7828

RECOMMENDED READINGS

Ackerman L: *Practical Canine Dermatology*. Goleta, CA, American Veterinary Publications, 1989.

Ackerman L: *Practical Feline Dermatology*. Goleta, CA, American Veterinary Publications, 1989.

Beale KM, Halliwell REW, Chen CL: Prevalence of antithyroglobulin antibodies detected by enzyme-linked immunosorbent assay of canine serum. *JAVMA* 196(5):745–748, 1990.

Beale KM, Keisling K, Forster-Blouin S: Serum thyroid hormone concentrations and thyrotropin responsiveness in dogs with generalized dermatologic disease. *JAVMA* 201(11):1715–1719, 1992.

Campbell L, Davis CA: Effects of thyroid hormones on serum and cutaneous fatty acid concentrations in dogs. *Am J Vet Res* 51(5):752–756, 1990.

Campbell KL, Small E: Identifying and managing the cutaneous manifestations of various endocrine diseases. *Vet Med* 86:118–135, 1991.

Chalmers SA, Medleau L: Identifying and treating sex-hormone dermatoses in dogs. *Vet Med* 85:1317–1330, 1990.

Feldman EC, Mack RE: Urine cortisol:creatinine ratio as a screening test for hyperadrenocorticism in dogs. *JAVMA* 200(11):1637–1641, 1992.

Fiorito DA: Hyperestrogenism in bitches. *Compend Contin Educ Pract Vet* 14(6):727–729, 1992.

Jensen RB, DuFort RM: Hyperadrenocorticism in dogs. *Compend Contin Educ Pract Vet* 13(4):615–620, 1991.

Lothrop CD: Adrenal and gonadal sex hormone disorders in dogs. Proceedings of the 10th ACVIM Forum, 1992, pp 677–678.

Nachreiner RF, Refsal KR: Radioimmunoassay monitoring of thyroid hormone concentrations in dogs on thyroid replacement therapy: 2,674 cases (1985–1987). *JAVMA* 201(4):623–629, 1992.

Nelson RW, Feldman EC, Ford SL: Topics in the diagnosis and treatment of canine hyperadrenocorticism. *Compend Contin Educ Pract Vet* 13(12):1797–1805, 1991.

Nelson RW, Ihle SL, Feldman EC, Bottoms GD: Serum free thyroxine concentration in healthy dogs, dogs with hypothyroidism, and euthyroid dogs with concurrent illness. *JAVMA* 198(8):1401–1407, 1991.

Panciera DL: Canine hypothyroidism. Part I. Clinical findings and control of thyroid hormone secretion and metabolism. *Compend Contin Educ Pract Vet* 12(5):689–701, 1990.

Panciera DL: Canine hypothyroidism. Part II. Thyroid function tests and treatment. *Compend Contin Educ Pract Vet* 12(6):843–857, 1990.

Peterson ME, Kemppainen RJ: Comparison of intravenous and intramuscular routes of administering cosyntropin for corticotropin stimulation testing in cats. *Am J Vet Res* 53(8):1392–1395, 1992.

Reimers TJ, Lawler DF, Sutaria PM, et al: Effects of age, sex, and body size on serum concentration of thyroid and adrenocortical hormones in dogs. *Am J Vet Res* 51(3):454–457, 1990.

Scott DW, Miller WH Jr: Probably hormonal hypersensitivity in two male dogs. *Canine Pract* 17(3):14–20, 1992.

Wilson SM, Feldman EC: Diagnostic value of the steroid-induced isoenzyme of alkaline phosphatase in the dog. *JAAHA* 28(3):245–250, 1992.

CHAPTER SEVEN
Cytology, Histopathology, and Immunopathology

*D*iagnostic techniques commonly used in animals with dermatologic disorders include:

- Cytologic evaluation—examination of the structure, function, and pathology of cells
- Histopathologic evaluation—examination of the microstructure, function, and pathology of tissues
- Immunopathologic evaluation—examination of the structural and functional changes associated with the immune response to disease

CYTOLOGY

Cytologic evaluation of specimens is a quick, efficient, and very useful diagnostic test. In most circumstances the procedure requires no anesthesia (local or general) and can be accomplished with little or no pain or risk to the patient.

Cytologic preparations often can be made and evaluated in the clinic before the animal is discharged. Alternatively, multiple samples can be collected; some are evaluated in house and others are sent to clinical pathologists for assessment.

The principal cytologic procedures useful for skin disorders are:

- Fine needle aspiration
- Impression smears
- Scrapings
- Swabs

Fine Needle Aspiration

Fine needle aspiration biopsies are excellent tools for collecting material from nodules, plaques, masses, and lymph nodes. They are easy to perform (see box on p. 152) and require only the following material:

- Syringe (6 to 12 ml)
- Fine needle (25 to 20 gauge)
- Microscope slides
- Regular hematologic stains

If smaller needles are used, sufficient numbers of cells likely will not be harvested. If larger needles are used, the sample is often contaminated with blood cells, core samples, and evidence of tissue trauma.

The procedure is performed by first swabbing the skin surface with alcohol or other antiseptics. If the material is to be used for microbial cultures, surgical preparation of the site is needed. Gloves should always be worn because the danger of contagion may not be evident (e.g., feline sporotrichosis, plague). Grasp the mass between thumb and forefinger to create a firm target and introduce the needle (with syringe attached) into the middle of the mass. When the needle is in place, withdraw the plunger of the syringe to the 8 to 10 ml mark, applying strong negative pressure on the tissue. If the mass is large, redirect the needle into different sections without removing the needle entirely from the mass or relaxing the negative pressure. It is important that the needle not be removed from the mass while negative pressure is being applied. A syringe holder can be purchased from a surgical supply facility and used to assist with this procedure.

When finished, relax the pulling pressure on the plunger and withdraw the needle. Often nothing is evident in the barrel of the syringe; the aspirated cells are located only in the hub of the needle. Failure to release the negative pressure

FINE NEEDLE ASPIRATION BIOPSY TECHNIQUE

Indications: To characterize cell type or contents of a mass (tumor, nodule) or cavity (cyst, vesicle, pustule) without surgical invasion

Procedure

1. Equipment and supplies: syringe (6 to 12 ml), hypodermic needle (25 to 20 gauge), clean glass slides, stain, microscope.
2. Carefully clip hair from lesion, avoiding trauma to surface.
3. Prepare biopsy site with surgical scrub.
4. Insert sterile needle attached to syringe into the lesion while creating a firm vacuum with syringe. (Needle and syringe sizes depend on size of lesion and density of tissue or content.) When material is aspirated into the syringe, withdraw the needle after allowing the pressure to equalize.
5. If initial aspiration is nonproductive, carefully move needle back and forth several times within the tissue while aspirating.
6. Place aspirate in the needle and syringe on the clean glass slides; spread it to make a thin film.
7. Select appropriate stain or send to reference laboratory.

on the plunger before withdrawing the needle results in aspiration of the cells into the barrel of the syringe rather than the hub. This can make recovery of those cells difficult or impossible.

Disconnect the needle from the syringe and load the syringe with air by pulling the plunger back to the 8 to 10 ml mark once again. Replace the needle onto the syringe and depress the plunger to expel the contents of the needle, one drop at a time, onto clean microscope slides. The sample can then be flattened onto the slide similar to blood-film preparation or by several techniques (e.g., squash or combination procedures), as outlined in cytology texts and handbooks. To perform the squash technique, place the aspirated material on a clean microscope slide and gently "squash" the material with another slide held perpendicular to the first. The aspirated material spreads between the slides naturally, and downward pressure need not be applied. For thick specimens

place a slide on top of another slide on which the aspirated material has been placed and then gently draw apart the two slides. Samples should be air dried immediately.

Impression Smears

Impression smears (see box on p. 153) are suitable for evaluating material that has been surgically removed or that is superficial, moist, and accessible. When lesions are biopsied or surgically excised, the cut surface can be blotted free of blood with a sterile gauze sponge and touched to reveal areas on a clean microscope slide. This creates an "imprint" of the cellular nature of the mass, which might provide valuable diagnostic information.

Impression smears of superficial oozing, pustular, or ulcerated lesions are quick, easy, and painless and provide a wealth of information. Gloves should be worn for collection of all samples and the skin surface swabbed with alcohol before sampling. Grasp the skin firmly between thumb and forefinger and apply pressure to exude material from fistulous tracts or sores. Lift scabs (crusts) and touch the moist surface with a clean microscope slide. Prick pustules and blisters with a needle to remove their fine epidermal covering and collect the liquid contents onto a clean microscope slide. The microscope slide should be touched to the tissue and lifted off directly, not pulled or dragged across the surface. The samples should then be air dried immediately, stained, and prepared for microscopic evaluation.

Scrapings

Scrapings can collect more surface material than most other procedures. Only superficial material is collected; thus the procedure is not suitable for deep lesions. Skin and nail (claw) scraping cytology is useful for patients suspected of having dermatophyte, yeast, or parasitic conditions, but any bacterial and inflammatory reactions probably reflect only the secondary superficial component of the condition and must be interpreted cautiously.

Scrapings are made with a dulled scalpel blade that is dragged perpendicular to the skin surface, removing superficial debris and skin cells. The material collected on the blade is transferred to a clean microscope slide, spread on the slide with the blade, air dried, appropriately stained, and evaluated microscopically.

Swabs

Swabs can be used to collect cells for evaluation, but this approach is inferior to impression smears or aspiration procedures. It is suitable for fistulous tracts or oral, nasal, conjunctival, rectal, or vaginal lesions where exposure is limited.

Sterile isotonic saline is used to first moisten the swab, which helps to minimize cell damage during sample collection. Then, the swab is gently touched to the exudate or tissue surface to harvest cells. After sample collection, the swab is gently rolled (not rubbed) on a clear microscope slide and prepared for microscopic evaluation.

Preparing Samples for Microscopic Examination

Regardless of the method of collection, preparation of cytologic specimens affects their diagnostic usefulness. Rough or inappropriate handling of samples can destroy or distort cells, complicating the diagnostic process. Only the edges of the slide should be touched because fingerprints on the slide contribute cells that could complicate the picture. The microscope slides should be precleaned or rinsed with alcohol and wiped dry prior to use. Air-dried smears should not be refrigerated, even in an attempt to preserve them for shipping to a diagnostic laboratory. This adversely affects cellular detail.

Once samples have been prepared on microscope slides, they need to be air dried before stains are applied. This helps to preserve the cells and to insure that they become fixed to the slides so that they do not rinse off during the staining procedure.

To air dry slides, briskly wave the slides in the air, which allows any liquid on the slides to evaporate. The result should be a single cell layer smear. Alternatively, gently pass the slide over a Bunsen burner or use the low setting on a hair dryer, being careful not to overheat the slides. Do not attempt to dry the slide by blowing on it, as this might introduce cells or microbes from the mouth.

For optimal detail, slides should be stained immediately after air drying. As a sample ages, cellular degeneration becomes more pronounced. Several types of stains can be used to highlight the cells and products collected. Most practical are the Romanowsky-type stains (e.g., Wright's, Giemsa, Diff-Quik) that are used for hematologic evaluation since they are already present in most veterinary clinics. If cancer is suspected, a new methylene blue (NMB) stain may also be used because it provides better nuclear and nucleolar detail at the expense of cytoplasmic features.

Several other stains may be used by cytologists; therefore nonstained, air-dried specimens should always be submitted in addition to stained samples. Papanicolaou-type stains are useful for examining some nuclear details but are not practical for routine use in veterinary hospitals. Immunocytochemical stains can identify cells precisely and are powerful diagnostic tools but are not yet routinely available to veterinarians.

Although the directions for each different type of stain should be closely followed, be aware that thicker specimens need a longer staining time than do thinner smears.

Microscopic Evaluation (see Figure 7-1)

A minimum of six suitably prepared slides should be available whenever cytologic collection has been done. Some of these smears can be read in house, while others are sent to veterinary laboratories for professional analysis.

Once the smear has been stained and air dried, it can be microscopically viewed "as is." (Alternatively, a drop or two of immersion oil can be added to the sample and then a coverslip applied. Although this often provides superior resolution, the sample must be examined shortly

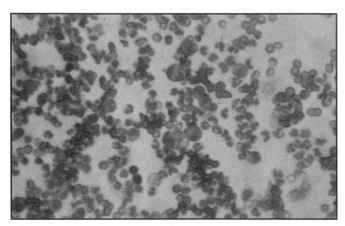

Figure 7-1. Direct smear of exudate with pyogranulomatous infiltration of neutrophils, histiocytes, and fibrin.

thereafter.) The sample is viewed on low magnification (4× to 10×) to assess areas that deserve further scrutiny and to determine the suitability of the staining. If the sample was poorly stained, another slide can be processed for evaluation. If samples were harvested optimally, there may be areas on the slide (e.g., edges, center) where staining is adequate for evaluation. This is usually a consequence of the thickness of the sample on different areas of the slide.

The sample is then viewed on intermediate magnification (10× to 20×), which usually provides information about the types of cells (e.g., leukocytes, round cells, epithelial cells, spindle cells) found in the sample. High-dry (40×) and oil immersion (100×) are used to evaluate nuclear and nucleolar features of cells and to identify most microbes and parasites.

A cytologic evaluation does not necessarily provide a diagnosis and prognosis for each case, but it may help differentiate inflammatory from neoplastic conditions or direct further diagnostic efforts. A major pitfall is that some cells are easier to harvest than others, and cells evaluated in samples may not necessarily be representative. For example, stromal tumors such as fibromas tend not to exfoliate well and so may contribute few if any cells to the preparation. A diagnosis of inflammatory dermatosis based on the accompanying cellular infiltrate would be erroneous.

All questionable cytologic preparations should be sent to a competent specialist for evaluation. Even if the specialist cannot arrive at a definitive diagnosis, he or she may be able to provide valuable diagnostic advice and suggestions.

Each cytologist usually has a preferred method of accepting samples, but some general guidelines follow:

- At least two air-dried, unfixed specimens and two air-dried, Romanowsky (Wright's, Giemsa, Diff-Quik) stained smears should be sent for evaluation.
- Specimens to be submitted to laboratories for cytologic examination by the Papanicolaou method (mostly in cases in which cancer is suspected) need to be wet fixed in special fixatives.
- The smears should be well labeled and accompanied by a complete patient history. Other valuable information includes the actual site of the lesion, sampling and fixation techniques, and the staining procedures used.
- If samples are to be mailed, care must be taken that breakage does not occur. Using bubble wrap and extensive padding is usually adequate. (Marking the packages with phrases such as "fragile" is helpful but may not influence the behavior of some mail handlers.)
- Do not mail cytology specimens together with formalin-preserved biopsy specimens because the formalin fumes can alter the staining and cellular characteristics of the cytologic preparations.

The diagnostic laboratory should be contacted for specific instructions.

Practical Information from Cytology

Even if a diagnosis is not rendered, cytologic findings should be reported in a manner that provides practical information. The very first distinction that needs to be made is between inflammatory and neoplastic conditions.

Inflammatory samples contain mainly white blood cells, especially neutrophils, lymphocytes, eosinophils, and macrophages (histiocytes; Figure 7-2). A few mast cells may be present in certain inflammatory conditions such as allergies, but they never constitute a large percentage of cells. In acute inflammatory conditions (e.g., bacterial infections, autoimmune diseases), the vast majority of cells are neutrophils. As time passes, the number of mononuclear cells (lymphocytes, macrophages) increases. In chronic inflammatory conditions over 50% of the cells recovered are macrophages (histiocytes). The accumulation of neutrophils (pus cells) and histiocytes (granuloma cells) frequently gives rise to chronic active dermatitis, or "pyogranuloma" which is common in

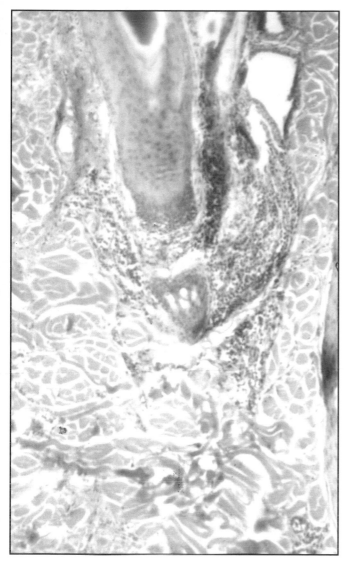

Figure 7-2. Sample of microscopic section with edema and dense perifolliculitis seen in deep pyoderma.

many deep, inflammatory conditions (see Plate VII-1). Macrophages (histiocytes) persistent in long-standing lesions are consistent with microbes, debris, or particulate matter that cannot be sufficiently eliminated by the immune system. This granulomatous response can be seen with bacterial (e.g., mycobacteriosis), fungal (e.g., blastomycosis; see Plate VII-2), immunologic (e.g., lupus profundus), foreign body (e.g., plant material such as thorns and sticks), and even cancerous (e.g., histiocytosis) processes. When numerous lytic neutrophils (characterized by swollen, pale-staining nuclei) are present, septic inflammation should be considered and cultures are advisable. Eosinophils are common in a number of inflammatory conditions including immunologic diseases (e.g., eosinophilic granuloma complex, pemphigus), folliculitis/furunculosis, parasitism, and even some cancers (e.g., mast cell tumor).

CYTOLOGIC FEATURES OF MALIGNANCY

Abnormal mitotic figures
Variable nuclear size
Increased nuclear/cytoplasmic ratio
Multiple nucleoli
Irregular nucleoli
Coarse chromatin patterns
Cytoplasmic basophilia and vacuolation

Eosinophils are a response to inflammation and are not specific to any one disorder.

If a sample can be identified as neoplastic based on cytologic findings (see box above), every attempt should be made to ascertain additional information; histopathologic evaluation of biopsies is needed in many cases. It is important to recognize malignant versus benign features. Identification of tumor types is also critical (see Plates VII-3 through VII-7):

- Epithelial tumors include squamous cell carcinoma, benign adnexal tumors, basal cell tumors, and perianal gland tumors.
- Mesenchymal tumors include fibroma/fibrosarcoma, lipoma/liposarcoma, hemangioma/hemangiosarcoma, and hemangiopericytoma. Mesenchymal tumors are usually the most difficult to diagnose with cytologic preparations because they are least likely to contribute cells as a result of the fibrous nature of these cancers.
- Round cell tumors include lymphocytic tumors, mast cell tumors, histiocytomas, and transmissible venereal tumors. Melanocytic tumors are also sometimes classified as round cell tumors.

No single criterion exists for differentiating hyperplastic inflammatory changes from some neoplastic features. A textbook or atlas of cytologic evaluation of cancers is mandatory for any individual intending to make a diagnosis based on these findings. More often than not, samples are sent to pathology/cytology laboratories for professional evaluation.

HISTOPATHOLOGY

Histopathologic assessment of biopsies is one of the most important diagnostic tests in dermatology. The skin is easily accessible and lends itself to

PUNCH BIOPSY TECHNIQUE

Indications: All types of solid skin lesions, if total excision is not indicated

All small lesions (up to 5 mm) that can be totally excised

Procedure

1. Equipment and supplies: 4 mm or 6 mm disposable biopsy punch, needle holder, skin suture, smooth thumb forceps, fine sharp-sharp scissors, 2 × 2 gauze sponges, formalin.
2. Carefully clip (fur only, not skin) near lesion only if needed, avoiding removal of scale or crust on surface.
3. Do not wash or disinfect the biopsy site because the diagnostic value of the specimen may be on the surface.
4. Inject 0.3 to 0.5 ml of local anesthetic subcutaneously.
5. Place biopsy punch on exact site to be biopsied and drill into tissue with rotary motion in one direction, applying moderate pressure. There will be less resistance when punch reaches subcutaneous tissue.
6. Withdraw punch. The plug should follow punch to surface if cut to an adequate depth.
7. Carefully lift plug with fine smooth forceps or a fine needle and cut base of plug including some fat with scissors or scalpel blade.
8. Close wound with one or two skin sutures.
9. Place specimen in 10% buffered formalin and submit to laboratory.

sampling for diagnostic purposes. Over the past 15 years or so, a multitude of new dermatoses have been described, and many of the descriptive breakthroughs have been the result of skin biopsies and sophisticated histopathologic analysis.

No simple rules can be followed to determine which skin conditions require biopsy. Common sense dictates that certain dermatoses are better candidates than others. Remember that biopsies should support or refute clinical impressions and not replace the veterinarian as diagnostician. If the diagnosis can be made by less invasive procedures such as skin scrapings or cytologic preparations, biopsies are not needed. When these other techniques do not allow a reasonably confident clinical diagnosis, biopsies can be invaluable (see

Plates VII-8 to VII-11). Similarly, biopsies are helpful when an animal is unresponsive to treatment and the tentative diagnosis needs to be reevaluated or when more than one problem may be involved. Biopsies should not be used as a last ditch diagnostic effort. The earlier that biopsies are taken in the course of a skin problem, the better are the chances of uncovering diagnostic changes. Older lesions become increasingly less specific as a result of the effects of time, inflammation, and drug therapy.

Skin biopsies are technically easy to perform, but insight into the selection of lesions is needed. Whenever possible, primary lesions should be selected (if they are a consistent part of the clinical presentation) because they are the most likely to yield diagnostic clues. The purpose of a biopsy may be to confirm a diagnosis or to suggest diagnoses for further consideration. A histopathology report that findings "are consistent with" a group of disorders is valuable, even if the diagnosis cannot be confirmed with a sample.

Histopathology findings are only part of a laboratory report, representing an image of a small piece of tissue at a particular point in time. They are not a crystal ball for diagnosing a problem and prescribing treatment.

Taking Biopsies

Although there are several different ways of taking biopsies, the use of biopsy punches has greatly facilitated the procedure in most cases. Punch biopsies are the preferred method of sampling inflammatory conditions in general practice (see box at left). For cancerous and very large noncancerous lesions, excisional, incisional, or core biopsy techniques are often used.

The selection of lesions is one of the most important aspects of the procedure. Unless a representative section is taken, histopathologic findings are not representative of the true problem. The temptation to sample the worst-looking lesions on an animal must be resisted. For instance, an allergic dog with traumatized and secondarily infected skin has sores, ulcerations, and crusts, but the primary problem is probably best represented by erythematous areas on the abdominal skin. To give another example, animals with bacterial or fungal folliculitis often develop bare areas after inflammation has subsided; sampling of these areas suggests inactive growth of hair, a situation more commonly associated with hormonal problems. Therefore it is critical to select areas with representative lesions (and not secondary changes) for sampling.

When appropriate lesions are identified, they should be circled with a marker for easy identification. At least two biopsies should be taken. The principal biopsy should be a sample of the center of the lesion. For cancerous conditions additional junctional biopsies also can be helpful. Samples from normal skin may identify features that are "normal" for an individual animal (e.g., mucinosis in a Chinese Shar pei). Junctional biopsies (half normal/half abnormal) cannot be relied on except in cases of suspected cancers, because sectioning in the laboratory (where half of each biopsy is processed and half is discarded) could eliminate all or a significant part of the lesion.

It is important that the skin not be shaved or "prepped" before biopsy because any manipulation might distort the changes evident on histopathology. A surgical scrub is only indicated when a deep portion of tissue is taken for microbial culture.

Local anesthesia is administered by injecting 0.3 to 0.5 ml of 2% lidocaine into the subcutaneous tissue immediately beneath the planned biopsy site. This is facilitated by the circling of sites beforehand. The site marking is also important because subtle erythematous lesions may blanch after the injection of local anesthetic, making them difficult to find otherwise. The inclusion of epinephrine in the local anesthetic aids in hemostasis and restricts the spread of the analgesia.

Because biopsy procedures are a routine part of general practice, a skin biopsy pack should be available. Contents should include:

- Biopsy punches (disposable punches can be sterilized and reused two to three times)
- Needle holder forceps
- Skin suture
- Forceps
- Fine sharp-sharp scissors
- Gauze sponges
- Formalin

A tray with cold sterilizer also should be available.

Biopsy punches come in two major forms:

- Disposable Baker biopsy punch
- Stainless steel Keyes biopsy punch

Most skin biopsies are made with a 6 mm punch, but a 4 mm punch is useful for samples from face and footpad areas and on mucous membranes. These punches have a sharp cookie cutter–like edge that allows a core of skin to be harvested.

The cutting edge is placed on the biopsy site and is gently but firmly rotated into the tissue. Once the punch has penetrated the subcutaneous tissue, it is removed and the small pedicle of fat attached is trimmed with scissors or a scalpel blade. The core of tissue remaining should include all layers of skin (i.e., the epidermis, dermis, and subcutaneous tissue; see Plate VII-12). Forceps can be used to pick up the core, but care is needed to lift only the edges, hairs, or the subcutaneous fat. Crushing damage done by inappropriately placed forceps can distort the tissue and seriously impair its diagnostic potential. The small wound in the skin can be closed with one or two interrupted sutures. Sutures are removed in 10 to 14 days.

The skin biopsy cores are gently blotted free of blood and immediately placed in vials of buffered neutral formalin (10%). Excessively bloody samples should first be rinsed with saline. All specimens should be fixed in *at least* 10 times their volume of fixative. If the outdoor temperature drops below freezing, specimens should be fixed overnight in formalin (indoors) to avoid being frozen. Alternatively, alcohol can be added to the solution to decrease the risk of ice crystal formation. The biopsy sample containers should be appropriately labeled and submitted to the pathology laboratory together with a detailed and thorough history (including diagnostic suspicions). Formalin-filled containers mailed to diagnostic facilities must be tightly sealed and wrapped with tape to avoid leakage. Government regulations regarding shipments of biohazardous materials should be checked.

Wedge biopsies are also useful in practice, especially for cancerous and large inflammatory lesions (see boxes on p. 158). An elliptical incision is made to obtain a large specimen that can then be easily oriented and trimmed by laboratory personnel. This method is preferred for cancerous conditions because the procedure may be able to provide a cure (surgical removal) as well as a diagnostic sample. Wedge biopsies are also preferred for disorders affecting the subcutaneous tissue (panniculus) or for fragile surface lesions (blisters) that might rupture with the shearing force of a biopsy punch.

The histopathologic interpretation of skin biopsies has become a subspecialty all its own. Because dermatopathology is such a complex and evolving discipline, it is often worthwhile to have

EXCISIONAL BIOPSY TECHNIQUE

Indications: Total removal of small nodules, cysts, vesicles, and tumors

Procedure

1. Equipment and supplies: sterile surgical pack (drape, scalpel handle and blade, hemostats, needle holder, suture needles, smooth thumb forceps, scissors, gauze sponges, suture), formalin.
2. Carefully clip hair from lesion and surrounding area, avoiding trauma to skin.
3. Clean surgical site with soap and water, rinse, and apply 70% alcohol, avoiding vigorous scrubbing.
4. Inject local anesthetic subcutaneously using ring block, or use general anesthesia.
5. Make an elliptical excision of the full depth of skin to the subcutis.
6. Close the wound in a routine manner.
7. Submit specimen in 10% buffered formalin.

INCISIONAL BIOPSY TECHNIQUE

Indications: To obtain a specimen for histopathologic examination from a large mass that cannot be totally excised because of size or location or for cosmetic reasons

Procedure

1. Equipment and supplies: sterile surgical pack (drape, scalpel handle and blade, hemostats, needle holder, suture needles, smooth thumb forceps, scissors, gauze sponges, suture), formalin.
2. Carefully clip hair from lesion and surrounding area, avoiding trauma to skin.
3. Clean surgical site with soap and water, rinse, and apply 70% alcohol, avoiding vigorous scrubbing.
4. Inject local anesthetic subcutaneously using ring block, or use general anesthesia.
5. Select a biopsy site on the basis of a representative tissue, access to biopsy site, and minimal postsurgical complications.
6. Be prepared to control excessive hemorrhage on large or active lesions.
7. Make a full-thickness incision to subcutaneous tissue in the form of a wedge or ellipse, removing a section at least 5 mm wide.
8. Close the wound in a manner to prevent postsurgical complications.
9. Submit specimen in 10% buffered formalin.

difficult or unusual cases evaluated by individuals with an interest in this area (see the Appendix on p. 160). Samples should be sent to veterinary dermatopathologists rather than human dermatopathologists because there are important species differences (e.g., a human dermatopathology specialist may incorrectly identify a canine histiocytoma as a malignant cancer, when, in fact, it would regress on its own without treatment).

When biopsy samples arrive at a pathology laboratory, they are removed from the fixative, trimmed to an appropriate size, and oriented optimally based on surface features and hairs. The specimens are placed in small cassettes and dehydrated in a series of alcohols of increasing strength. The fat (lipid) is then cleared with xylene, and the specimen is embedded in wax (paraffin). A microtome is used to cut the wax block into very thin sections, which are then placed on microscope slides and dried in a vacuum oven. The paraffin is then dissolved away, the tissue rehydrated with alcohols, and the tissue stained. The most common histologic stain used is hematoxylin and eosin (H&E) but many other stains are used for special purposes. For example, periodic acid–Schiff (PAS) stains are often used to highlight fungal organisms and toluidine blue may be used to highlight the granules of a mast cell tumor.

Often an absolute diagnosis cannot be made on the basis of histopathologic analysis. Many disorders cannot be "fingerprinted" with biopsies, which demonstrate consistent but not absolute findings. Biopsies are never "negative"; they may not confirm a diagnosis, but they always show something, even if it is just normal skin. For convenience, inflammatory conditions are often grouped based on their inflammatory "pattern" (see box on p. 159, left). For example, a histopathologic report may describe a superficial perivascular dermatitis (pattern) and say it is consistent with an immediate-type hypersensitivity reaction (presumptive diagnosis). Nevertheless, a histopathologic analysis cannot conclusively differentiate between inhalant allergies, food allergies, and flea bite hypersensitivity. All reports must be interpreted in light of clinical findings and other diagnostic information. Do not confuse

DERMATOLOGIC PATTERNS OF INFLAMMATION	
Pattern	**Example**
Perivascular	Inhalant allergy
Vasculitis	Immune-mediated vasculitis
Intraepidermal vesicular/pustular	Pemphigus
Subepidermal vesicular/pustular	Pemphigoid
Perifollicular/Follicular	Bacterial folliculitis
Nodular/Diffuse	Mycobacteriosis
Panniculitis	Vaccine reaction
Resting follicles	Hypothyroidism

PREPARING MICHEL'S SOLUTION
1. Mix 2.5 ml of 1 M potassium citrate pH 7 with 5 ml of 0.1 M magnesium sulfate.
2. Add 5 ml of 0.1 M N-ethyl maleimide.
3. Add 87.5 ml of distilled water.
4. Add 55 g ammonium sulfate.
5. Adjust pH to 7.0 with 1 M KOH.

pattern analysis with diagnosis. For example, panniculitis and vasculitis are descriptions of inflammatory reactions and neither is specific for any one diagnosis.

IMMUNOPATHOLOGY

Immunopathologic techniques include direct immunofluorescent testing and immunoperoxidase testing. These specialized tests use immunologic markers to detect antibodies (immunoglobulins) and/or complement present in tissues. The pattern of antibody deposition can support a diagnosis, but it is not foolproof. In humans the tests are much more useful because they can be diagnostic over 90% of the time. Unfortunately, this is not the case in animals. In dogs and cats these tests are only positive in about 50% to 60% of confirmed cases, severely limiting their usefulness. Also, biopsies submitted from nose or footpad tissues may have immunoglobulin deposition (usually IgM) in the absence of any clinical disease; positive test results in these tissues must be evaluated carefully.

Biopsies for immunopathologic assessment are collected similarly to those intended for histopathology with some important exceptions. When pustules, vesicles, or ulcers are evident, damage in these regions causes reactions that destroy immunoglobulins in tissue; the biopsies should be taken from normal-appearing skin adjacent to lesions. For inflammatory areas the biopsies can be taken from the involved areas.

Samples taken for direct immunofluorescence cannot be preserved with buffered formalin. They must be added to Michel's solution, a transport medium that preserves tissue proteins. The medium can be purchased commercially from laboratory suppliers, acquired from testing laboratories, or prepared from stock ingredients (see box above).

Immunoperoxidase testing can be done on paraffin-imbedded specimens and is suitable for use on animal tissues. It is not commonly used in many laboratories. This procedure uses a special dye that has an affinity for immunoglobulins. It is less specific than direct immunofluorescence testing in some cases, depending on the immunoglobulin involved.

Patterns and Immunopathology

Immunopathology is used to detect the presence of antibodies in tissues. The results of these tests are not specific for any one condition. They are significant when immunoglobulin is found in tissues (positive) and can provide further information, depending on where antibodies are located. Immunoglobulin deposition is usually found in the intercellular spaces between epidermal cells and the basement membrane zone separating the epidermis from the dermis and around the blood vessels of the dermis.

Immunopathologic deposition in the intercellular spaces is most consistent with the variants of pemphigus, although it may be a false-positive finding in other conditions. Conditions that result in staining at the basement membrane zone include bullous pemphigoid, cicatricial pemphigoid, the different variants of lupus erythematosus, linear IgA disease, and dermatitis herpetiformis. Staining around blood vessels is associated with all of the potential causes of vasculitis.

APPENDIX:
DERMATOPATHOLOGY CONTACTS

FACILITY	PATHOLOGIST
A & E Clinical Laboratories 11518 Pico Boulevard Los Angeles, CA 90064	Dr. Emily Walder
Department of Pathology College of Veterinary Medicine Michigan State University East Lansing, MI 48824	Dr. Robert Dunstan
Department of Veterinary Medicine School of Veterinary Medicine University of California Davis, CA 96616	Dr. Anthony Stannard
Dermatodiagnostics c/o HCS 1254 West Pioneer Way, Suite E Oak Harbor, WA 98277	Dr. Ann Hargis
Dermopathology & General Pathology Consultants 694 Panchita Way Los Altos, CA 94022	Dr. James Hill
Derm-Path Consulting Services 4725 Cornell Rd. Cincinnati, OH 45241	Dr. Gary Johnson
DVM Pathology Laboratory P.O. Box 10246 Prescott, AZ 86304	Dr. James Conroy
Histovet Veterinary Histopathology Consultants 309 Edinburgh Road South Guelph, Ontario, Canada N1G 2K3	Dr. Julie Yager Dr. Brian Wilcock
Institut für Tierpathologie University of Bern Bern, Switzerland	Dr. Claudia von Tscharner
Laboratory of Pathology School of Veterinary Medicine University of Pennsylvania 3800 Spruce Street Philadelphia, PA 19104	Dr. Michael Goldschmidt
Veterinary Pathology Consultants Dermopathology Service 3911 West Capital Avenue West Sacramento, CA 95691	Dr. Thelma Gross
Western College of Veterinary Medicine Department of Veterinary Pathology University of Saskatchewan Saskatoon, Saskatchewan, Canada S7N 0W0	Dr. Ted Clark

RECOMMENDED READINGS

Austin VH: Skin biopsies: When, where and why. *Compend Contin Educ Pract Vet* 2(7):531–536, 1980.

Cowell RL, Tyler RD: *Diagnostic Cytology of the Dog and Cat.* Goleta, CA, American Veterinary Publications, 1989.

Gross TL, Ihrke PJ, Walder EJ: *Veterinary Dermatopathology: A Macroscopic and Microscopic Evaluation of Canine and Feline Skin Disease.* St Louis, Mosby–Year Book, 1992.

Yager JA, Wilcock BP: Skin biopsy: Revelations and limitations. *Can Vet J* 29:969–972, 1988.

CHAPTER EIGHT
Specific Therapies

*T*his chapter focuses on management of a number of important skin disorders, including:

- Acanthosis nigricans
- Acral lick dermatitis
- Anal sac disorders
- Claw (nail) disorders
- Eosinophilic granuloma complex
- Keratinization disorders
- Cutaneous lymphoma
- Mast cell tumors
- Necrolytic dermatitis
- Otitis externa
- Panniculitis
- Pododermatitis
- Solar dermatitis

ACANTHOSIS NIGRICANS

The pathogenesis of acanthosis nigricans has never been well defined. Clearly, some cases have a hereditary or familial incidence whereas most others are secondary phenomena:

- The familial primary form of the disease is seen mainly in dachshunds.
- The secondary form features regional hyperpigmentation and can result from allergies, hormonal problems, frictional changes (e.g., intertriginous dermatitis), and other conditions.

Although acanthosis nigricans is often an indicator of internal malignancy in humans, this is not the case in dogs.

Clinical Signs

The appearance of acanthosis nigricans is quite distinctive and involves thickening and hyperpigmentation in the axillae and groin area (see Plate VIII-1). The first indication is often a brown patch in the axillary regions. As the disease progresses, larger, thickened, hyperpigmented, and lichenified plaques are seen. Pruritus may or may not occur, but secondary keratinization disorders (seborrheic changes) are common.

Diagnosis

Recognizing acanthosis nigricans is not difficult but differentiating primary from secondary disease is more challenging. Allergy tests and thyroid profiles are usually indicated. Biopsies are not specific for this condition but might help uncover or exclude specific primary causes.

Treatment

Early in the course of the disease, affected animals usually respond to low dose corticosteroid therapy. Prednisone at 0.5 mg/kg is given daily for 14 days and then on alternate days for another 14 days. If the response is encouraging, the dose can be reduced and maintained on an alternate day basis. Mild topical therapies (0.5% hydrocortisone in a moisturizing base) are also helpful. Vitamin E (200 IU bid) should be administered to dachshunds, many of which benefit from the supplementation.

Once the tissue has reached the plaque stage, however, corticosteroids have a less profound effect. Antibiotics may be required as secondary pyoderma is common. Frequent antiseptic and antiseborrheic shampooing is indicated to control the associated secondary keratinization disorder and the infection. Melatonin,[a] a pineal gland extract, has been used experimentally in the management of acanthosis nigricans. A dose of 2 mg is given every other day for four treatments and then every 2 to 4 weeks as needed. Melatonin can be dissolved in absolute ethanol (2 to 3 ml) and 90% dimethyl sulfoxide (DMSO; 2 to 3 ml).

> **TOPICAL THERAPY FOR ACRAL LICK DERMATITIS**
>
> 1. Add 3 ml of Banamine® to a bottle of Synotic®.
> 2. Apply several drops to affected areas twice daily.

ACRAL LICK DERMATITIS

Acral lick dermatitis (also known as lick granuloma) has always been difficult to manage in the dog. The actual cause is not known but it is suspected that a neurologic (including behavioral) component is involved. There are some striking similarities to obsessive-compulsive disorder seen in humans. Doberman pinschers, Great Danes, German shepherds, Labrador retrievers, and Irish setters are most commonly affected.

Clinical Signs

Dogs with acral lick dermatitis lick and chew at a body part (usually the legs) for no apparent reason. The constant licking removes the hair, induces inflammation, and removes layers of skin (see Plate VIII-2), sometimes down to the bone. The resulting irritation further stimulates the dog to lick and chew at the area. Lesions tend to recur at the same or different sites.

Diagnosis

Diagnostic efforts are critical because many other disorders can mimic this condition, including dermatophytosis (ringworm), bacterial infection, and some cancers. An appropriate diagnostic workup involves the following:

- Histopathologic evaluation of biopsies
- Skin scrapings
- Microbial cultures
- Radiography of the limb

Further diagnostic tests may be warranted once biopsy findings are available.

Treatment

Because the condition is not well understood, therapeutic success is variable. Treatment of underlying or coexisting problems are critical. The best approaches to symptomatic treatment have involved anti-inflammatory therapy and mood-altering medications. Antibiotics are frequently helpful (e.g., oxacillin, cephalexin, trimethoprim-sulfa); although bacteria are unlikely to be the primary cause, treatment of bacterial complications of cellulitis and ulceration often needs to be given for 2 to 3 months.

The most effective topical therapy to date has been a mixture of flunixin meglumine (Banamine®—Schering-Plough Animal Health) with flu-ocinolone acetonide in DMSO (Synotic®—Syntex Animal Health) as described in the box above. Although some reports herald this therapy as a major breakthrough in treatment, results are extremely variable. In addition, there are concerns regarding the long-term use of a corticosteroid-DMSO mixture, which could lead to iatrogenic Cushing's syndrome.

Systemic therapy has provided the most reproducible results. The most interesting work has been done with antiobsessional drugs and narcotic antagonists. Research on humans with obsessive compulsive disorder has shown that certain new antidepressant drugs (serotonin re-uptake inhibitors) are very beneficial. Antiobsessional drugs such as clomipramine (1 to 3 mg/kg/day) also have shown promise in dogs. Recent work with pimozide (Orap™—Gate Pharmaceuticals), a drug used to treat delusions of parasitosis in humans, has also been encouraging. Amitriptyline (2.2 mg/kg bid), fluoxetine (1 mg/kg/day), and pentazocine (2.2 mg/kg bid) have also been shown to be helpful in some cases.

Another line of research has evaluated narcotic antagonists in the treatment of acral lick dermatitis. Naltrexone (2.2 mg/kg sid-bid) has been used with good results. Unfortunately, it is awkward to administer and expensive. Hydrocodone (Hycodan®—Du Pont Pharmaceuticals; 0.25 mg/kg tid) has also shown some success.

Early in the course of the condition, other therapies may be beneficial. Intralesional injections of triamcinolone acetonide or methylpred-

---

[a]Melatonin can be acquired for experimental use from Rickards Research Foundation, 18001 Euclid Ave., Cleveland, Ohio 44112.

nisolone acetate may reduce inflammation and manage the situation before it becomes indolent. Radiation therapy (600 rad for three treatments on alternate days) can also be helpful at this time. Finally, protective covering of lesions or the use of Elizabethan collars or muzzles may be useful, although they cannot eliminate the problem on their own.

ANAL SAC DISORDERS

The anal sacs (often incorrectly referred to as anal glands) are present on either side of the rectum and have ducts that serve as conduits to the surface. The sacs are also supplied by glands (anal sac glands). The pathogenesis of anal sac disease is poorly understood. Dogs tend to have many more anal sac problems than do cats.

Predisposition to anal sac disease may be associated with the following:

- Thick secretions of large quantity
- Abnormally small duct system
- Anal irritation
- Changes in muscle tone
- Changes in fecal form
- Recent diarrhea or estrus

It is believed that anal sac impaction is followed by bacterial fermentation of the discharge. Several bacteria are associated with anal sac disease, including *Streptococcus fecalis, Escherichia coli, Clostridium welchii, Proteus* spp., micrococci, *Staphylococcus* spp., and diphtheroids. Conditions that affect the anal sacs include abscessation, anal sacculitis, conditioned hyperirritability (autosensitization), and cancer.

Clinical Signs

Most dogs with anal sac problems scoot their hind ends on the floor and bite or lick at the area. Often diarrhea has occurred 1 to 3 weeks before the onset of problems. Anal sac disorders are not evident (without palpation) unless there is concurrent abscessation (see Plate VIII-3), fistulous tracts, or tumorous masses.

Diagnosis

Distended anal sacs can be palpated at the 4 and 8 o'clock positions, relative to the anus. Occasionally, it is necessary to palpate the sacs during the rectal examination to appreciate impaction.

Difficulty in expressing the contents of the sacs is highly suggestive of impaction.

Normal anal sac fluid is pale yellow or straw-colored, serous, clear to translucent, slightly viscous, and granular with a pungent odor. Abnormal fluid color may be greenish-yellow (pus), red, brown, clay, or black. Infected anal sacs are often associated with an opaque, thick, reddish- or greenish-colored fluid with a fetid odor. Impacted anal sacs are characterized by clay- or black-colored contents that are dry or pasty and have minimal odor.

Evaluation of anal sac disease should include:

- *Direct microscopic evaluation of anal sac secretions.* Evaluation of normal anal sac secretions by direct smear reveals cellular debris and a few leukocytes, whereas secretions from diseased anal sacs yield a large number of leukocytes and numerous bacteria.
- *Bacterial culture and antibiotic sensitivity testing.* Culture and sensitivity testing is indicated in chronic, nonresponsive, or recurrent anal sac infections.
- *Biopsy.* Occasionally, when neoplasia is suspected, biopsies are performed.

Apocrine and anal sac gland tumors are rare. They occur more commonly in aged females but have no breed predilection. Perianal swelling is the primary complaint. Ulceration of the perianal skin is observed in approximately 50% of animals with anal sac tumors. These tumors can result in hypercalcemia. Metastasis to lumbar, iliac, and sacral lymph nodes occurs frequently.

Treatment

Impacted anal sacs can be painful and lead to more severe anal sacculitis and abscessation. Gentle expression of the contents from the sacs results in symptomatic relief and provides material for evaluation. Excessive force should be avoided to prevent anal sac rupture and resultant cellulitis. If the contents are dry and cannot be expressed with gentle pressure, a softening or ceruminolytic agent (e.g., hexamethyltetracosane, mineral oil) can be instilled into the sacs with a blunt needle or lacrimal cannula. If purulent material is expressed, the sacs should be irrigated with a mild antiseptic solution (e.g., 0.5% chlorhexidine, 10% povidone-iodine solution). After the sacs are emptied and/or flushed, they can be infused with an antibiotic solution (e.g., chloramphenicol cream, nitrofurazone lotion, corticosteroid-antibiotic ointment).

When an anal sac abscess is present with cellulitis but without rupture, a hot pack should be applied several times a day until the abscess is ready for drainage. The abscess is then lanced, and the contents are expressed by rectal and external pressure. The anal sac duct must be opened, which often requires cannulation. After the abscess has ruptured or has been surgically opened, it should be flushed with 10% povidone-iodine or chlorhexidine daily until it closes. Systemic antibiotics should be administered and hot packs should be applied until inflammation resolves.

For chronic, recurrent, and poorly responsive anal sac disease, surgical removal of the anal sacs (anal sacculectomy) should be contemplated. Several surgical protocols are suitable. Care must be taken not to damage nerves in the area, or incontinence may result.

CLAW (NAIL) DISORDERS

Disorders of the nails (more correctly termed claws) and nailbeds are uncommon in dogs but are difficult to manage when encountered. They can result from a number of unrelated causes, including microbial infections, autoimmune disorders, inherited defects, nutritional imbalances, cardiopulmonary disease, and parasitism. Broken nails occur frequently from trauma, bite wounds, and environmental causes.

Clinical Signs

Although nail disorders are frequently regarded as one syndrome, several different manifestations are possible. Bacterial infections (paronychia), fungal infections (onychomycosis), and yeast infections (*Candida* paronychia) of the nail or nailbeds have all been recognized. Dermatophytosis, blastomycosis, cryptococcosis, and sporotrichosis have also been implicated in nail diseases.

Onychorrhexis (brittle nails) is most commonly caused by chronic low grade infections or may be the result of genetic or nutritional factors. It is most commonly seen in young German shepherds, Rhodesian ridgebacks, dachshunds, and cocker spaniels. Onychorrhexis may also be an incidental finding in geriatric dogs and cats.

Onychomadesis is sloughing of the horny claw caused by clefting within the keratinizing layers of the claw. The most common causes are immune-mediated diseases (e.g., pemphigus, bullous pemphigoid, lupus erythematosus, "lupoid" syndrome, vasculitis, cold agglutinin disease, and drug eruption), but trauma, bacterial infection, dermatophytosis, metabolic conditions, neoplasia, and hypothyroidism have also been implicated.

Diagnosis

A careful workup is needed to pinpoint the exact cause of the problem. Initial diagnostic procedures should include the following:

- Scrapings
- Direct microscopic examination
- Microbial cultures
- Routine hematologic and biochemical profiles
- Antinuclear antibody (ANA) test

Cats should also be evaluated for infection with feline leukemia virus and feline immunodeficiency virus.

Scrapings taken from the ungual folds can be viewed microscopically for the presence of parasites, especially *Demodex* mites. Scrapings from the hard surface of the nail also can be appropriately stained and evaluated for the presence of fungi, especially dermatophytes and yeasts. Additional material can be collected for fungal culture.

Sampling exudate from the ungual fold can be very enlightening. The material is applied to a clean microscope slide, heat fixed, and appropriately stained (e.g., with Wright's or Gram's stain). Inflammatory cells, microbes, or cells suggestive of a disorder (e.g., acantholytic keratinocytes) may be revealed.

Microbial cultures must be carefully evaluated because contaminant growth is likely. For this reason the exudate should be evaluated cytologically so that valid comparisons can be made.

Because many different systemic disorders cause nail diseases, affected individuals should be examined carefully and hematologic and biochemical profiles and ANA findings should be scrutinized for evidence of internal involvement. Radiographic evaluation of the affected digits may also be of value.

If a diagnosis cannot be rendered from these tests, the entire distal digit should be surgically removed and submitted for histopathologic evaluation. This is needed for most congenitohereditary problems (e.g., mechanobullous diseases), cancers (e.g., squamous cell carcinoma, metastatic bronchial adenocarcinoma), most immune-mediated diseases, and metabolic problems.

Treatment

Treatment is aimed at correcting the underlying problem and providing symptomatic relief with soothing baths. Soaks with diluted chlorhexidine or povidone-iodine for 5 to 10 minutes twice daily can be used to successfully manage most surface infection. Griseofulvin or ketoconazole is usually selected for dermatophyte infections, which are often caused by *Trichophyton mentagrophytes* in dogs and *Microsporum canis* in cats. Treatment for these infections may last for 9 to 12 months and should continue for at least 2 months beyond an apparent cure. Systemic mycoses are usually treated with ketoconazole, and immune-mediated disorders are managed with appropriate immunosuppressive therapy.

Antibiotic therapy is common in nail disorders because of the frequent secondary involvement of microbes. Bactericidal antibiotics such as oxacillin or cephalexin are often used for 6 to 8 weeks.

Many nutritional therapies have been tried, with variable results. Gelatin (Knox gelatin added to food at one packet/15 lb body weight daily) and zinc methionine are usually involved in these remedies. Ultimately, therapy directed at the primary cause of the problem is the most effective.

EOSINOPHILIC GRANULOMA COMPLEX

Eosinophilic granuloma complex is a confusing collection of feline disorders, which include eosinophilic ulcer, eosinophilic plaque, and linear (collagenolytic) granuloma. In reality, these conditions have many more dissimilarities than similarities. The involvement of eosinophils (which are known to downgrade immunologic responses) in the inflammatory process in each of these conditions is apparently enough to group these conditions together as a complex.

There are two common mechanisms by which cats develop these conditions:

- Allergic reactions
- Hereditary means

Allergic reactions are the most common reason for onset of lesions. Linear (collagenolytic) granuloma can result from mosquito bite hyper-sensitivity, and it is presumed that reactions to flea and black fly bites could also induce lesions. Inhalant allergies and adverse food reactions have been implicated as well. The pathogenesis of eosinophilic ulcer is not as clear. Some cases may be associated with feline leukemia virus infection. Another speculation is that lesions could result from constant irritation, perhaps related to the rough tongue or sharp canine teeth.

Clinical Signs

The signs for each of the major diseases in this complex are as follows:

- Eosinophilic (indolent) ulcers are usually nonpruritic, ulcerative lesions found principally on the lips (see Plate VIII-4), but they can occur on any part of the body and, occasionally, in the oral cavity (see Plate VIII-5). They may gradually resolve without therapy, but most cases are unrelenting.
- Eosinophilic plaques are localized, raised, and often pruritic lesions found principally on the abdomen (see Plate VIII-6) and medial thighs, but they can occur anywhere on the body or in the oral cavity. The surface of the lesions is often moist, ulcerated, and exudative.
- Linear (collagenolytic) granuloma is characterized by well-circumscribed, raised, firm, dermal masses, which are occasionally arranged in a linear pattern. The masses are found principally on the back of the hind legs (see Plate VIII-7), but they can occur on the footpads and in the oral cavity. The surface is usually dry and yellow to pink in color.

Diagnosis

In cats suspected of having eosinophilic granuloma complex, diagnostic efforts include the following:

- Skin scrapings
- Direct microscopic examination of cytologic preparations
- Complete blood count
- Viral profiles for feline leukemia virus and feline immunodeficiency virus

Whenever possible, biopsies should be performed to provide tissue for histopathologic assessment and microbiologic studies, if needed.

Cytologic preparations can be made quickly and are very helpful in making an appropriate diagnosis. Eosinophils are usually plentiful in preparations. Because some tumors resemble the nodules or ulcers seen in these conditions, an alternate diagnosis also might be correct. Blood eosinophilia is often associated with eosinophilic plaques, but it is not usually observed in the other types of lesions. Tissue eosinophilia is prevalent in eosinophilic plaques but is uncommon in indolent ulcer and is only associated with collagenolysis in linear granuloma.

Hypoallergenic diet trials and intradermal allergy testing are warranted in all cases of eosinophilic granuloma complex. Several insect allergens (e.g., mosquito, black fly, flea) should be included with the inhalant allergens in testing. The hypoallergenic diet trial should be performed for a minimum of 4 weeks.

Histopathologic assessment of biopsies is the single most valuable test to confirm the diagnosis. It not only supports a diagnosis in the majority of cases, but it also may reveal alternate diagnoses not originally considered.

Treatment

Treatment is always more effective if the underlying cause can be determined and corrected or appropriately managed:

- For cats with inhalant allergies hyposensitization is often successful, especially when combined with other allergy therapies such as antihistamines and omega-3 and omega-6 fatty acid preparations.
- Cats with adverse food allergies can be challenge-fed to determine problem foods or maintained on commercial hypoallergenic diets.
- In cases of insect hypersensitivity strict insect control on the cat and in the environment is needed. Safe topical preparations (e.g., Skin-So-Soft—Avon) or commercial insect repellents can be used. For cats with mosquito bite hypersensitivity, sleeping in a cage covered with mosquito netting may dramatically reduce the number of new lesions.

If no specific cause can be determined, the treatment of choice is anti-inflammatory doses of corticosteroids. Injectable methylprednisolone acetate can be given intramuscularly or subcutaneously and is safe and effective in most cases. An

initial dose of 20 mg is given and repeated twice at 2 week intervals. If remission occurs, injections can be repeated every 6 to 12 weeks as needed. Routine hematologic and biochemical profiles should be performed annually. Alternatively, anti-inflammatory doses of oral prednisone can be given on a daily or alternate day basis. Initially, daily doses of 2 to 4 mg/kg are administered to effect remission, followed by maintenance doses of 1 to 2 mg/kg on alternate days. This regimen is often less desirable for owners who have difficulty giving pills to their cats on a regular basis.

Megestrol acetate was once a common treatment for eosinophilic granuloma complex but has fallen into disfavor because of its many side effects. Medroxyprogesterone acetate carries the same risks and warnings. Neither can be recommended for treatment of these conditions.

Other therapies deserve mention. In some cases remission of lesions has been achieved with antibiotic therapy, even when no primary bacterial disease was suspected. Reports of success with trimethoprim-sulfonamides, cefadroxil, and amoxicillin clavulanate have been made. Surgery, cryosurgery, and carbon dioxide laser therapy have also been effective in the management of these patients. Radiation therapy (four to eight weekly treatments with 300 to 400 rad per session) has been used to treat solitary lesions of indolent ulcer refractory to corticosteroids and progestational compounds.

Nonspecific immunostimulants—such as levamisole (2.2 mg/kg three times weekly), mixed bacterins, thiabendazole (5 mg/kg three times weekly), and thymus gland extracts—have recently been advocated for cases of eosinophilic granuloma complex. Unfortunately, levamisole and thiabendazole can have severe side effects and are not recommended for routine therapy. The use of bacterins probably may be of the most benefit, but protocols need to be developed for general use.

KERATINIZATION DISORDERS

Keratinization disorders (seborrhea, erythroderma, exfoliative dermatitis; see Chapter 1) refer to several different disorders that upset the balance in epidermal cell renewal. The vast majority of cases are secondary to underlying disease processes. Dozens of different disorders with different causes and different treatments have been lumped together under the heading "seborrhea," but this is a poor term for these conditions. A better descriptive term is "disorder of keratinization," which implies a problem with epidermal cell turnover. This discussion examines only scaly, dry, or greasy dermatoses for which a specific diagnosis cannot be rendered.

Clinical Signs

Scaling, crusting, greasiness, and hair loss are the primary clinical signs of canine keratinization disorders. Secondarily, variable degrees of inflammation, scratching, self-trauma, and bacterial dermatitis are present in some cases. The normal cutaneous bacterial flora of 100 to 200 colonies/cm² increases to an average of 16,000 colonies/cm² on skin with a keratinization defect. Ceruminous otitis externa and hyperplasia of the tail gland are also commonly noted. Lesions on dogs can vary from dry to greasy, but most dogs have "combination skin" that has some greasy areas and other areas that are dry.

The most common clinical signs associated with feline keratinization disorders are generalized dry skin and haircoat with excessive scaling. Excessive oiliness is rare in cats but can be associated with feline leukemia, liver disease, neoplasia, congenitohereditary disorders, or immune-mediated diseases.

Diagnosis

The most common causes for secondary keratinization disorders in dogs are allergies, parasites, and endocrine disorders. If allergies are suspected, hypoallergenic diet trials and intradermal allergy testing are warranted. Multiple skin scrapings are indicated in all cases. Blood should be collected for hematologic, biochemical, and thyroid profiles in dogs and for hematologic, biochemical, and viral (feline leukemia virus and feline immunodeficiency virus) profiles in cats.

Histopathologic analysis of biopsies is often extremely valuable because it can direct further diagnostic efforts. Several causes of keratinization disorders have suggestive histologic patterns, such as vitamin A–responsive dermatosis (follicular hyperkeratosis and dyskeratosis), zinc-responsive dermatosis (parakeratotic hyperkeratosis), pemphigus (acantholysis), and T-cell lymphoma (Pautrier's microabscesses).

Treatment

Treatment is most often successful when the primary problem has been identified and corrected. When it cannot be identified, aggressive and long-term treatment is needed in many cases. For this reason diagnostic efforts must be vigorous enough to discover the underlying cause when possible.

Topical therapy is imperative for the symptomatic control of keratinization disorders. The frequency of application can range from three times weekly to once every 2 to 3 weeks, depending on the severity of the problem. Common antiseborrheic ingredients include:

- Sulfur
- Salicylic acid
- Selenium sulfide
- Tar
- Quaternary ammonium surfactants
- Benzoyl peroxide

Owners must understand that shampoo therapy does not cure the condition. It merely removes the surface scale and grease, which will recur over time.

Antiseborrheic shampoos have different advantages and disadvantages (Table 8-1). Keratolytic agents damage the epidermal cells so that the cells swell and are easier to shed. Keratoplastic agents "normalize" the epidermal cell cycle, usually by their cytostatic effect on the basal cell layer.

Dry, scaling skin responds best to emollient shampoos (e.g., HyLyt—DVM; Allergroom®—Allerderm/Virbac) or the use of after-bath rinses (e.g., Skin-So-Soft—Avon) or humectants. Sulfur-salicylic acid combinations are suitable for more severe, dry, scaling conditions. Tars, selenium sulfides, and benzoyl peroxides are drying and should not be used on skin that is already dry and scaling.

Oily or greasy skin responds best to drying agents such as tar, selenium sulfide, or benzoyl peroxide. As soon as the problem has been managed, however, it is important to switch to less irritating products such as sulfur-salicylic acid shampoos. If pyoderma is a concurrent problem, chlorhexidine shampoo (e.g., Nolvasan®—Fort Dodge) is preferred to benzoyl peroxide or tar.

Contact time of the shampoo with the skin is critical. Most medicated shampoos must have between 5 and 15 minutes contact with the skin to reach full effect. A clock should be used to judge the time interval because 15 minutes seems deceptively long when bathing a dog or cat. Owners should also be informed that the shampoo must reach the skin to be effective. In long-haired animals, routine clipping of the coat tends to make the process easier and more effective.

TABLE 8-1

MEDICATED SHAMPOOS

INGREDIENTS	ADVANTAGES	DISADVANTAGES	EXAMPLES
Sulfur	Safe; keratolytic; keratoplastic; antipruritic; antifungal; antibacterial	Nondegreasing; malodorous; may stain coat; may dry skin	Sebolux® (Allerderm/Virbac) Sebalyt (DVM) Micro Pearls (Evsco) Sebbafon® (Upjohn)
Selenium disulfide	Keratolytic; mildly degreasing	Weak antiseborrheic	Seleen® Plus (Sanofi Animal Health) Selenium (Vet Derm)
Salicylic acid	Mildly antibacterial; astringent; mildly antipruritic	Weak antiseborrheic	Medi-Clean® (Lambert Kay) Cerbinol® (Pitman-Moore) Soothing Medicated (Vet Derm)
Tar	Keratolytic; keratoplastic; degreasing; antipruritic	Poorly standardized; can stain coat; contact sensitivity; irritating; possibly carcinogenic	Allerseb-T® (Allerderm/Virbac) Lytar® (DVM) Clear Tar™ (VRx Products) Mycodex® Tar & Sulfur (SmithKline Beecham Animal Health)
Benzoyl peroxide	Keratolytic; keratoplastic; antibacterial; mildly antipruritic; degreasing	Very drying; stains coat; may irritate skin; possibly carcinogenic; bleaches fabrics	Pyoben® (Allerderm/Virbac) Oxydex® (DVM) Vet-Derm® (Vet Derm) Sulf/Oxydex (DVM) Benoxyderm® (Coopers Animal Health)

Whenever possible, veterinary shampoos, rather than products marketed for humans, should be used on dogs and cats. The thickness of the skin, its pH, and the types of hair follicles present are different in animals than in humans.

Omega-3 and omega-6 fatty acid supplements (e.g., DermCaps—DVM; EFA-Z Plus®—Allerderm/Virbac) may also be beneficial in an animal with a keratinization defect. Eicosapentaenoic acid has been used to alter arachidonic acid metabolism and help normalize the epidermal cell cycle. These supplements should be used regularly in any animal given long-term treatment for a keratinization disorder. Other sources of linoleic acid (e.g., sunflower oil, safflower oil, flaxseed oil) can also be helpful. Following supplementation with oral sunflower oil (1.5 ml/kg/day) for 30 days, cutaneous fatty acid profiles can return to near normal values in seborrheic dogs. Thus some of the clinical signs of seborrhea in dogs may be partly attributed to a localized deficiency of linoleic acid and/or elevated levels of arachidonic acid in the skin.

In particularly severe keratinization disorders, synthetic derivatives of vitamin A (retinoids) may be beneficial. Vitamin A has long been known for its normalizing effects on the skin, as well as for its potential for toxicity. Etretinate (Tegison®—Roche Laboratories) and isotretinoin (Accutane®—Roche Laboratories) are commercially available, but they are not licensed for use in dogs and cats. Etretinate is useful in surface-scaling conditions; its main indication for use in humans is psoriasis. Etretin (Soritane®—Roche Laboratories), a less toxic metabolite of etretinate, will soon be commercially available. Isotretinoin, on the other hand, acts on hair follicle epithelium and is licensed for the treatment of severe nodulocystic acne in humans.

Both etretinate and isotretinoin have been used experimentally in dogs and cats. Etretinate

(0.75 to 1.5 mg/kg/day) is more effective in managing idiopathic seborrhea, lamellar ichthyosis, and epidermal dysplasia, whereas isotretinoin (1 to 2 mg/kg/day) is better used in cases of schnauzer comedo syndrome and sebaceous adenitis.

Dogs generally have a higher tolerance for the retinoids than do humans and experience minimal side effects. These products should not be used in breeding animals, however, because of the teratogenic effects of vitamin A and the retinoids. Clients administering these drugs to their pets must also understand the risks of accidental ingestion by other family members. These products are expensive, and treatment needs to be continued for 2 months before success can be determined. All animals maintained on retinoid therapy should have periodic tests to evaluate blood counts, basic biochemistries (including liver function, cholesterol, and triglycerides), urinalysis, and tear production. These tests should be performed monthly for the first 3 months and then every 3 to 6 months while on maintenance therapy. For dogs experiencing bone pain, radiography is indicated or, alternatively, the long bones should be palpated every 6 months for signs of sensitivity. Bone pain usually disappears after discontinuation of the drug.

Vitamin A alcohol (retinol) also can be used in dogs (750 IU/kg/day) and is far less expensive. Unfortunately, it is also less effective in most keratinization disorders, except for the vitamin A–responsive dermatoses reported in cocker spaniels, miniature schnauzers, and Labrador retrievers.

CUTANEOUS LYMPHOMA

Cutaneous lymphoma (lymphosarcoma) is a malignant disorder of lymphocytes. Several different forms occur in the dog and cat, including:

- T-cell lymphoma
- B-cell lymphosarcoma
- Pagetoid reticulosis
- Plasmacytoma

In most cats with cutaneous lymphoma, tests for feline leukemia virus infection are negative.

Clinical Signs

B-cell lymphosarcoma is relatively rare in dogs and elderly male dogs are most likely to be affected. This condition may manifest itself as a strictly cutaneous disorder (characterized by nod-ules, plaques, or a maculopapular rash; see Plate VIII-8), or it may result in systemic involvement (leukemia or enlargement of the liver, spleen, and lymph nodes). Affected cats have solitary or multiple cutaneous lesions, masses, or a rash; as the disease progresses, systemic involvement occurs.

T-cell lymphoma (mycosis fungoides) is a slightly less malignant process in which lesions evolve from a red, scaly, exfoliative rash (erythroderma) through a plaque stage to large cutaneous nodules. This process can take months or years. Associated leukemia (Sézary syndrome) has also been noted. When more than one lesion is present, it should be presumed that systemic spread has occurred. Pruritus may or may not develop.

Pagetoid reticulosis (Woringer-Kolopp disease) is believed to be a form of T-cell lymphoma. Affected animals have scaling and plaques with a site predilection for the mouth and footpads. This disorder is extremely rare.

Cutaneous plasmacytomas (plasma cell tumors) may arise as primary tumors or may represent metastasis of primary osseous multiple myeloma. These dome-shaped nodules may become ulcerated and are most frequently seen on the lips, digits, and ears. Mucocutaneous plasmacytomas are usually seen in the mouth and rectum.

Diagnosis

Lymphomas may be suspected clinically, but confirmation requires cytologic or histopathologic assessment. Tumors of lymphocytes and plasma cells display neoplastic round cells with basophilic cytoplasm. Fine needle aspirates of nodules and lymph nodes or impression smears of ulcerated lesions or excised tumors might result in a quick diagnosis.

Biopsies for histopathologic analysis are needed for confirmation of specific diagnosis and for grading of tumors. An appropriate prognosis can then be given.

In all animals in which lymphoma is suspected, blood should be collected for hematologic and biochemical profiles for evidence of systemic involvement, including leukemia. Circulating neoplastic T-lymphocytes (Sézary cells) tend to have convoluted nuclei.

Treatment

The treatment of lymphoma depends on the specific disorder involved. For example, cutaneous plasmacytomas are generally benign,

---

CVP CANCER PROTOCOL

Cyclophosphamide—2.2 mg/kg PO 3 to 4 days per week

Vincristine—0.025 mg/kg or 0.5 mg/m² weekly for 3 weeks and then every 3 weeks

Prednisone—2.2 mg/kg daily for 1 week and then 1.1 mg/kg daily

---

although recurrence is occasionally reported; in contrast, mucocutaneous tumors of the mouth and rectum are often invasive and are associated with a poor prognosis.

B-cell lymphomas are responsive to various types of chemotherapy and immunotherapy; chemotherapy is more commonly used. Prednisone is often given initially and is capable of maintaining remission in some dogs. Unfortunately, dogs maintained initially on corticosteroids are less likely to respond to combination chemotherapy, the mainstay of treatment for systemic lymphoma. Primary cutaneous lymphomas may respond to chemotherapy with cyclophosphamide, vincristine, and prednisone (CVP; see box above) plus cytosine arabinoside or CVP plus doxorubicin. Doxorubicin (30 mg/m² IV every 3 weeks for a maximum of five to eight cycles) is indicated in animals with thymic or multicentric lymphosarcoma. These dogs can have median survival times of over 1 year.

One of the main problems with chemotherapeutic agents is that they pose a health risk for animals and health care professionals alike. Accidental exposure to even small amounts of these drugs during preparation and administration is extremely dangerous. They are not only irritating to skin and mucous membranes, but they may be carcinogenic to exposed hospital staff. Chronic exposure to small amounts of these drugs is associated with chromosome abnormalities, liver damage, malformed or aborted offspring, and cancer. Innocuous procedures such as withdrawing a drug-filled syringe from a vial, expelling air bubbles from a syringe, clipping drug-contaminated needles, and crushing tablets could lead to exposure of hospital staff. Therefore chemotherapeutic agents should only be handled by experienced and well-trained individuals.

An alternative to conventional chemotherapy is immunotherapy involving the use of biologic response modifiers. Autologous tumor cell vac-

cines are most successful once dogs are already in remission and help prolong survival times. A mouse-derived anti–canine lymphoma monoclonal antibody therapy is currently being evaluated. These immunotherapies are not yet commercially available.

T-cell lymphomas (including pagetoid reticulosis) are managed similarly to B-cell lymphomas. It is questionable, however, whether any treatment prolongs survival time because of the prolonged course (months to years) of disease. Treatment is likely only to improve clinical features associated with the disease. Corticosteroids or topical mechlorethamine (nitrogen mustard) may be of some benefit. Mechlorethamine is potentially very toxic and should be mixed by a licensed pharmacist.

MAST CELL TUMORS

Mast cell tumors (mastocytomas) are relatively common in dogs but somewhat uncommon in cats. The boxer, Boston terrier, English bulldog, English bull terrier, fox terrier, Staffordshire terrier, Labrador retriever, dachshund, and weimaraner have an increased incidence.

Benign mast cell tumors grow slowly over a period of months to years. In contrast, malignant mast cell tumors rapidly increase in size.

Clinical Signs

Cutaneous canine mastocytoma is usually benign. Solitary or multiple tumors may be seen that range in size from one to several centimeters in diameter (see Plate VIII-9). Benign tumors are firm, circumscribed, and encapsulated and are attached to the epidermis.

In contrast, malignant tumors in dogs are nonencapsulated and extend deep into subcutaneous tissue. Ulceration, erythema, edema, and inflammation are common in the surrounding tissue. Metastasis to regional lymph nodes usually occurs. Systemic signs of duodenal and gastric bleeding, bleeding tendencies (coagulopathies), and inflammatory kidney disease have all been associated with these tumors.

Systemic mastocytosis is an uncommon sequela to cutaneous mast cell tumor. Anorexia, vomiting, and diarrhea are seen in about half of affected dogs. The lymph nodes, spleen, and liver are most commonly involved.

Feline mast cell tumors may be benign or malignant. Cutaneous tumors have a variable clinical presentation. Most cats have multiple tumors in the head and neck region (see Plate VIII-10). Small papules and ulcerated plaques are other clinical presentations. Splenomegaly, hepatomegaly, and metastasis to regional lymph nodes and lungs are evidence of an aggressive disease process.

Older male cats (more than 4 years of age) appear to be predisposed to the condition. A second subtype occurs in younger cats (less than 4 years of age); Siamese appear to be predisposed to this type, which tends to spontaneously regress.

Diagnosis

The diagnosis of mast cell tumors can often be made while the patient is in the office as cytologic preparations are usually quite distinct. Mast cell tumors exfoliate readily, and representative cells are easily identified on fine needle aspirates. Typical hematologic stains (e.g., Wright's stain) are suitable for diagnostic purposes. (Alternatively, mast cell granules can be visualized by briefly air drying the prepared smear on a microscope slide, fixing it in 10% formalin for 5 to 10 seconds, washing in distilled water, and staining for 5 to 10 seconds in 0.1% toluidine blue solution.) Mast cells are round cells with nuclei often obscured by cytoplasmic granules. They are approximately one to three times the size of neutrophils. Eosinophils are often plentiful among the mast cells. Occasionally, mast cell granules do not stain adequately with quick staining methods.

All suspected mast cell tumors should be biopsied for grading of the tumor. The organization of the tumor and the degree of differentiation of the neoplastic cells are of prognostic significance. Poorly differentiated mast cell tumors are more aggressive and associated with a shorter survival time than are well-differentiated tumors. In dogs tumors are graded as follows:

- Grade I tumors are anaplastic, immature, and poorly differentiated and carry a mean survival time of about 18 weeks following diagnosis.
- Grade II tumors are intermediate in their differentiation and carry a mean survival time of about 28 weeks.
- Grade III tumors are well differentiated and offer a mean survival time of about 52 weeks.

In suspected cases of mast cell tumor, buffy coat smears, hematologic and biochemical pro-

---

PERFORMING A BUFFY COAT SMEAR

1. Collect whole blood in microhematocrit tube.
2. Centrifuge sample.
3. Break tube at level of buffy coat.
4. Express buffy coat onto clean microscope slide.
5. Heat fix for 3 to 5 seconds.
6. Apply series of hematologic stains.
7. Apply one or two drops of immersion oil to dried slide.
8. Evaluate microscopically for mast cells.

---

files, occult blood tests on stool, and survey radiography should also be done. In cats evaluation of viral profiles (feline leukemia virus, feline immunodeficiency virus) is needed as this can affect the prognosis.

Buffy coat smears (see box above) can be made by centrifuging a microhematocrit tube of blood, breaking it at the level of the buffy coat, expressing the buffy coat onto a microscope slide, and evaluating for circulating mast cells. The presence of these cells is an indicator of systemic disease and a poor prognosis.

Heparin released from mast cells can cause bleeding irregularities; thus finding of occult blood on fecal evaluation provides additional evidence of systemic disease. Finally, abdominal and thoracic radiographs may reveal evidence of metastasis.

Treatment

Treatment is variable depending on the distribution and grade of mast cell tumor. Young cats affected with mast cell tumors sometimes experience a spontaneous remission.

Solitary tumors should be excised, whereas multiple benign tumors usually require some form of chemotherapy. Recurrence of mast cell tumors at the excision site is common, and the surgical site should be reevaluated every 6 months. Cryosurgery has been useful, especially for multiple small skin tumors. A wide margin of normal tissue must be frozen to lessen the chance of recurrence.

Corticosteroids are often administered for systemic disease (prednisone [initially 1 mg/kg/day, which is then tapered]) or are injected into the tumors (triamcinolone). Cimetidine (Tagamet®—SmithKline Beecham Pharmaceuticals), an

H_2-specific antihistamine is often given at 4 mg/kg qid if there is evidence of gastrointestinal bleeding.

Where available, radiation therapy (10 equal treatments of 400 rad each for 3 days per week) is used for lesions not amenable to complete excision. Radiation therapy is an effective treatment of mast cell tumor in dogs. Surgical debulking of the tumors is usually done before irradiation.

Immunotherapy is an exciting process for the management of systemic mast cell tumors. Intralesional injections of preparations of *Propionibacterium acnes* (ImmunoRegulin®—ImmunoVet) or mycobacteria (Regressin®—Vetrepharm) may result in tumor regression after 3 to 4 months.

NECROLYTIC DERMATITIS

Canine superficial necrolytic dermatitis is a confusing metabolic condition that has been receiving increasing attention. It bears many similarities to necrolytic migratory erythema in humans, a condition seen primarily in patients with a glucagon-secreting pancreatic tumor. In dogs, however, pancreatic tumors are rarely the cause. More often, affected dogs have underlying diabetes mellitus, liver disease, kidney disease, pancreatic disease, or other metabolic disorders. Reports in the veterinary literature list the condition variably as superficial necrolytic dermatitis, necrolytic migratory erythema, diabetic dermatopathy, hepatocutaneous syndrome, and glucagonoma syndrome.

The lesions of superficial necrolytic dermatitis are thought to be manifestations of nutritional abnormalities. Although deficiencies of zinc or essential fatty acids may complicate the condition, its primary cause appears to be a blood amino acid deficiency (secondary to liver disease) that results in depletion of epidermal protein.

Clinical Signs

Most affected dogs have a history of recent weight loss. Skin lesions consist of erythema, erosions, ulcerations, and crusts. Primary areas affected include the muzzle, lips, nose, feet, and perineum. Hyperkeratosis of the footpads may also be noted.

Diagnosis

The diagnosis may be suspected on the basis of clinical findings and routine hematologic and biochemical profiles, but confirmation requires histopathologic assessment. Normochromic, normocytic, nonregenerative anemia is a common finding. Increased levels of alanine transaminase and other liver enzymes are present in most cases, and elevations of glucose are also common. Rarely, glucagon levels support a diagnosis of islet cell tumor in affected dogs. Percutaneous liver biopsies might reveal degenerative, fibrotic, and nodular changes, but these findings are not diagnostic.

Skin biopsies for histopathologic assessment are the diagnostic method of choice. The findings are very specific for this condition.

Treatment

No one therapy is effective in all dogs with this condition. Corticosteroids may be beneficial in the short term but are poor choices when dogs have overt liver disease or diabetes mellitus. Supplementation with zinc or essential fatty acids is not helpful in most cases. Temporary resolution of the condition may be achieved with intravenous amino acid preparations, but a long-term cure does not seem likely. Treatment of the underlying liver disease appears to be the best option in the majority of cases. The prognosis is poor.

OTITIS EXTERNA

Otitis externa is very common in dogs but somewhat less so in cats. Contributing factors include a long, relatively narrow ear canal, pendulous ears, and hair growth within the ear canal. Otitis externa is also commonly associated with allergic, immune-mediated, parasitic, bacterial, and fungal conditions, as well as with keratinization disorders, nutritional disorders, environmental causes, some endocrine and neoplastic processes, and foreign body reactions. Otitis externa is rarely a primary event. In most dogs and cats with otitis externa, other problems need to be addressed if management is to be optimal.

Clinical Signs

Signs of otitis externa include head shaking, erythematous pinnae, pain, and/or an exudative process. Ear canal involvement needs to be differentiated from pinnal involvement to help direct diagnostic efforts. Repeated trauma to the ears by shaking and rubbing can result in aural hema-

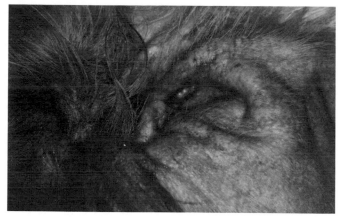

Figure 8-1. Otitis externa associated with a keratinization disorder.

toma, a condition in which a blood pocket forms between the cartilage of the ear and the overlying skin.

Diagnosis

Whenever possible, diagnostic efforts should be based on the clinical presentation, as many different disorders result in otitis externa:

- Extensive inflammatory involvement of the pinnae in otitis externa should prompt consideration of systemic problems, including allergies, food intolerance, ear margin dermatosis, cutaneous vasculitis, pemphigus, lupus erythematosus, dermatomyositis, lichenoid-psoriasiform dermatosis, and keratinization disorders (Figure 8-1).
- Hair loss confined to the pinnae without inflammation is more suggestive of pinnal alopecia (seen most commonly in dachshunds, chihuahuas, and whippets), periodic alopecia (seen in poodles), and congenito-hereditary disorders.
- Hormonal disorders (hypothyroidism, hyperestrogenism), dermatophytosis, demodicosis, and alopecia areata may or may not be associated with inflammation.
- Otitis externa with ear canal disease and minimal pinnal involvement is more likely to involve foreign bodies, parasites (ear mites, *Demodex* mites), bacteria, fungi, or yeasts (*Malassezia*).

The most important diagnostic test is a thorough examination of the ear canal to the level of the eardrum (tympanum). Heavy sedation or general anesthesia is usually required because the examination is very painful if severe ear canal inflammation is present. This procedure can be complicated by the presence of foreign bodies, polyps, hyperplastic tissue, or tumors within the ear canal. Undiagnosed rupture of the eardrum is one of the most common reasons for treatment failure.

Otitis media, a common sequela to otitis externa, usually follows eardrum rupture, but it can occur even when the eardrum is intact. The major clinical sign of otitis media is pain; difficulty with balance and other vestibular deficits do not occur until the inner ear is compromised. Diagnosis of otitis media can be presumed with eardrum rupture, but radiographic studies and surgical exploration may be necessary for confirmation. Radiographic studies confirm the diagnosis of otitis media in about 75% of cases.

If the ear is full of debris, appropriate samples should be collected for cytologic evaluation. The color of the discharge may provide further clues (e.g., mites often produce a black discharge; gram-positive bacteria are often associated with a brown exudate, and gram-negative infections are often associated with a yellow exudate). A smear can be stained (e.g., with Gram's or Wright's stain) to facilitate visualization of yeasts, bacteria, inflammatory cells, and wax. It is important to note whether the microbes seen were found within the white blood cells or in the extracellular debris. Unstained smears are best to determine whether parasites are present. Samples should be collected for microbial culture before any materials such as cleansers are instilled into the ear canal; these can be discarded later if they are not needed. Culture and sensitivity tests of ear exudates are less productive because opportunistic bacteria and yeasts are invariably present in the ear canal, which is simply a modified region of skin, containing all the same microbes. Staphylococci, alpha-hemolytic and nonhemolytic streptococci, *Micrococcus*, *Corynebacterium*, *Malassezia pachydermatis*, and, occasionally, coliform bacteria are commonly recovered for the ear canals of normal dogs. Sensitivity testing is only worthwhile when oral administration of antibiotics is being considered, especially if the eardrum has ruptured. Organisms of significance in the inflamed ear include *Staphylococcus intermedius*, beta-hemolytic streptococci, *Pseudomonas*, *Proteus*, coliform bacteria, and, occasionally, yeasts.

For careful otoscopic examination, the ear first must be thoroughly but gently irrigated to remove debris and waxy deposits. This not only aids in diagnosis but also allows medication to penetrate to the real site of the problem. Moreover, antibacterial agents (e.g., gentamicin) become inactivated in the presence of pus and debris.

Treatment

The underlying cause of otitis externa must be addressed if management is to be successful over the long term. Only rarely is the condition the result of a primary microbial infection. The important aspects of symptomatic therapy are to keep the ear canals flushed clean, instill appropriate anti-inflammatory and antibacterial medications, and effectively manage the underlying problem.

All debris and hairs should be removed from the inflamed ear canal. Removal of debris can be accomplished with flushing and antiseptics (e.g., chlorhexidine, povidone-iodine) and wax-dissolving substances (e.g., propylene glycol, dioctyl sodium sulfosuccinate, aluminum acetate). Before any materials are placed in the ear canal, it is important to determine if eardrum rupture has occurred because some medications are toxic to the cochlea and/or vestibular apparatus. Ototoxicity is common with topical aminoglycosides, especially gentamicin and neomycin, but these are common ingredients in many topical ear medications. Polymyxin B and chloramphenicol are also problematic. Contrary to earlier findings that suggested chlorhexidine was also ototoxic, it appears to be a safe antiseptic to use for flushing ears, even in the event of eardrum rupture.

Debris must not be removed from the ear canal with swabs. A swab can pack the material deeply into the ear canal. Rather, flushing should be used to remove the material from bottom to top. A swab or cotton ball can then be used to remove excess liquid, or suction can be gently applied to the canal. Although hair removal from the ear canal has been controversial, it improves air circulation and aids in preventing attachment of earwax (cerumen). The hair can be removed by manual plucking or by chemical depilatories. Manual plucking can result in significant trauma. Chemical depilatories (e.g., Nair—Carter-Wallace) can be instilled into the ear canal with a soft rubber urinary catheter and left in place for 10 minutes. The canal is then flushed with saline or a dilute povidone-iodine solution. Few adverse effects have been reported. Dogs without otitis externa *do not* require routine removal of hair from the ear canals.

In animals with otitis externa with mild inflammation, administration of a moderate topical corticosteroid (e.g., triamcinolone) for 5 to 7 days and then a milder product (e.g., hydrocortisone) for maintenance should be beneficial. Stronger or more prolonged therapies should not be used as research has shown that otic administration of corticosteroids for as little as 3 weeks can affect liver function tests. Combinations of corticosteroids and antimicrobial products are overused in general. Most bacteria and yeasts are susceptible to safe antiseptics (e.g., chlorhexidine) or agents that create a more acidic environment (e.g., vinegar and water in a 1:1 or 1:2 ratio) without the risks of adverse effects or resistance.

Long-term use of potent antibiotics within the ear canal can lead to drug resistance and may also cause allergic drug reactions and overgrowth of yeasts and resistant bacteria. Treatment with products such as vinegar and water, antiseptics, or drying agents greatly reduces the incidence of adverse effects, making long-term treatment safer. Antibiotics are best given systemically for a week or so in the treatment of otitis externa, especially if the eardrum is ruptured. Apparently, systemic therapy is less likely to interfere with the normal flora of the ear canal. Of course, elimination of the underlying cause is best, if possible.

In chronically affected ears surgical alternatives need to be considered. A lateral ear resection (Zepp or Lacroix procedure) is beneficial in about 50% of patients. Chronically inflamed and scarred ears or those in which the horizontal ear canal has been markedly narrowed show the least favorable results. The procedure is inadequate for cases of end stage otitis. Vertical ear canal resection has the advantage of removing all inflamed tissue with the exception of the short segment of remaining horizontal canal while providing a route of drainage for the infected middle ear. Finally, ear canal ablation combining bulla osteotomy and curettage can be used for dogs with chronic non-responsive otitis externa and/or otitis media, tumors of the horizontal portion of the ear canal, or failed previous procedures.

PANNICULITIS

Panniculitis, an uncommon inflammatory disease of the subcutaneous fat in dogs and cats, is caused by a variety of underlying disorders. Most cases of panniculitis involve immune-mediated mechanisms but microbial, nutritional, metabolic, and drug-induced causes have been reported.

The type of degenerative changes seen in the

adipose tissue depends on whether the arterial or venous supply has been compromised:

- Interference with the arterial supply results in diffuse degeneration of the fat lobules (lobular panniculitis).
- Venous disorders result in alterations of the fibrous septae and the peripheral portions of the fat lobules (septal panniculitis).

Clinical Signs

Lesions can be localized or generalized, can vary in size up to several centimeters, and are sometimes painful. They often become evident as deep subcutaneous nodules occurring singly or in groups. The nodules can subsequently ulcerate and drain, which can result in pronounced scarring.

Benign (juvenile) panniculitis occurs in young dogs, although older animals display similar syndromes. The most commonly affected breeds are dachshunds, toy poodles, collies, and wire-haired fox terriers. The nodules rupture, discharging an oily, purulent material, or they regress spontaneously.

Connective tissue panniculitis results from disorders that compromise the blood vessels and connective tissues, such as lupus erythematosus, dermatomyositis, and scleroderma. Lupus profundus, a variant of lupus erythematosus, is characterized by ulcerating subcutaneous nodules (see Plate VIII-11).

Pancreatic panniculitis results when pancreatic enzymes cause digestion of the subcutaneous fat. Most cases occur as a sequela to pancreatitis or pancreatic cancer. The condition is characterized by enlarging papules and nodules that rupture and leave deep subcutaneous ulcers.

Immune-mediated panniculitis, such as erythema nodosum, results from hypersensitivity reactions to infectious agents or medications (including vaccines). In addition to the presence of subcutaneous nodules, the syndrome is associated with fever, depression, and joint pain. Remission is usually spontaneous. Vaccine site panniculitis is associated with the subcutaneous injection of killed rabies vaccine. This recently recognized disorder is characterized by a round patch of hairless skin at the vaccination site. Scarring can occur secondarily and result in permanent hair loss. Poodles appear to be more prone to developing this condition than are other breeds.

Steatitis results from a vitamin E deficiency in cats. This condition is often associated with diets containing high levels of fish (especially red tuna), which contain large amounts of highly unsaturated fatty acids. Improper processing or prolonged storage of fish-based foods or dietary deficit can also result in a relative deficiency of vitamin E in cats. In affected cats the fat becomes firm and yellow-orange. They lose their appetites, have high fevers, are reluctant to move, and sometimes experience pain.

Chronic relapsing panniculitis is a general term describing cases of panniculitis that elude specific diagnosis or recur following cessation of therapy. These cases might represent the yet undescribed versions of a number of human conditions, or they may inexplicably test false-negative for the conditions already discussed.

Finally, subcutaneous nodules occur in a variety of other conditions, including bacterial infections, fungal infections, skin tumors, cutaneous cysts, foreign body penetration, trauma, and reactions to injections.

Diagnosis

Because many different conditions result in panniculitis, a systematic diagnostic approach should be taken. Blood should be collected for hematologic and biochemical profiles and ANA testing. Pancreatic enzyme levels and ANA findings are particularly useful.

Fine needle aspiration should be performed on all subcutaneous nodules. Impression smear cytology is a valuable adjunct whenever draining tracts or ulcerated surfaces are noted. The findings may be suggestive but often are not specific enough to confirm a particular diagnosis.

Biopsies are critical to uncovering the exact cause of the problem. Often, the pattern of the inflammatory infiltrate is helpful in diagnosis (e.g., erythema nodosum involves a septal panniculitis and lupus profundus often is associated with both a lobular and septal panniculitis). Microbial infections, such as mycobacteriosis or systemic fungal infections, usually have characteristic patterns, even if the organisms cannot be specifically identified in sections. Microbial cultures should be harvested from biopsy specimens rather than from surface discharge.

Treatment

The treatment of panniculitis must be individualized to the specific cause. This gives the best chance for success. For example, benign (juvenile) panniculitis usually responds completely to a 2 week course of corticosteroids (2.2 mg/kg/day). Erythema nodosum may clear spontaneously in weeks or months. Vaccine site panniculitis requires no therapy because it does not constitute a medical threat.

On the other hand, the immune-mediated causes of panniculitis often require long-term immunosuppressive therapy (see Chapter 5). When no cause can be determined for the panniculitis and it is not associated with bacterial, fungal, or viral infections, a therapeutic trial with corticosteroids may be indicated.

PODODERMATITIS

Pododermatitis refers to an inflammatory condition of the feet and interdigital spaces and results from myriad causes. Although animals with this disorder are commonly seen in general practice, they tend to be incompletely evaluated and the result is a poor response to treatment. Most cases are presumed to involve bacterial infections, but many studies refute this. Other causes are allergic (contact, inhalant, food, drug eruption) disorders, fungal (dermatophytosis, *Candida, Malassezia,* eumycotic mycetoma) diseases, parasitic (e.g., demodicosis, *Pelodera,* hookworm, tick) disorders, and neoplastic conditions (e.g., squamous cell carcinoma, melanoma, mast cell tumor, cysts). Trauma, foreign body reactions, immunodeficiency, immune-mediated disturbances (e.g., pemphigus, pemphigoid, lupus erythematosus, eosinophilic granuloma complex, plasmacytic pododermatitis), nutritional imbalances (e.g., zinc-responsive dermatosis), and neurologic problems (e.g., acral lick dermatitis, acral mutilation syndrome) must also be considered.

Clinical Signs

Pododermatitis has two major presentations:

- Interdigital pododermatitis
- Footpad pododermatitis

With interdigital pododermatitis there is evidence of inflammation in the interdigital spaces. Inflammation can be as mild as the erythematous interdigital dermatitis of allergy, or the thick, nodular, and exudative lesions of sterile pyogranuloma can occur (Figure 8-2).

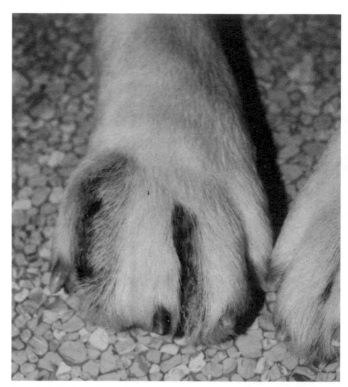

Figure 8-2. Pododermatitis associated with sterile pyogranuloma.

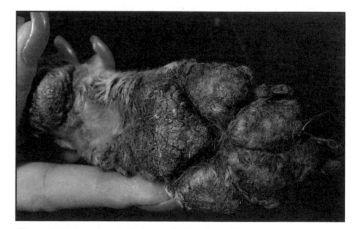

Figure 8-3. Hyperkeratotic footpads in a dog with pemphigus foliaceus.

Signs of footpad pododermatitis also vary and include the ulcerative process of a contact eruption, the swollen nature of plasmacytic pododermatitis, and the hyperkeratotic presentation of zinc-responsive dermatosis or pemphigus foliaceus (Figure 8-3).

Diagnosis

The most common cause of pododermatitis associated with licking and chewing at the feet is allergy. Dogs suspected of having the condition should undergo hypoallergenic diet trials and intradermal allergy testing. Any nodular, pustular, or ulcerative form of interdigital pododermatitis warrants histopathologic assessment of biopsies, which can provide more information than microbial cultures or routine blood tests. Other immediate tests should include skin scrapings and cytologic preparations. More specific testing can be conducted once the biopsy results are available. In cats tests for feline leukemia virus infection, feline immunodeficiency virus infection, and diabetes should be performed in addition to the tests listed above. A higher incidence of neoplastic pododermatoses is found in cats than in dogs, and histopathologic evaluation in suspected feline cases is critical.

Biopsy of the footpads is sometimes technically difficult but invariably rewarding, even if it serves to refute a supposed diagnosis. Rare diagnoses such as lethal acrodermatitis or tyrosinemia would not likely be uncovered by other routine diagnostic tests.

Treatment

Most cases of interdigital pododermatitis can be effectively managed if the underlying problem is identified. Concurrent infection is likely, and bactericidal antibiotics (e.g., oxacillin, cephalexin) are usually prescribed in such a case. Although *Staphylococcus intermedius* is the primary bacterial isolate in canine cases, secondary opportunistic bacteria include *Proteus* spp., *Pseudomonas aeruginosa*, and *E. coli*. Once established in the tissues, gram-negative organisms can cause chronic or recurrent problems. Scarring, granuloma formation, and fibrosis often result and make it difficult to eliminate bacterial infection from the tissues. In severe cases surgical procedures such as fusion podoplasty may provide alternatives for long-term control.

For footpad disorders, hyperkeratotic areas can be pared down with a surgical blade to normal pad tissues. Alternatively, keratolytic preparations (e.g., KeraSolv—DVM) can be applied to hydrate the scale, making it easier to remove. For ulcerative lesions on the pads, topically applied aloe vera often works better than antibiotic preparations. In all circumstances, identification and correction of the underlying problem offer the best guarantees of suitable recovery.

SOLAR DERMATITIS

Solar dermatitis (photodermatitis) is the adverse effect of ultraviolet light that occurs on white, depigmented, or sparsely haired skin. Certain breeds and individual animals with lightly colored or sparsely haired skin have an increased risk. Ultraviolet exposure, coupled with a genetic predisposition, are thought to play major roles in the cause of solar dermatitis. Although the cause of the skin damage is not completely known, evidence suggests that ultraviolet rays alter DNA synthesis and repair in the epidermis.

Dalmatians and white bull terriers have a higher incidence than do other dog breeds. White-furred cats also have an increased incidence. Although not directly caused by exposure to sunlight, dogs and cats with cutaneous (discoid) or systemic lupus erythematosus may develop a facial dermatitis that worsens in direct sunlight.

Clinical Signs

Common sites of involvement are:

- Dorsal muzzle (in dogs)
- Tips and margin of the pinnae (in cats)

There is a geographic trend in that incidence is increased in areas with long periods of intense sunlight. The Australian shepherd is the breed at most risk for nasal solar dermatitis. Many cases of "collie nose," which once were thought to be sun induced, are now recognized to have an immune-mediated basis.

Solar-induced dermatitis can also be observed in dogs that enjoy sunbathing. Breeds at risk include white bull terriers, American Staffordshire terriers, German short-haired pointers, dalmatians, white boxers, whippets, and beagles. The damage usually occurs on the underside or flanks, but, occasionally, facial lesions are noted. Early in the course of the condition, the skin becomes pink and edematous, the equivalent of a sunburn. In time, these areas become thickened, eroded, or ulcerated. Actinic keratoses, squamous cell carcinomas, or hemangiosarcomas can develop on chronically affected skin.

In feline solar dermatitis there are initial inflammatory changes of the ear tips, which later lose hair and become encrusted. The eyelid margins, lips, and nares may also be affected in chronic cases. Squamous cell carcinoma can develop after several years of sunlight exposure. Neoplastic lesions are characterized by persistent, ulcerative, locally invasive lesions of the pinnae.

Diagnosis

In the early stages the erythematous changes may be suggestive of inhalant allergies, contact eruptions, or sunburn. With chronic exposure permanent skin damage results.

Histopathologic assessment of biopsies is important because it can determine the amount of damage done, comment on solar elastosis or other changes evident, and identify cancerous or precancerous changes.

Treatment

Several different treatments have been suggested to control the lesions associated with solar dermatitis, including the following:

- Confinement to an indoor or shady environment during peak daylight hours
- Application of topical sunscreens
- Protective clothing
- Administration of beta-carotene
- Administration of topical and systemic corticosteroids

Tattooing the nose with black ink may halt the clinical manifestations of solar exposure but does little to protect the epidermis from actinic damage. Temporary pigmentation can be created by use of a black felt-tipped marker.

Topical sunscreens with a SPF of 15 or greater can be helpful if the animal allows it to be applied. Sunscreens should be reapplied every 12 hours. Topical hydrocortisone preparations (0.5% to 1%) can also be applied to help reduce inflammation; during acute bouts they can be safely used for approximately 1 week.

With sunbathers that are prone to solar dermatitis, a cotton T-shirt or other form of protective clothing may be adequate to halt solar damage. Beta-carotene (30 mg twice daily) and synthetic vitamin A derivatives have been used experimentally in the treatment of solar dermatitis with mixed results. Etretinate (Tegison®—Roche Laboratories) has also been used in dogs with precancerous lesions or squamous cell carcinoma at doses of 1 to 2 mg/kg/day. Any response should be noted in 6 to 12 weeks.

In cats surgery is sometimes required when the ear tips become necrotic or affected by squamous cell carcinoma. These tumors are usually slow to metastasize, and early excision might resolve the problem permanently. After surgery it is critical to keep these cats out of direct sunlight.

RECOMMENDED READINGS

Beckman SL, Henry WB Jr, Cechner P: Total ear canal ablation combining bulla osteotomy and curettage in dogs with chronic otitis externa and media. *JAVMA* 196(1):84–90, 1990.

Campbell KL, Uhland CF, Dorn GP: Effects of oral sunflower oil on serum and cutaneous fatty acid concentration profiles in seborrheic dogs. *Vet Dermatol* 3(1):29–35, 1992.

Clinkenbeard KD: Diagnostic cytology: Mast cell tumors. *Compend Contin Educ Pract Vet* 13(11):1697–1704, 1991.

Goldberger E, Rapoport JL: Canine acral lick dermatitis: Response to the antiobsessional drug clomipramine. *JAAHA* 27(2):179–182, 1991.

Guaguere E, Hubert B, Delabre C: Feline pododermatoses. *Vet Dermatol* 3:1–12, 1992.

Hahn KA, Morrison WB: Safety guidelines for handling chemotherapeutic drugs. *Vet Med*, pp 1094–1099, Nov 1991.

Hammond DL, Conroy JD, Woody BJ: The histological effects of a chemical depilatory on the auditory canal of dogs. *JAAHA* 26(5):551–554, 1990.

Hendrick MJ, Dunagan CA: Focal necrotizing granulomatous panniculitis associated with subcutaneous injection of rabies vaccine in cats and dogs: 10 cases (1988–1989). *JAVMA* 198(2):304–305, 1991.

Kwochka DW: Retinoids and vitamin A therapy, in Griffin CE, Kwochka KW, MacDonald (eds): *Current Veterinary Dermatology—The Science and Art of Therapy.* St Louis, Mosby–Year Book, 1993, pp 203–210.

Mansfield PD: Ototoxicity in dogs and cats. *Compend Contin Educ Pract Vet* 12(3):331–337, 1990.

McCarthy RJ, Caywood DD: Vertical ear canal resection for end-stage otitis externa in dogs. *JAAHA* 28(6):545–552, 1992.

Meyer DJ, Moriello KA, Feder BM, et al: Effect of otic medications containing glucocorticoids on liver function test results in healthy dogs. *JAVMA* 196(5):743–744, 1990.

Miller WH Jr: Topical management of seborrhea in dogs. *Vet Med*, pp 122–131, Feb 1990.

Miller WH Jr, Scott DW, Buerger RG, et al: Necrolytic migratory erythema in dogs: A hepatocutaneous syndrome. *JAAHA* 26(6):573–581, 1990.

Remedios AM, Fowler JD, Pharr JW: A comparison of radiographic versus surgical diagnosis of otitis media. *JAAHA* 27(2):183–188, 1991.

Rosenkrantz W: Eosinophilic granuloma complex (confusion). *Vet Focus* 1(1):29–32, 1989.

Rosenthal RC, MacEwen EG: Treatment of lymphoma in dogs. *JAVMA* 196(5):774–781, 1990.

Rosenthal RC, Michalski D: Storage of expensive anticancer drugs. *JAVMA* 198(1):144–145, 1991.

Rosychuk RA: Nail diseases of the dog and cat. Proceedings of the 10th ACVIM Forum, San Diego, May 1992, pp 125–127.

Scott DW, Miller WH Jr: Disorders of the claw and

clawbed in cats. *Compend Contin Educ Pract Vet* 14(4):234–239, 1992.

Swaim SF, Lee AH, MacDonald JM, et al: Fusion podoplasty for the treatment of chronic fibrosing interdigital pyoderma in the dog. *JAAHA* 27(3):264–274, 1991.

Swaim SF, Riddell KP, McGuire JA: Effects of topical medications on the healing of open pad wounds in dogs. *JAAHA* 28(6):499–502, 1992.

White SD: Pododermatitis. *Vet Dermatol* 1:1–18, 1989.

White SD: Naltrexone for treatment of acral lick dermatitis in dogs. *JAVMA* 196(7):1073–1076, 1990.

CHAPTER NINE
Client Counseling

*D*ermatology is often a frustrating discipline for veterinarians and owners alike. Most conditions cannot be cured but can be controlled, and owner education and compliance are critical in providing ongoing care to animals. Owners must understand that safe management—and not just "doing something"—is the most important goal. Overtreatment often results in worse consequences than conscientious neglect; although it may resolve a particular problem, it may lead to a potentially more dangerous condition later on.

Providing optimum veterinary care involves more than just dispensing pills and giving injections. Owner education is also important and is the entire staff's concern. The informed owner is the preferred client; he or she understands the options and can make intelligent choices. The uninformed client is often an accident waiting to happen. This client wants the pet to receive the same treatment (e.g., the little white pills it has been getting for years or the "allergy shot" it gets every month or so), without even realizing what drugs are involved.

Practicing medicine is always more rewarding when veterinarians, hospital staff, and pet owners work on the same team. It is not unusual for owners to leave a veterinary clinic and not fully understand what has just transpired. Sometimes they do not ask what they perceive to be "stupid" questions, and other times they do not realize how little they know until questioned by family members at home.

Any opportunity to educate a client is time well spent. Often, however, the subject matter can be too overwhelming to be completely digested by the client all at once.

The collection of client handouts that follows may be useful in your general practice. Client handouts are very helpful because they serve as resource material that owners can refer to as needed. They also indicate to clients that you are sincerely interested in their pet's problem and that you want to provide them with as much information as possible. More often than not, clients perceive that their pet's ailment is rare—that you never have dealt with a similar case before. It may be reassuring to them that they are not alone and that there are options for them to consider.

Reducing Itchiness in the Allergic Dog and Cat

In managing allergic dogs and cats, our goal is to provide safe and effective products that help relieve itching. We must make pets comfortable without causing unwanted side effects. Although the methods listed below are not always effective individually, combining two or more of the treatments may significantly reduce itchiness.

Immunotherapy (allergy injections) is the best and safest long-term way of managing allergies. Treatment is formulated on the basis of allergy tests (similar to those done in people). At present, skin tests are superior to blood tests in the diagnosis of allergy. Immunotherapy is successful in about 75% of cases, and 6 to 8 months of injections are needed before any benefits are evident.

Bathing the allergic pet is an excellent way to relieve itchiness, but the effect is short lived. Animals should be bathed in cool water with an appropriate medicated shampoo to relieve itchiness. These shampoos contain a variety of ingredients and should be chosen based on the individual pet's coat condition. These ingredients include sulfur and salicylic acid (e.g., Sebolux, SebaLyt), selenium (e.g., Seleen), and oatmeal (e.g., Epi-Soothe). Dry coats can be further moisturized after bathing by using sprays (e.g., Humilac, HyLyt) or cream rinses (e.g., Epi-Soothe, HyLyt). Hypoallergenic shampoos are not designed for allergic pets but for animals with sensitive skin that cannot tolerate other products. Medicated shampoos should be used regularly and frequently.

Antihistamines may be helpful in relieving itchiness in perhaps one-third of allergic patients. Dogs respond best to clemastine (Tavist), diphenhydramine (Benadryl), chlorpheniramine (Chlor-Trimeton), hydroxyzine (Atarax), and terfenadine (Seldane). Cats often do best on chlorpheniramine (Chlor-Trimeton). Some antihistamines are only available by prescription, while others are over-the-counter preparations. They have few side effects, except for drowsiness (which may help pets get a good night's sleep).

Dietary supplements (including specific essential fatty acids known as omega-3 and omega-6 fatty acids) are completely safe products that have anti-inflammatory effects to counteract itchiness. These prescription items are different than over-the-counter dietary supplements designed to make the coat glossy. Products such as DermCaps and EFA-Z Plus are effective in perhaps 20% of allergic pets.

Environmental management is important when the source of allergies (e.g., house dust mites, molds, or specific foods) can be identified. The pet's exposure to the allergic source should be reduced as much as possible. For example, using electronic air cleaners and dehumidifiers and changing filters regularly decreases the population of molds and house dust mites. Vacuuming is another important aid in removing allergens from the environment.

Corticosteroids are very effective at relieving itching, but they have a variety of side effects and should only be used sparingly. Products that combine low levels of prednisone with antihistamines (e.g., Temaril P, Vanectyl P) are probably the safest forms available. Injectable corticosteroids may be suitable for cats, but are the least suitable form of treatment for allergic dogs.

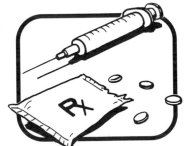

Environmental Control for Allergic Pets

Pets with an inhalant allergy (or "hay fever") can benefit from many medications, but there are also some things that you can do around the home.

Pollen Allergies: If your pet is allergic to pollen, keep the animal indoors most of the day. You may not realize that pollens can travel up to 30 miles in the wind and the pollen source does not have to be in the pet's immediate environment to cause a problem.

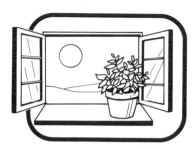

Though air conditioners do little to remove airborne allergens, they limit pollen exposure because doors and windows are kept closed when they are in use. Periodically clean humidifiers, vaporizers, dehumidifiers, and air conditioners, which may develop growths of mold.

Mold Allergies: Depending on the type of mold, spores may be dispersed by rainfall, humidity, or winds. When the sun warms the air during the day, most airborne spores are carried high into the atmosphere, only to descend again with the cool night air. The condition of many pets with mold allergy tends to worsen at night, unless they also spend their days in such mold-rich environments (e.g., damp basements or outside with their nose to the ground). Usually, there are just as many molds inside a home as there are outside.

If your dog or cat is allergic to mold, you should remove all houseplants because they harbor large numbers of molds. If plants cannot be removed, their mold content can be reduced by covering the soil surface with aquarium tank filter charcoal bits.

Dust Allergies: It is impossible to completely eradicate house dust and house dust mites from a home, but they can be controlled. Control measures should be most stringent in areas where the allergic pet spends most of its time. The stuffing of any pet bedding should be of a synthetic material; kapok, feathers, wool, and horsehair should be avoided. Vacuuming is an important way of removing dust from the environment. Unfortunately, most upright vacuum cleaners have bags through which dust particles and mites can pass. Newer allergy management bags have a smaller pore size through which fewer dust particles can escape.

Control of house dust and house dust mites is an important component of therapy for dust allergy. Electrostatic filters help reduce the amount of dust in the air by about 80%, but they do not produce a dust-free environment. In addition, they produce ozone, which may cause headaches in some individuals. High efficiency particulate air (HEPA) filters can clear over 95% of pollens, molds, yeasts, bacteria, and viruses from the air and, when coupled with a charcoal filter, can remove practically all of the dust.

Because house dust mites cannot reproduce at humidities less than 60% and mold growth is negligible near 30%, maintain relative humidity between 30% to 50%. Pets themselves can act as dust magnets, and animals allergic to dust are also likely to be more affected when they share a home with other animals. Keep pets well groomed to minimize this problem.

Antihistamine Therapy in the Dog and Cat

Antihistamines are not a cure-all for the allergic patient, but they provide an alternative to steroids for symptomatic relief. Antihistamines appear to work well in about one-third of allergic dogs and cats. They can also be combined with other safe forms of therapy, such as fatty acid supplements and medicated baths. If necessary, they can also be used to lessen the amount of cortisone (steroid) needed to control a problem.

To determine whether an antihistamine is effective, try one for a minimum of 7 to 10 days. You may need to try three or four different products before finding one that is effective. Just because one product doesn't work, don't assume that none will.

Most antihistamines are relatively safe for routine use. Be aware, however, that most preparations intended for human use have not been approved for use in animals.

*　　*　　*

In the chart below, several available antihistamine products are listed. To use the chart, follow these steps:

1. Choose a product from the chart.
2. Find the proper dose for your pet's body weight. If there is more than one dose, start with the lowest dose first and increase the dose only if there is no improvement after 1 week.
3. Find out how many times a day to give the antihistamine by looking under the daily doses column. If there is a choice, begin at the smallest number of doses and increase the number only if the pet does not improve after 1 week.

GENERIC NAME	TRADE NAME	FORMS	DOSE (BY BODY WEIGHT)					DAILY DOSES
			1–5 kg	5–10 kg	10–15 kg	15–25 kg	>25 kg	
Diphenhydramine hydrochloride	Benadryl	2.5 mg/ml oral liquid	½–1 tsp	1–2 tsp	—	—	—	2–3
		25 mg capsule	—	—	1 capsule	—	—	
		50 mg capsule	—	—	—	1 capsule	2 capsules	
Clemastine	Tavist	1 mg tablet	—	½ tablet	1 tablet	1½ tablets	2 tablets	2
Chlorpheniramine	Chlortrimeton Chlortripolon (in Canada)	0.5 mg/ml oral liquid	1 tsp	—	—	—	—	2–3
		4 mg tablet	—	1	2	2½	3	
Brompheniramine	Dimetapp	0.4 mg/ml oral liquid	1 tsp	—	—	—	—	2–3
		4 mg tablet	—	1	2	2½	3	
Trimeprazine tartrate	Temaril Panectyl (in Canada)	2.5 mg tablet	½ tablet	1 tablet	—	—	—	2–3
		5 mg tablet	—	—	1 tablet	—	—	
		10 mg tablet	—	—	—	1 tablet	2 tablets	
Terfenadine	Seldane	6 mg/ml oral liquid	½–1 tsp	—	—	—	—	2
		60 mg tablet	—	½ tablet	1 tablet	2 tablets	3 tablets	
Astemizole	Hismanal	2 mg/ml oral liquid	½–1 tsp	—	—	—	—	1–2
		10 mg tablet	—	½ tablet	1 tablet	2 tablets	3 tablets	
Hydroxyzine	Atarax	10 mg capsule	1 capsule	—	—	—	—	3
		25 mg capsule	—	1 capsule	—	—	—	
		50 mg capsule	—	—	1 capsule	2 capsules	3 capsules	

Adverse Food Reactions

Adverse food reactions are relatively common in both dogs and cats. Although the term "food allergy" is frequently used when discussing this problem, other conditions may be involved. Pets can also have food intolerance, just as people do.

A dog or cat with food allergy or food intolerance can have many different problems, including signs of digestive disorders such as vomiting, diarrhea, or flatulence. In many cases, however, only skin problems result. These might include recurrent ear infections, itchy skin, dermatitis, and "hot spots."

You may think that a food allergy can't occur in a pet that has eaten the same food without problems for years, but this is not true. Like people, pets can develop adverse food reactions even after having eaten certain foods for many weeks, months, or years. Surveys show that most food-allergic pets eat the same food for over 2 years before problems start.

Diagnosis—the hypoallergenic diet trial: The diagnosis of adverse food reactions is best made with a hypoallergenic diet trial, which involves limiting a pet's diet to food ingredients that it has never

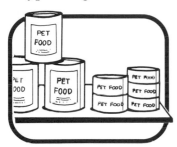

eaten before. Unfortunately, you can't just buy a different commercial diet or buy a commercial food with a novel ingredient such as lamb. Commercial hypoallergenic diets are not foolproof, and their results are incorrect about 20% of the time. For a proper diet trial, homemade meals must be prepared for a minimum of 4 weeks.

Providing a hypoallergenic diet trial may not be convenient, but there are no easy tests to diagnose food-related problems. Blood tests have been developed, but research has shown them to be exceptionally unreliable and they cannot be recommended at this time. The best test we have is

the hypoallergenic diet trial, where the ingredients fed to pets are restricted and the pets are observed for any signs of improvement.

Preparing the hypoallergenic diet: Try to select foods that have never been in a commercial food or in table scraps fed to the pet. If your pet has never eaten lamb before, this is a convenient source of protein. There is nothing magical about lamb; it is selected because many dogs and cats in North America have never been exposed to it. Other suitable ingredients are deer, rabbit, moose, and sometimes fish. Rice or potatoes are usually suitable as a carbohydrate source. During the trial pets must not receive any treats, chew toys, or even flavored vitamin-mineral mixes or medications.

Boil the ingredients and mix them in a ratio of one part protein to two parts carbohydrate. Although this diet is not nutritionally balanced, it will cause no harm in the 4 weeks necessary to complete the trial. The goal of the test is to determine if food is involved in the problem. If food does have a role, improvement should be evident by the end of the trial.

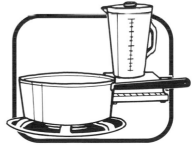

If improvement on the food trial is seen, it doesn't mean you will have to prepare homemade meals for the rest of your pet's life. The next step is to determine which ingredients (e.g., beef, soy, milk, corn, wheat) is causing the adverse reaction and to find an appropriate diet that excludes any problem-causing items.

Fleas

Fleas have been pestering dogs and cats for millions of years. Our best strategy to combat fleas is to understand how they cause problems and where they are most vulnerable to attack.

Flea bites are not only irritating; they can cause allergic reactions as well. In flea-hypersensitive dogs and cats the bite of one flea can cause itchiness for 5 to 7 days. A pet with a flea problem is not necessarily loaded with fleas. In fact, animals that have had heavy flea burdens since they were young are unlikely to be allergic to fleas. Most flea-allergic pets have only been exposed to fleas intermittently. It may be difficult to find evidence of even a single flea on these animals, which can complicate identification of the problem. Flea feces (also known as "flea dirt"), which are tiny, black, comma-shaped particles on the skin and hair-coat, may be the only sign of flea infestation.

In the past it was believed that fleas spent 90% of their time in the environment and only 10% on the pet. This is probably true for the rat flea but not for fleas commonly found on dogs and cats. These fleas spend 100% of their adult life on the pet, unless they are removed by scratching, rubbing, or bathing. Flea eggs are laid on the animal but fall into the environment where the immature fleas hatch and develop further. Since a single female flea can lay hundreds of eggs within a week, there are many more flea eggs in the home than fleas on the pet. This is why environmental control is so important.

Flea control is a family project. All animals in the household must be treated, even if they show no problems. It doesn't do any good to treat the dog but not the cat that roams outdoors. Also, you shouldn't just treat pets and neglect the carpets and floor surfaces in the household where flea eggs hatch.

Flea Control on the Pet: Flea combs are excellent tools for locating hard-to-detect fleas and for removing them from the pet. The best areas to concentrate on are the hindquarters, belly, neck, and armpits.

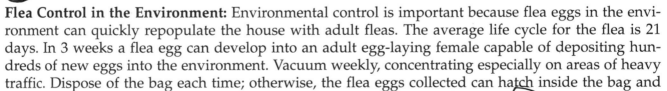

When fleas are located, they should be deposited in a jar of alcohol, which kills them quickly.

Shampoos and safe dips are also important in flea control. Pyrethrins, which are derived from chrysanthemums, are the safest ingredients, but they must be reapplied often. The organophosphates are the most potent and last the longest, but they are also the most dangerous. You should be aware that a dog or cat can pick up a new crop of fleas immediately after being bathed.

Flea Control in the Environment: Environmental control is important because flea eggs in the environment can quickly repopulate the house with adult fleas. The average life cycle for the flea is 21 days. In 3 weeks a flea egg can develop into an adult egg-laying female capable of depositing hundreds of new eggs into the environment. Vacuum weekly, concentrating especially on areas of heavy traffic. Dispose of the bag each time; otherwise, the flea eggs collected can hatch inside the bag and the adults can escape into the environment. After vacuuming, apply an insecticide (especially a safe product like pyrethrin or pyrethroid) as well as an insect growth regulator to the carpets. (Most insect growth regulators come already formulated with an insecticide.) The insecticide kills adult fleas, and the insect growth regulator stops flea eggs and larvae from developing further. Because insect growth regulators themselves are not insecticides, they are exceptionally safe for home use.

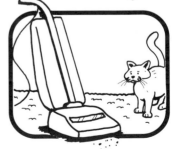

For the outdoor environment, concentrate on the edges of the patio and the garden. Fleas do not survive well in exposed areas. Apply appropriate products to sheltered areas and other spots where pets spend most of their time.

You as a pet owner must be extremely diligent in your control efforts for the products to work properly. The key is not to apply stronger and stronger insecticides but to use the safest ones to best advantage.

Natural Flea Control

As people are becoming more conscious of the environment and the impact of insecticides and other chemicals on nature, it is sensible to consider natural approaches to flea control. It has never been easier to control fleas with safe and natural products.

Any rational approach to flea control must include management of the pet, the home, and, to some extent, the outdoor environment as well. Contrary to popular belief, the common flea of dogs and cats spends all its adult life on the animal; it does not willingly jump off into the home environment, although it may be knocked off by biting, scratching, and grooming. The flea eggs that are laid on the animal do fall off into environment, where the fleas hatch and develop further.

Shampoos/Dips: Any shampoo is effective at cleansing the skin and removing fleas, eggs, and flea feces. Adding soothing shampoos that contain oatmeal or sulfur and using cool water also helps to reduce some of the itchiness caused by fleas. Natural flea-killing ingredients include pyrethrins (from chrysanthemum flowers) and d-limonene (from citrus). A natural flea dip can be made by adding sliced lemons to a pot and steeping the concoction for at least 12 hours; the solution is sponged on to the pet on a daily basis, as needed.

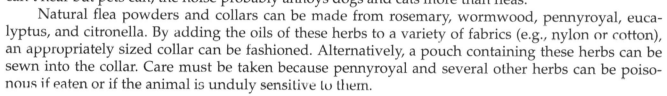

Flea Collars: Commercial insecticidal flea collars and electronic flea collars are best avoided by the health conscious pet owner. Most flea collars contain strong insecticides (carbamates, organophosphates) that can be toxic to pets as well as fleas. Electronic flea collars emit a tone that people can't hear but pets can; the noise probably annoys dogs and cats more than fleas.

Natural flea powders and collars can be made from rosemary, wormwood, pennyroyal, eucalyptus, and citronella. By adding the oils of these herbs to a variety of fabrics (e.g., nylon or cotton), an appropriately sized collar can be fashioned. Alternatively, a pouch containing these herbs can be sewn into the collar. Care must be taken because pennyroyal and several other herbs can be poisonous if eaten or if the animal is unduly sensitive to them.

Flea Repellents: Currently, there is no universal flea repellent. Brewer's yeast, thiamine, and garlic have been regarded for years as flea deterrents, but this could not be confirmed in scientific studies. That doesn't mean that they are ineffective in all cases, only that they could not consistently reduce flea populations in controlled experiments. Skin-So-Soft (an Avon product) diluted with water (5 parts Skin-So-Soft to 95 parts water) can be effective in reducing numbers of fleas found on pets.

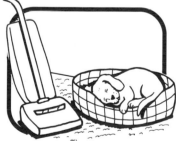

Environmental Control: Vacuum frequently to rid the carpets of fleas, larvae, cocoons, and eggs. Concentrate on high traffic areas and places where the pet sleeps. The inside of the house should be re-treated every few weeks. Pyrethrins, derived from chrysanthemums, are the safest and most effective insecticides to use indoors. They should be coupled with an insect growth regulator to get rid of eggs and larvae. Insect growth regulators are not insecticides. These natural insect hormones stop flea eggs and larvae from developing into adults. They are extremely safe and essentially nontoxic to all mammals. They represent a major breakthrough in safe and natural flea control.

Borax (boric acid, polyborate) is also a relatively safe and natural product that is effective for flea control. Its best use at present is in homes where at least 40% of the floor surfaces are covered with carpets. This compound is also effective against cockroaches. Other products such as diatomaceous earth have also been used for indoor flea control but are not as safe as the other products listed here.

Ringworm (Dermatophytosis)

Contrary to its name, "ringworm" is not caused by a worm and it rarely results in ring-shaped markings. It is actually a fungal infection, similar to athlete's foot in people. As such, it can be spread among cats, dogs, and people, and some people and animals are more susceptible to infection than others. The proper term for ringworm is "dermatophytosis," meaning a fungal infection caused by specific types of fungi called dermatophytes.

Diagnosis: The most common tests for dermatophytosis are Wood's lamp evaluation, direct microscopic examination, and fungal cultures. In the Wood's lamp evaluation a special ultraviolet light is used to identify dermatophytes, which may appear fluorescent green under this light. Although this test is quick and easy, it fails to detect infection at least half of the time. Therefore a negative Wood's lamp test does not mean that dermatophytes aren't present.

In direct microscopic examination, suspicious-looking hairs are plucked and examined with a microscope for any evidence of fungi. This test isn't foolproof either because fungus will not be found on every hair. It is quick, however, and sometimes allows a fast diagnosis.

Fungal culture is the most accurate way of identifying dermatophytes. On the special culture medium used, fluffy white colonies that change the color of the medium from yellow to red are good evidence of dermatophytosis. Occasionally, it takes 2 weeks for the fungi to grow. Confirmation of dermatophytosis requires examining the growth microscopically for characteristic spores.

Treatment: Dermatophytosis can be effectively cured, but the treatment process is often complicated. First, it is important to clip the haircoat as short as possible, because the fungi actually live in the hair follicles (pores). Clipping the hair gives the fungi fewer places to hide. Special antiseptic dips that kill the fungi on contact are used weekly or twice weekly for about 6 weeks. Creams and ointments may be adequate to control ringworm in people, but pets have too much hair and spot treatment alone is usually ineffective. The fungi just move into and infect the surrounding untreated hair.

Oral medications are often given to dogs and cats with dermatophytosis to help kill the fungi from the inside out. This also requires about 6 weeks because the drugs are slow to make their way from the bloodstream to the hair follicles where the fungi are located. These drugs make some pets sick, especially cats; pets being given these medications should be carefully monitored for any evidence of side effects.

Environmental Control: One of the difficulties in treating dermatophytosis is that once in the home fungal spores can survive for a year or more. Pets do not become immune to dermatophytes, and the infection can recur if the environment is not disinfected. Vacuuming is helpful but can't eliminate all of the spores. Even steam cleaning cannot generate enough heat to positively kill all spores. Nevertheless, every effort must be made to clean the environment as best as possible.

Ear Mites

Ear mites are tiny parasites that can cause infestations in the ears of dogs and cats. These highly contagious mites are transferred between animals when an infested pet comes into contact with a susceptible dog or cat.

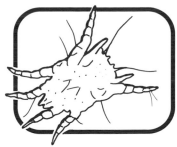

Some animals are intensely bothered by these mites, while others don't seem to notice their presence. Affected animals may have a dark brown or black discharge in the ears. A pet can often spread ear mites just by shaking its head in response to the irritation.

Diagnosis: The diagnosis is confirmed by visualizing the mites. When a veterinarian examines the ear canals with an otoscope, the mites sometimes come into view. More often, discharge from the ear canal is put on a glass slide and examined under the microscope. The mites are very classic in their appearance, resembling small crabs.

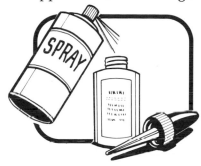

Treatment: For therapy to be effective, all pets (dogs and cats) need to be appropriately treated. In addition to instilling ear drops in the pet's ears, it is also advisable to use an insecticidal spray or powder on the rest of the body. Otherwise, the mites can migrate out of the ear canals to other parts of the body; after the effect of the ear drops wears off, they can return in full force. To eliminate the problem permanently, the entire body surface of all pets in the household should be treated.

Demodectic Mange

Demodectic mange (also called "demodicosis") is caused by tiny cigar-shaped mites (*Demodex* mites) that live in the hair follicles. They are present in small numbers on all dogs, cats, and humans. Problems occur when the number of mites become excessive and crowd out the hairs in the follicles (pores), causing hair loss. Skin can become red and inflamed when the mites cause the follicles to burst and release their contents within the sensitive tissue of the skin.

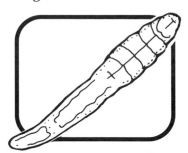

Since *Demodex* mites are found in the hair follicles of all normal animals, why do these mites cause a problem in particular animals? The most common reason is that *Demodex* mites increase in number when the body's resistance is suppressed. Low levels of resistance are associated with inherited problems in the immune system, diseases or therapies that suppress the immune system, or chronic disease processes or stressors that interfere with the effective functioning of the immune system. Demodectic mange is a signal of an underlying immune problem that must be addressed.

Diagnosis: Demodectic mange is diagnosed when characteristic mites are found on deep scrapings of the skin surface. Occasionally, the mites are embedded so deeply that only a surgical biopsy can provide a suitable sample for evaluation. In normal dogs or cats *Demodex* mites are very hard to find, even with multiple scrapings.

Treatment: Most young dogs with demodectic mange outgrow their disease when they reach immunologic maturity, usually around 18 months of age. To provide suitable care for these dogs, feed them nutritious diets, make sure that they have no other parasites, and use cleansing antiseptic baths on a regular basis. You may also apply mild antiparasitic products (e.g., rotenone) on individually affected patches of skin.

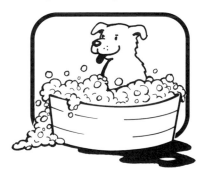

Only about 10% of dogs with generalized demodectic mange cannot be controlled with the simple procedures given above. These animals likely have more severe immune system–related problems. In these cases special medicated dips (e.g., containing amitraz [Mitaban]) are needed to kill the mites. The dips are repeated every week or two until scrapings reveal that no mites remain. Treatment may need to be given for several weeks or a lifetime, depending on the state of the immune system. Newer methods, including high doses of some heartworm preventive medicines, are also being explored as treatment alternatives for resistant cases.

Skin Biopsy

A skin biopsy is a surgical procedure in which a small portion of skin is removed, most often to provide tissue for pathologists to examine. The skin biopsy has the advantage of providing all layers of the skin (epidermis, dermis, and subcutaneous fat) and hair follicles for analysis and allows the whole architecture of the skin structure to be evaluated. In contrast, a skin scraping only provides some of the superficial dead cells of the skin.

Procedure: The first and most important part of the skin biopsy involves selection of the appropriate tissue. This is critical, because the pathologist's evaluation of the specimen can be based only on the material sent. To increase the chances for an accurate diagnosis, multiple biopsies may be taken if suitable tissue is available. The surgery itself is painless, and a local anesthetic is used to deaden the sensations in the area.

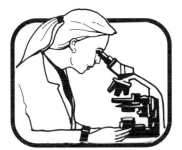

If suitable, a skin biopsy punch is often used to collect the specimens. This punch has a cookie-cutter edge that cuts the skin neatly and cleanly, yielding a solid round core. There is usually very little, if any, bleeding and no pain, even hours after the procedure. The tiny hole that is left is closed with one or two stitches.

The small cores of skin taken are blotted free of any blood and added to a vial of formaldehyde and sent to the pathologist for evaluation. After the tissue is preserved and treated (or "fixed"), it is embedded in a block of paraffin wax and then cut into very thin slices. The slices are placed on microscope slides, and a variety of stains are added to the samples to highlight different aspects of the skin. The slices are then examined microscopically.

*   *   *

The skin biopsy is one of the most important diagnostic tests for skin disorders because it allows the pathologist to examine the whole depth of the skin, not just its surface. Just as a doctor may want to take an X-ray to see if a bone is broken, the skin biopsy provides the pathologist with information about what's going on beneath the skin surface.

Seborrhea

Seborrhea, a term that is commonly used in veterinary medicine, does not refer to just one problem. Seborrhea is part of a whole group of disorders that result in scaling, greasiness, or dryness of the skin. These disorders are more correctly referred to as "keratinization disorders," because they usually represent some problem with the orderly turnover of epidermal cells (keratinocytes) into dead surface scale (keratin).

In a normal dog the skin cells are continually growing and evolving and are finally shed from the skin surface as dead skin cells. Usually, it takes about 3 weeks for cells to migrate from the deepest skin layers to the skin surface; the cells then remain on the skin surface for another 3 weeks before being shed. In dogs with keratinization defects, this cycle is greatly accelerated. Cells may replenish themselves in 3 to 4 days rather than 3 weeks. As a result, the skin becomes thicker and more scaly and greasy and is a perfect target for bacteria and yeasts. These microbes ordinarily do not cause problems on normal skin, but on skin with keratinization defects their populations grow because of the increased surface debris on which they can feed.

Diagnosis: Keratinization disorders can be inherited, but they can also result from inflammatory diseases (e.g., allergies), nutritional problems (e.g., zinc-responsive dermatosis), parasitism (e.g., mite infestations), or metabolic disorders (e.g., hypothyroidism). An appropriate diagnosis must be made before therapy is started. Tests designed to look for allergies, parasites, specific blood levels, and skin biopsy findings may be performed.

Treatment: Treatment can only be effective when a correct diagnosis has been made. Obviously, a thyroid deficiency only responds to appropriate thyroid hormone therapy. A parasite-related problem only resolves when the parasite has been eradicated. A dog with allergies cannot improve unless the allergic condition is correctly managed.

Bathing is important symptomatic therapy for pets with keratinization disorders, although it is not a cure. Medicated shampoos can loosen and remove the dead surface skin. Appropriate shampoos and conditioners can rehydrate the skin to make it less dry, which may also help in reducing the amount of itchiness.

A pet that has a keratinization disorder needs frequent and routine baths. If the skin cycle takes only 3 to 4 days instead of the normal 3 weeks, the animal should be bathed twice a week. As the condition improves, you can increase the interval between baths.

Many medicated ingredients—including sulfur, selenium, salicylic acid, and tar—are considered "anti-seborrheic." Sulfur and salicylic acid are best for dry skin, while selenium and tar are good for removing greasy scales.

Hypothyroidism

Hypothyroid animals have an insufficient amount of circulating thyroid hormones. Hypothyroidism is the most common form of endocrine (hormonal) disease in the dog. Although many people can remember goiter being a problem, this manifestation of hypothyroidism is extremely rare in dogs. Most (95%) cases result from a thyroid problem and not an iodine deficiency. Many of these cases have a hereditary component, and the disorder definitely runs in certain families of dogs.

There is not one universal picture for hypothyroidism. The most common manifestation is ongoing or recurrent infections. A lowered level of activity is also common. Obesity, which many believe to be a common finding, is only occasionally linked to hypothyroidism. Hair loss is also seen in some but not all cases of hypothyroidism. Problems are not usually evident until late in the course of the disease.

Diagnosis: Ideally, the diagnosis should be made before any signs of disease are apparent. The diagnosis of hypothyroidism is the subject of much controversy; although many of the common tests are quick and easy, they do not detect the condition in its early stages. Probably the best test currently available is one that measures levels of hormones and thyroid autoantibodies (i.e., antibodies produced by the animal to its own thyroid tissue). The autoantibody levels are useful because they may predict animals that are at risk even before their hormone levels become abnormal. A stimulation test can also be done to measure the highest output of hormone the body is capable of.

What is the best approach for breeds at risk of becoming hypothyroid? At this point, it would seem prudent to perform a blood count, a biochemical profile (including cholesterol) and a thyroid hormone profile at 1 year of age and annually thereafter. For certain breeds (e.g., Great Danes, Old English sheepdogs, and Irish setters) it would also be advisable to measure thyroid autoantibody levels. For breeds that are not at high risk, thyroid hormone levels should be measured at 5 to 7 years of age and annually thereafter as part of a typical geriatric profile.

Treatment: Treatment is simple, straightforward, and relatively inexpensive. Thyroid hormone is given daily to compensate for its lack of production in the body. Initially, it is given twice a day; at 6 weeks the thyroid levels are rechecked. Generally, the blood sample is collected 4 to 6 hours after the morning pill is given when thyroid levels are at their highest. If the levels are in the high normal range, the dosage may be reduced to once daily. If the levels are in the low normal range, treatment continues to be given twice daily. If the levels have not reached normal, further investigation is warranted.

Ticks

Ticks not only annoy dogs and cats by their bites but also transmit several important blood-borne diseases, including Lyme disease and tick fever. Although not every tick carries disease, pets parasitized by ticks have a genuine risk of acquiring a blood-borne infection.

Most ticks parasitize small animals other than pets (e.g., rodent, rabbits), which serve as a reservoir for ticks in nature. Ticks require surface cover such as leaves or long grass in which to reproduce. By limiting ground cover around homes and yards, the risk of tick bites can be greatly reduced. Some ticks (e.g., brown dog ticks) can survive in sheds, garages, attics, and kennels. If ticks are discovered in any of these areas, professional exterminators should be called.

Tick Control: Flea and tick collars can be quite effective in limiting the number of ticks on dogs and cats. A new collar impregnated with amitraz causes ticks to withdraw, even after they have attached themselves to the pet. This greatly reduces the risk of tick-related disease.

Insect repellents that contain "DEET" (e.g., Off) are often effective in warding off ticks, but these products are sometimes poisonous to children as well as dogs and cats and must be used carefully.

Most ticks are susceptible to **insecticidal dips** but only if the preparation actually comes into contact with the tick itself. Bathing alone is usually not sufficient. The insecticide needs to be worked into the skin to maximize the chances of killing ticks. Special medicated ear drops are usually necessary when ticks are present in the ear canals. Most dips are too irritating to be applied to this sensitive area.

Tick Removal: After all outings and walks, check pets thoroughly for ticks, concentrating on the ears, neck, and between the toes. Because ticks carry diseases that are transmissible to people as well as pets, appropriate caution should be taken. If ticks are located, remove them carefully. *Do not use bare fingers.* Use special tick tweezers or put a glove or plastic wrap over your hand. Grasp the body of the tick firmly and apply gentle traction until the tick releases its grasp. Breaking off the body from the head can lead to infection, inflammation, and disease transmission so *do not rush.* After the tick is removed, dab antiseptic on the bite area. Dispose of the tick by flushing it down the toilet or placing it in a jar of alcohol.

Pyoderma

Bacteria are normally found on the skin surface of all animals. These normally harmless bacteria cause problems when their numbers increase beyond the body's ability to control them. This can happen when the immune system defenses are not functioning optimally or as a result of some other ongoing disease process (e.g., allergies, hypothyroidism).

POSSIBLE CAUSES:

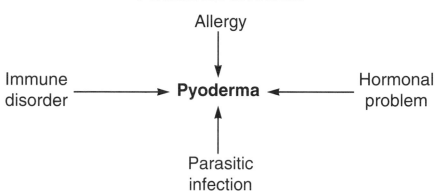

Pyoderma is derived from the Latin roots for pus ("pyo") and skin ("derma"). It is used to describe most bacterial infections of the skin, regardless of cause.

Diagnosis and Treatment: Pyoderma is *not* a specific diagnosis, and therefore no one treatment can be given for all cases.

Because the skin is meant to accommodate a certain number of bacteria, the goal of treatment of pyoderma is to correct the underlying problem. An antibiotic may kill all the bacteria present, but, unless the underlying problem is addressed, the problem will resume when the effect of the antibiotic is over and new bacteria colonize the skin surface. In the long run, it is always easier to address the root of a problem rather than to try to correct it with temporary solutions.

While searching for the true cause of the problem, antibiotics are often dispensed to control the bacteria temporarily, usually for about 2 to 6 weeks. During this time medicated baths are helpful, especially if they contain an antiseptic that kills bacteria on contact.

TEMPORARY MEASURES:

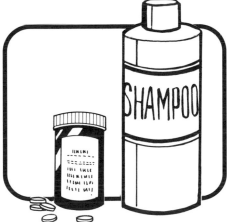

Searching for the underlying cause sometimes is simple and straightforward, but in other cases many tests are needed before the answers are found. The search is worthwhile, however; if no cause can be determined, antibiotics will likely need to be continued. Prolonged antibiotic administration is expensive and increases an animal's risk of side effects from the medications.

Antibiotic Therapy

Antibiotics are medications that help treat infections, especially those caused by bacteria, yeasts, or fungi. Available antibiotics include natural, synthetic, or semi-synthetic compounds, and new products are continually being developed.

Antibiotics must be used properly to combat infection and decrease the risk of side effects. Although antibiotics are generally regarded as safe, any drug can cause problems if given over a long period or if used inappropriately.

Antibiotics *must* be administered for the entire period prescribed and not just until the animal "seems better." If the harmful bacteria are not completely eliminated, strains resistant to the antibiotic are likely to develop after treatment is discontinued. If the same antibiotic is used again, it will not be as effective against these resistant strains. More powerful (and more expensive) drugs are then needed to eliminate the infection.

An animal with a skin infection is usually given antibiotics for at least 2 to 4 weeks. This period allows the antibiotic to penetrate the layers of the skin to combat the many different types of bacteria that may be present. To augment the effects of the antibiotic, shampoos and skin cleansers with antibacterial properties can be used. Some medicated ingredients that are satisfactory for this purpose include chlorhexidine, hexachlorophene, triclosan, povidone-iodine, and benzoyl peroxide. To keep the bacterial population on the skin surface under control, apply these skin cleansers daily or several times a week.

If your pet has a bacterial infection, the best way to eliminate it is to follow your veterinarian's directions *exactly*. This helps prevent drug resistance, lessens the need to prescribe stronger and stronger drugs, and decreases the risk of side effects from antibiotic therapies.

Corticosteroid Therapy

Corticosteroids have the ability to combat inflammation in the body. In high doses they can even suppress the immune system.

Corticosteroids are used frequently in dermatology. At certain doses corticosteroids effectively reduce itchiness caused by allergies and many other conditions. High doses of corticosteroids are used to combat immune-mediated diseases like systemic lupus erythematosus or rheumatoid arthritis.

Corticosteroids are not the same as the anabolic steroids used by weight lifters and athletes. Anabolic steroids tend to increase muscle mass. Corticosteroids do not promote muscle mass; their job is to symptomatically reduce inflammation.

Corticosteroids are not a cure; they just relieve symptoms. As such, they are very handy in relieving itchiness, but they do not solve the underlying problem. Whenever possible, corticosteroids should be used for temporary relief until the root of the problem can be eliminated.

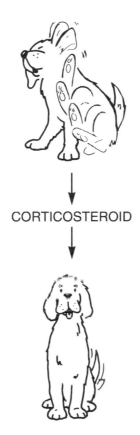

CORTICOSTEROID

SYMPTOMATIC RELIEF ONLY

The most common oral corticosteroid preparations are prednisone/prednisolone and triamcinolone. These products are the safest to use for long-term treatments. Ideally, they should be administered daily for a short course (5 to 14 days) and then given on an every-other-day basis. The off day gives the body a chance to produce its own form of cortisone. This is important because long-term daily treatment can "shut down" the body's ability to make cortisone and discontinuation of treatment can result in serious withdrawal symptoms.

Corticosteroids are very useful products, but they are not without risk. They decrease resistance to infection, promote the development of diabetes mellitus, cause fat to collect in the liver, and are associated with numerous other problems. However, in the proper hands and with the proper care, corticosteroids are an important tool in the management of many skin problems.

Condensed Glossary of Dermatologic Disorders

Abscess A cavity filled with pus.

Acanthosis nigricans A disorder in which the armpit and groin areas become hyperpigmented and thickened. Most common in the dachshund.

Acne A localized area of cellulitis or infection, most commonly located in the chin area. A keratinization disorder and not a bacterial infection appears to be primarily responsible.

Acral lick dermatitis (lick granuloma) A disorder in which dogs lick at and traumatize their legs for no apparent reason. May be due to sensory neuropathy, stereotypical behavior patterns, or other initiating factors.

Acral mutilation syndrome A congenitohereditary disorder in which there is a sensory neuropathy of the limbs. The feet become mutilated as they are chewed upon by affected pups. Most common in pointers. Probably inherited as an autosomal recessive trait.

Acrodermatitis (lethal acrodermatitis) A fatal skin disorder of bull terriers, associated with thymic hypoplasia and inherited as an autosomal recessive trait. Similar to lethal trait A46 in cattle and acrodermatitis enteropathica in humans.

Actinic keratosis A premalignant change in the skin as a result of overexposure to ultraviolet light. Scaling is associated with dysplastic changes of the epidermis.

Actinomycotic mycetoma An atypical bacterial infection characterized by lumps (tumefaction), draining tracts, and "grains" of bacterial filaments. Most often caused by the actinomycetes such as *Actinomyces, Nocardia,* or *Streptomyces.*

Adverse food reactions Clinical problems following ingestion of foods caused by hypersensitivity reactions or food intolerance.

Albinism An extremely rare, hereditary lack of pigmentation. Supposedly transmitted as an autosomal recessive trait.

Allergic contact dermatitis A contact hypersensitivity caused by a variety of substances, such as plants, medications, collars, fibers, leathers, disinfectants, carpet deodorizers, and plastics.

Allergic inhalant dermatitis (atopy, hay fever) Allergies to substances that are inhaled, such as pollens, molds, house dust, and danders.

Allergy A heightened sensitivity to substances normally encountered. The initiating substance is known as the allergen.

Alopecia Hair loss.

Alopecia areata An area of hair loss resulting from immune-mediated attack on growing hair follicles.

Anal furunculosis (perianal fistulae, perianal pyoderma) A deep infection around the rectum characterized by the appearance of draining tracts. Most common in German shepherds and Irish setters. The cause is unknown.

Anal sacculitis Inflammatory disorder of the anal sacs.

Ancylostomiasis Infection caused from the hookworm *Ancylostoma caninum.*

Apocrine cyst A cavity filled with apocrine secretions, caused by occlusion of the excretory duct of an apocrine gland.

Apocrine gland adenocarcinoma A malignant cancer of apocrine sweat glands.

Apocrine gland adenoma A benign tumor of the apocrine sweat glands.

Aspergillosis A form of hyalohyphomycosis caused by various species of *Aspergillus* fungi.

Atopy *See* allergic inhalant dermatitis.

Atypical mycobacteriosis Infection caused by species of mycobacteria other than the species causing tuberculosis and leprosy. These mycobacteria are usually common soil and water inhabitants that contaminate wounds.

Aural hematoma A blood-filled cavity on the ear flaps (pinnae) caused by some form of trauma, such as pronounced head shaking.

Autoimmune skin diseases Skin disorders in which the immune system targets the skin for damage.

Autosensitization reactions (id reactions) A generalized hypersensitivity reaction that develops from specific lesions. Dermatophytes are a common source of antigens, but anal sac material also has been implicated.

Bacterial granuloma An infection in which microorganisms are walled off from the body's immune system. The disorder may be caused by several different bacteria such as mycobacteria or staphylococci.

Bacterial hypersensitivity (pruritic pyoderma, pruritic superficial folliculitis) A bacterial infection with associated pruritus.

Basal cell tumor A benign tumor of epidermal basal cells found predominantly in middle-aged dogs.

Basosquamous carcinoma A rare, malignant subset of basal cell tumor with aggressive behavior and metastatic potential.

Black hair follicular dysplasia A developmental hair growth abnormality confined solely to areas with black haircoat.

Blastomycosis A systemic fungal infection caused by *Blastomyces dermatitidis*. Exists in a hyphal or spore stage in nature and as a budding yeast in tissue.

Botryomycosis A deep granulomatous infection.

Bullous pemphigoid A variant of pemphigoid in which autoantibodies are found in the junction between the dermis and epidermis. There is a generalized distribution of lesions, which are most commonly found on the mucous membranes, axillae, groin, and neck areas.

Calcinosis circumscripta (tumoral calcinosis) An unusual condition in which there is calcification in the skin that is not associated with defects in calcium metabolism or renal disease.

Calcinosis cutis Calcium deposits in the skin. Most commonly associated with hyperadrenocorticism (Cushing's disease) or the percutaneous absorption of calcium salts.

Callus A localized area of skin thickening. Most commonly found on the elbows and hocks of large breeds of dogs and on the sternum of others (e.g., dachshunds).

Callus pyoderma An infected callus, often the result of the traumatic inoculation of hairs and debris into the dermis and subcutaneous tissues.

Candidiasis An infection caused by the yeast *Candida albicans*.

Cellulitis Inflammation of the connective tissue that does not form a discrete abscess.

Cheyletiellosis ("walking dandruff") Infestation with *Cheyletiella* mites.

Cicatricial pemphigoid A relatively benign variant of pemphigoid usually limited to the mucous membranes of the mouth and eyes.

Clear cell hidradenocarcinoma An extremely rare malignancy of eccrine sweat glands.

Coccidioidomycosis (valley fever) A systemic fungal infection caused by *Coccidioides immitis*. Exists in spore stage in nature and as a yeast in tissue.

Color dilution alopecia (color mutant alopecia) A congenitohereditary disorder characterized by a patchy, poor haircoat in areas of abnormally colored hairs. Usually associated with blue color dilutions but occasionally also seen with fawn and red varieties.

Conditioned hyperirritability A dermatitis on one area of the body that results in a more generalized inflammatory skin condition.

Cryptococcosis A systemic fungal infection caused by

Cryptococcus neoformans and related species. Exists as a budding yeast in nature as well as in tissue.

Cushing's disease (hyperadrenocorticism) An endocrine disorder characterized by high circulating levels of cortisol. Caused by a pituitary tumor, an adrenal tumor, or corticosteroid administration.

Cutaneous asthenia (Ehlers-Danlos syndrome) A congenitohereditary disorder characterized by skin fragility and extreme extensibility. Caused by several different biochemical disorders of collagen.

Cutaneous hamartoma *See* nevus.

Cutaneous horn *See* proliferative keratosis.

Cutaneous lupus erythematosus (discoid lupus erythematosus) A variant of lupus erythematosus that is limited to the skin. Most commonly causes a chronic facial rash.

Cuterebriasis A nodular condition in dogs in which larvae of the botfly *Cuterebra* are found in the subcutaneous tissue.

Cyclic hematopoiesis A congenitohereditary disorder seen in collie pups born with a silver-grey haircoat. Associated with cyclic neutropenia and rebounding neutrophilia.

Dalmatian bronzing syndrome A nutritionally related and metabolic disorder seen in dalmatians caused by an inherited defect in the metabolism of uric acid.

Deep pyoderma An infection that tends to involve the deeper aspects of the dermis and subcutaneous tissues. Most commonly caused by extension of an intermediate pyoderma.

Demodicosis A skin disorder resulting from an overpopulation of *Demodex* mites in the hair follicles and stratum corneum. Often categorized as either localized or generalized.

Dermatitis Any inflammatory process involving the skin.

Dermatitis herpetiformis An immune-mediated disorder associated with gluten sensitivity.

Dermatomyositis A congenitohereditary disorder seen primarily in collies, Shetland sheepdogs, and their crossbreeds. Affected animals may have abnormalities of muscle as well as of skin.

Dermatophytosis (ringworm) Cutaneous infection due to three genera of fungi: *Microsporum, Trichophyton,* and *Epidermophyton.*

Dermoid cyst An epidermal cyst in which adnexal structures are associated with the epithelial lining.

Dermoid sinus An abnormal congenital tract that connects the skin surface with the underlying supraspinous ligament or dura mater of the spine. Most commonly seen in Rhodesian ridgebacks.

Diabetic dermatopathy A rare metabolic dermatosis often associated with increased glucagon levels and, at least in some cases, a glucagon-secreting tumor.

Dirofilariasis Heartworm infection. When microfilariae are found in the dermis, the condition is referred to as cutaneous dirofilariasis.

Discoid lupus erythematosus *See* cutaneous lupus erythematosus.

Dracunculiasis A helminth-related skin disorder caused by *Dracunculus insignis.*

Drug eruption An immune-mediated reaction to a medication. The eruption may be seen after the drug has been given for days or years or even after the drug has been withdrawn for a few days. The most common causes are antibiotics, vaccines, parasiticides, topical preparations, hormones, tranquilizers, and antineoplastic agents.

Eccrine adenoma A very rare but benign tumor of eccrine sweat glands.

Ehlers-Danlos syndrome *See* cutaneous asthenia.

Eosinophilic granuloma An immune-mediated disorder of dogs associated with collagen breakdown and tissue eosinophilia.

Eosinophilic granuloma complex A trilogy of inflammatory conditions (indolent ulcer, eosinophilic plaque, and linear [collagenolytic] granuloma) in cats, which is associated in some fashion with tissue eosinophilia.

Epidermal cyst A cyst derived from the epidermis or the outer root sheath of hair follicles.

Epidermolysis bullosa A family of mechanobullous diseases in which trauma to the skin results in tearing and cleft formation in the skin.

Epidermolysis bullosa simplex A congenitohereditary disorder most commonly reported in collies and Shetland sheepdogs.

Erythema multiforme A presumably immune-mediated reaction to a drug, microbe, or other inciting agent. The disorder is self-limiting if the initiator is removed. A severe form is called Stevens-Johnson syndrome or erythema multiforme major.

Erythema nodosum A rare form of panniculitis thought to be a hypersensitivity reaction to an infectious agent or medication.

Eumycotic mycetoma A deep granulomatous fungal infection characterized by lumps (tumefaction), draining tracts, and "grains" of fungal mycelia. Most commonly due to *Curvularia, Pseudoallescheria (Petriellidium), Acremonium,* and *Madurella.*

Fatty acid deficiency A nutritional problem in which the diet is poor or deficient in the essential fatty acids, particularly linoleic acid. This is most common in dry foods in which the amount of fat that can be added is limited.

Fibroma A benign tumor of fibrocytes (connective tissue cells).

Fibrosarcoma A malignant tumor of fibrocytes (connective tissue cells).

Fibrous histiocytoma (nodular fasciitis) A granulomatous disorder, now thought to be immune-mediated rather than cancerous. (Ophthalmologists may refer to the condition as nodular granulomatous episcleritis.)

Follicular cyst (pilar cyst) A cyst derived from follicular epithelium. Further subclassified as trichilemmal or proliferating based on histologic features.

Follicular dysplasia A congenitohereditary disorder characterized by developmental abnormalities of hair growth. The condition is characterized by alterations in size, shape, and orientation of hairs.

Folliculitis Infection of the hair follicles.

Food allergy (food hypersensitivity) An adverse reaction to a food with an immunologic basis.

Food intolerance An adverse reaction to a food not due to an immunologic cause. Can result from idiosyncracy, toxicity (food poisoning), pharmacologic reactions, and metabolic reactions.

Furunculosis Inflammatory reaction that results from rupture of an infected hair follicle.

Generic dog food disease A nutritionally related skin problem associated with the feeding of generic dog foods. A zinc imbalance caused by the high cereal (fiber, phytates) content of generic dog foods may be responsible.

Giant cell tumor (malignant fibrous histiocytoma) A rare malignancy believed to be of histiocytic origin.

Glucagonoma syndrome A metabolic dermatopathy associated with diabetes mellitus and a glucagon-secreting tumor.

Granuloma An inflammatory condition in which histiocytes (members of the mononuclear phagocyte system) are prominent.

Grey collie syndrome *See* cyclic hematopoiesis.

Growth hormone–responsive dermatosis An endocrine disorder originally thought to be related to abnormal growth hormone levels. Dehydroepiandrosterone or other adrenal sex hormone levels are now believed to be involved.

Hay fever *See* allergic inhalant dermatitis.

Hemangioma A benign tumor of blood vessels.

Hemangiopericytoma A benign tumor originating from the tissue around blood vessels.

Hemangiosarcoma A malignant tumor of blood vessels.

Hepatocutaneous syndrome A metabolic dermatosis caused by liver disease. May be associated with aberrations in amino acid levels.

Hepatoid gland adenoma (perianal adenoma) A benign tumor of modified sebaceous glands commonly found around the anus. The tumor cells resemble normal hepatic cells.

Hepatoid gland adenocarcinoma (perianal adenocarcinoma) The malignant counterpart of hepatoid gland adenoma.

Histiocytoma A common benign tumor that often clears spontaneously. Behaves more like an inflammatory nodule than a tumor. Seen in younger dogs predominantly.

Histiocytosis An aggressive accumulation of histiocytes in tissue. Cutaneous histiocytosis waxes and wanes regardless of treatment. Malignant (systemic) histiocytosis is a rapidly progressive and fatal condition most commonly seen in Bernese mountain dogs.

Histoplasmosis A systemic fungal infection caused by *Histoplasma capsulatum*. Exists as fungal spores in nature and as a yeast in tissue.

Hormonal hypersensitivity A very rare condition caused by a hypersensitivity reaction to sex hormones, including estrogen, progesterone, and testosterone.

Hyalohyphomycosis An intermediate fungal infection characterized histologically by septate nonpigmented mycelia and associated inflammation. Most commonly caused by infection with *Aspergillus, Penicillium, Paecilomyces,* and *Chrysosporium.*

Hyperadrenocorticism *See* Cushing's disease.

Hypereosinophilic syndrome A rare and potentially fatal disorder in cats characterized by persistent unexplained eosinophilia and diffuse infiltration of various organs by mature eosinophils.

Hyperestrogenism An endocrine condition presumably caused by increased levels of estrogen. Previously known as ovarian imbalance type I.

Hypersensitivity A heightened reaction to substances. The four classic hypersensitivity reactions are immediate (type I; e.g., allergic inhalant dermatitis); cytotoxic (type II; e.g., pemphigus); immune complex (type III; lupus erythematosus), and delayed or lymphokine mediated (type IV; contact allergy).

Hyperthyroidism An endocrine disorder characterized by an increase in circulating thyroid hormones.

Hypothyroidism An endocrine disorder characterized by a decrease in the amount of circulating thyroid hormones.

Hypotrichosis A rare ectodermal defect resulting in patchy, poor hair growth or baldness at birth. Poodles and basset hounds may be predisposed.

Ichthyosis A congenitohereditary condition in which the surface of the skin is covered with a thick, tenacious scale. There are likely several varieties reflecting different keratinization defects and modes of inheritance.

Id reactions *See* autosensitization reactions.

Immune-mediated skin diseases Skin diseases initiated by an abnormal response of the immune system. Often used synonymously with autoimmune skin diseases, although immune-mediated skin disorder is a more general term.

Impetigo A term used for the superficial bacterial infection often seen on the underside of puppies. Not related to human impetigo, which is a contagious disease.

Interdigital pyoderma Inflammation between the toes caused by a variety of etiologies.

Intermediate mycosis Fungal infections caused by several genera of opportunistic environmental fungi that cause problems when inoculated into the skin. Subdivided by several criteria into such families as aspergillosis, hyalohyphomycosis, and phycomycosis.

Intermediate pyoderma Skin infections involving the hair follicles (folliculitis) and surrounding adnexa (perifolliculitis). More severe than superficial pyoderma and less severe than deep pyoderma.

Intracutaneous cornifying epithelioma A benign tumor consisting of a keratin-filled cavity lined by stratified squamous epithelium. Lesions may be solitary or multiple. Previously referred to as keratoacanthoma.

Juvenile cellulitis A presumably immune-mediated disorder in which the face and head of young pups become inflamed and swollen. Responds to short-term immunosuppressive therapy; relapse is uncommon.

Keratinization disorder Condition that results in

increased layers of scale on the skin surface. Often referred to as seborrhea.

Keratosis A condition characterized by an accumulation of keratin (scale).

Kerion reaction An inflammatory response to dermatophytes (ringworm fungi).

Leishmaniasis A rare protozoal disease caused by five species of nonmotile flagellated protozoa of the genus *Leishmania*. More common in the Mediterranean, but enzootic pockets have been found in parts of North America.

Lentigo A rare congenitohereditary condition in which there is focal increase in pigmentation of the skin. The most common breed affected is the pug. Inheritance is thought to be autosomal dominant.

Lethal acrodermatitis *See* acrodermatitis.

Leukocytoclastic vasculitis An inflammatory disorder of blood vessels in which neutrophils surrounding the vessels are broken down.

Lichenoid dermatosis A condition that can be described clinically as regional clusters of papules or histologically as mononuclear cell infiltrates that tend to hug the junction between the dermis and epidermis.

Lichenoid keratosis Groups of plaques usually found on the ears that are associated with scaling and lichenoid dermatosis.

Lichenoid-psoriasiform dermatitis A congenitohereditary disorder peculiar to springer spaniels characterized by the appearance of asymptomatic plaques, usually on the pinnae.

Lick granuloma *See* acral lick dermatitis.

Lipoma A benign tumor of fat cells.

Lipomatosis A proliferative disorder in which fat cells infiltrate or replace muscle or collagen.

Liposarcoma A malignant tumor of fat cells.

Lupus erythematosus A disorder characterized by the presence of autoantibodies. The two variants in dogs and cats are systemic lupus erythematosus and cutaneous (discoid) lupus erythematosus.

Lupus profundus A form of lupus erythematosus that presents as panniculitis, a connective tissue disorder in the subcutaneous fat.

Lymphomatoid granulomatosis A rare lymphohistiocytic proliferative disorder associated with vascular and granulomatous lesions. Most of these lesions are confined to the lungs or viscera but cutaneous cases have been reported. The clinical presentation involves ulcers, crusts, erosions, and lymphadenomegaly. This condition has a poor prognosis.

Lymphosarcoma A malignant disorder of lymphocytes. The tumorous lymphocytes may be of B-cell (B-cell lymphosarcoma) or T-cell (e.g., cutaneous T-cell lymphoma, mycosis fungoides, Sézary syndrome, pagetoid reticulosis) origin.

Majocchi's granuloma A deep granulomatous infection caused by dermatophytes (ringworm fungi).

***Malassezia* dermatitis** Infection caused by the yeast *Malassezia pachydermatis* (previously known as *Pityrosporon canis*).

Malignant fibrous histiocytoma *See* giant cell tumor.

Mange A clinical disorder caused by mites.

Mast cell tumor A potentially malignant tumor of dermal mast cells, which are related to basophils in the blood. Systemic mastocytosis is an uncommon sequela to mast cell tumor.

Melanoma A tumor of the pigment-producing cells, the melanocytes. As a general rule, tumors arising on the skin are more likely to be benign than those originating on mucous membranes.

Metabolic dermatosis A skin disease associated with a metabolic defect. Diabetes mellitus, hepatobiliary disease, renal disease, neoplasia, and defects of bile acid, tyrosine, and uric acid metabolism have all been implicated. Individually referred to as superficial necrolytic dermatitis, diabetic dermatopathy, hepatocutaneous syndrome, glucagonoma syndrome, necrolytic migratory erythema, etc.

Miliary dermatitis A descriptive term for dermatitis in cats characterized by papules and crusts. The underlying problem is most often allergy.

Morphea The cutaneous variant of scleroderma characterized by a localized scarring patch of skin. In the early stages there is lymphocytic infiltration of the deep dermis and subcutaneous fat.

Mucinosis A rare skin condition caused by the accumulation of mucin in focal areas of skin. Most commonly reported in Chinese Shar peis and Doberman pinschers.

Mucopolysaccharidosis A group of rare diseases that results from defects in the metabolism of glycos-aminoglycans. Mucopolysaccharidosis VI (Maroteaux-Lamy syndrome) and mucopolysaccharidosis I (Hurler syndrome) have both been reported in cats.

Mycosis A disorder caused by fungi.

Mycosis fungoides A form of T-cell lymphoma characterized by a red scaly rash that evolves into cutaneous tumors. Named because the clinical appearance of these tumors in humans was said to resemble mushrooms.

Myiasis A clinical condition in which flies lay their eggs in wounds; maggot infestation.

Myxoma A benign tumor of the connective tissue cells that produce mucin.

Myxosarcoma A malignant tumor of the connective tissue cells that produce mucin.

Nasal pyoderma An inflammatory condition of the nose and snout area. Not a specific diagnosis.

Nasodigital hyperkeratosis A poorly understood condition in which excessive scale accumulates on the nose and footpads.

Necrolytic migratory erythema A metabolic dermatosis reported in dogs based on the description of the human condition of the same name. In humans it is often associated with glucagonoma syndrome. In dogs liver impairment is more often implicated.

Neurodermatitis (psychogenic alopecia) A poorly described condition involving cats that lick the fur until bald patches develop. Thought to occur in "emotional" breeds of cat such as the Siamese, Burmese, Himalayan, and Abyssinian. Most cases have an underlying allergic etiology. The response of some cases to dopamine antagonists supports the involvement of a behavioral component in some cases.

Nevus (cutaneous hamartoma) A well-demarcated developmental defect in the skin. Categorized by tissue of origin (e.g., sebaceous, collagenous, epidermal, vascular, melanocytic, organoid).

Nodular dermatofibrosis A tumor of densely packed fibrous connective tissue, which has been associated with malignant kidney cancer. Seen most commonly in German shepherds. Its main significance is that it is the first skin disorder recognized as a "marker" of internal malignancy.

Nodular fasciitis *See* fibrous histiocytoma.

Nodular panniculitis An inflammatory reaction in the subcutaneous fat.

Onychomycosis A fungal infection of the nails.

Oomycosis *See* pythiosis.

Otitis externa Infection of the external ear canal.

Otitis interna Infection of the inner ear.

Otitis media Infection of the middle ear.

Otodectic mange Infestation with *Otodectes cynotis*, the common ear mite.

Ovarian imbalance Previously used term for skin diseases presumed related to abnormal levels of the female sex hormone estrogen. Ovarian imbalance type I is now called hyperestrogenism. Ovarian imbalance type II is now called estrogen-responsive dermatosis.

Paecilomycosis An intermediate fungal infection caused by various species of *Paecilomyces*.

Pagetoid reticulosis (Woringer-Kolopp disease) A rare form of T-cell lymphoma.

Panniculitis An inflammatory reaction in the subcutaneous fat that results from several known, and possibly many more unknown, causes.

Papilloma A common skin tumor frequently referred to as a wart. This tumor is not induced by viruses like those that cause papillomatosis.

Papillomatosis An oral proliferative disorder caused by a virus (papovavirus).

Parapsoriasis Large plaque parapsoriasis refers to a focal exfoliative dermatitis with similarities to the human condition. It does not appear to be pruritic or painful. Corticosteroid therapy is usually an effective means of control.

Paronychia A microbial infection of the nailbeds.

Pediculosis Infestation by lice.

Pemphigoid An autoimmune skin disease in which autoantibody is deposited in the junction between the epidermis and the dermis. The two varieties are bullous pemphigoid and cicatricial pemphigoid.

Pemphigus An autoimmune skin disease in which autoantibodies lodge in the epidermis and cause damage. Pemphigus is derived from the Greek word for "blister," but blisters are rarely seen in dogs and cats because of the thinness of the epidermis in these species. The four variants are pemphigus foliaceus, pemphigus erythematosus, pemphigus vulgaris, and pemphigus vegetans.

Penicillinosis An intermediate fungal infection caused by various species of *Penicillium*.

Perianal adenoma *See* hepatoid gland adenoma.

Perianal adenosarcoma *See* hepatoid gland adenocarcinoma.

Perianal fistulae *See* anal furunculosis.

Perianal pyoderma *See* anal furunculosis.

Periappendageal dermatitis A general term for inflammatory disorders of the follicular adnexa.

Phaeohyphomycosis An intermediate fungal infection characterized by the presence of pigmented fungal hyphae in the tissue. Most common causes are *Dreschlera* and *Phialophora*.

Phycomycosis An intermediate fungal infection caused by members of the orders Mucorales and Entomophthorales (e.g., *Rhizopus, Mucor, Absidia, Mortierella, Conidiobolus, Basidiobolus).* Many cases in dogs and cats previously referred to as phyco-mycosis were actually caused by *Pythium* spp. *(see also* pythiosis).

Pilar cyst *See* follicular cyst.

Pilomatrixoma A generally benign tumor thought to originate from cells of the hair matrix. Malignant variants are rare but have been reported.

Plasma cell pododermatitis A rare disorder of cats in which there is nonpainful swelling of multiple footpads. An immune-mediated etiology is believed to be involved.

Plasmacytoma A tumor of plasma cell origin that may arise as a primary tumor or as an extension of multiple myeloma.

Pododermatitis An inflammatory condition of the feet and toes resulting from a number of different underlying causes.

Proliferative keratosis (cutaneous horn) An accumulation of scale that may overlay an underlying tumor, virus-induced lesion, or another keratosis.

Pruritic pyoderma *See* bacterial hypersensitivity.

Pruritic superficial folliculitis *See* bacterial hypersensitivity.

Psychogenic alopecia *See* neurodermatitis.

Pyoderma A skin condition characterized by the influx of neutrophils (pus cells). Generally used to describe any form of skin infection.

Pythiosis (oomycosis) Infection with *Pythium*. Previously described as phycomycosis; however, *Pythium* is not a fungus.

Renal cystadenocarcinoma A malignant kidney tumor associated with nodular dermatofibrosis.

Rhabditis dermatitis A previously used term for the condition caused by the nematode *Pelodera (Rhabditis) strongyloides*.

Rhinosporidiosis An intermediate fungal infection caused by *Rhinosporidium seeberi*. Most common clinical manifestation involves nasal polyps.

Ringworm *See* dermatophytosis.

Sarcoptic mange Infestation with sarcoptid mites.

Schnauzer comedo syndrome A keratinization disorder seen in schnauzers in which keratin plugs develop in hair follicles.

Scleroderma A rare connective tissue disease characterized by thickening and firmness of the skin. There are systemic and cutaneous variants in humans, but only the cutaneous variant (morphea) has been described in dogs and cats.

Sebaceous adenitis A poorly understood disorder thought to be a congenitohereditary as well as an immune-mediated member of the periappendageal family of disorders. In classic sebaceous adenitis, such as seen in poodles, the sebaceous glands are inflamed and then destroyed by the process, leaving patches of hairless and scaly skin.

Sebaceous gland carcinoma A rare malignancy of sebaceous glands.

Sebaceous gland hyperplasia A common proliferative disorder of sebaceous glands. Frequently referred to incorrectly as warts.

Seborrhea Keratinization disorder of the sebaceous glands. Commonly (but incorrectly) used to describe any skin condition that is dry, greasy, or scaly

Sertoli cell tumor A testicular tumor that can secrete female sex hormones and can result in hyperestrogenism in male dogs.

Sézary syndrome A form of T-cell lymphoma in which there are circulating malignant T-lymphocytes (Sézary cells).

Sjögren's syndrome An autoimmune disorder characterized by dry eyes (keratoconjunctivitis sicca), dry mouth (xerostomia), and an autoimmune connective tissue disease. There may be a clinical overlap between this disorder and lupus erythematosus.

Spiculosis A hair shaft disorder in which hairs are brittle, thick, and shiny. Most commonly reported in Kerry blue terriers.

Sporotrichosis An intermediate fungal infection caused by *Sporothrix schenckii*. This organism is transmissible from cats to humans.

Squamous cell carcinoma A malignant epithelial tumor. Most are locally invasive but slow to metastasize.

Staphylococcal hypersensitivity Bacterial hypersensitivity to staphylococci.

Sterile eosinophilic pustulosis A rare pustular disease in which eosinophils are found within pustules of the epidermis and hair follicle epithelium.

Sterile pyogranuloma A nonbacterial and presumably immune-mediated form of pododermatitis in which nodules and draining tracts are found between the toes. Most common in Great Danes, St. Bernards, Newfoundlands, dachshunds, and English bulldogs.

Stevens-Johnson syndrome A severe form of erythema multiforme.

Subcorneal pustular dermatosis A rare pustular disease of uncertain cause. An immune-mediated cause is considered most likely. Miniature schnauzers appear to be predisposed.

Superficial necrolytic dermatitis *See* metabolic dermatosis.

Superficial pyoderma (surface pyoderma) Skin infection involving only the superficial aspects of the epidermis and hair follicles.

Systemic lupus erythematosus A variant of lupus erythematosus in which circulating autoantibodies cause tissue damage. The most common clinical findings are arthritis, fever unresponsive to antibiotics, kidney disease, anemia, and skin disease.

Systemic mycoses Also known as deep mycoses, these fungal infections are acquired by inhaling infectious spores. Most common causes are *Blastomyces dermatitidis, Coccidioides immitis, Cryptococcus neoformans,* and *Histoplasma capsulatum.*

Telogen defluxion (telogen effluvium) Hair loss following stressful events such as pregnancy or illness.

Toxic epidermal necrolysis A life-threatening disease involving the mucous membranes and skin. The most common initiating factor is an adverse reaction to a drug. The toxic reaction results in destruction of the tissue (necrolysis). May be a severe manifestation of erythema multiforme.

Transmissible venereal tumor A contagious tumor of dogs transmitted by sexual contact and direct contact associated with social behavior.

Trichoepithelioma A benign tumor of hair matrix cells.

Trombiculiasis Infestation with chiggers.

Tuberculosis Infection caused by microbes of the genus *Mycobacterium*. The most common cause is *M. bovis*, but *M. avium* and *M. tuberculosis* have also been implicated.

Tumoral calcinosis *See* calcinosis circumscripta.

Tyrosinemia A rare metabolic disorder caused by an inherited defect of tyrosine metabolism. Shares similarities with tyrosinemia II or Richner-Hanhart syndrome in humans. Diagnosis is based on elevated serum and urine levels of tyrosine. Skin biopsies stained with Millon's stain may reveal orange-staining dermal granules. Treatment is supportive and includes a low phenylalanine, low tyrosine diet.

Uveodermatologic syndrome (Vogt-Kayanagi-Harada syndrome) An autoimmune disorder in which the pigment-producing melanocytes are targeted. Results in loss of pigment in affected tissues. When the eyes are involved (granulomatous panuveitis), blindness can result.

Valley fever *See* coccidioidomycosis.

Vasculitis An inflammatory condition of the blood vessels. This may occur secondary to a number of processes, including infections, drug reactions, adverse reactions to foods, arthropod bites, immune-mediated disorders, and many chronic diseases.

Vitamin A–responsive dermatosis A nutritionally related skin disorder in dogs. Responsive to high doses of supplemental vitamin A. Does not involve a vitamin A deficiency. Synthetic vitamin A preparations (retinoids) are used in the treatment of keratinization disorders and acne in humans and dogs.

Vitiligo An inherited or acquired patchy loss of pigment. Nongenetic causes include autoimmune diseases, some cancers, and postinflammatory changes.

Vogt-Koyanagi-Harada syndrome *See* uveodermatologic syndrome.

"Walking dandruff" *See* cheyletiellosis.

Woringer-Kolopp disease *See* pagetoid reticulosis.

Xanthomatosis A rare disorder of cats characterized by accumulation of lipids in large foam cells in the skin or other tissues. Primary xanthomatosis is associated with inherited disorders of lipid metabolism. Secondary xanthomatosis follows disorders that alter cholesterol or triglyceride metabolism, such as diabetes mellitus, hypothyroidism, or disease of the liver, kidney, or pancreas.

Zinc-responsive dermatosis A nutritionally related skin problem due to either dietary deficiency, poor absorption, or competitive inhibition of zinc. There is a genetic predisposition in the sled dog breeds. Rapidly growing dogs given high calcium diets or supplements can also be affected. High fiber, high phytate diets also bind zinc, decreasing its availability in the body.

Index

Note: Tables, boxes, and figures are indicated by *t*, *b*, or *f*, respectively, following the page number. Material presented in Chapter 9 is indexed by the handout number (i.e., Handout 1, Handout 2, etc.).